Inorganic Chemistry
of Vitamin B$_{12}$

Inorganic Chemistry of Vitamin B₁₂

J. M. PRATT

I.C.I. Petrochemical and Polymer Laboratory, Runcorn, Cheshire, England.

1972

ACADEMIC PRESS · London · New York

CHEMISTRY

ACADEMIC PRESS INC. (LONDON) LTD
24/28 Oval Road,
London NW1

United States Edition published by
ACADEMIC PRESS INC.
111 Fifth Avenue
New York, New York 10003

Library of Congress Catalog Card Number: 77-172363
ISBN: 0 12 564050 1

PRINTED IN GREAT BRITAIN BY
WILLIAM CLOWES & SONS LIMITED
LONDON, COLCHESTER AND BECCLES

PREFACE

The rapid increase over the last decade in our knowledge of the co-ordination chemistry of the cobalt corrinoids, together with the stimulus this has given to the study of other cobalt complexes, has created the need for a source of reference on the subject. It is hoped that the present work will help to fill that need. For most sections of the book the literature has been covered up to the end of 1969; several additional papers published before September 1971, which provide substantial or significant new material, are mentioned in the Appendix. Some errors will doubtless have escaped detection and certain relevant items have been inadvertently omitted; I should be grateful if readers would let me know of any such errors or omissions.

I owe a debt of gratitude to a great many people; in particular to Dr. R. J. P. Williams, under whose supervision I carried out my D.Phil. research and began my interest in vitamin B_{12}; to Professor Dorothy Hodgkin and Drs. R. Bonnett, M. A. Foster, L. Mervyn and E. Lester Smith, who gave me the benefit of their advice on certain chapters; to Mr. S. C. Dyke for allowing me to make use of unpublished material on the history of pernicious anaemia; to two of my former research students, Drs. R. A. Firth and R. G. Thorp, who not only produced some of the experimental results recorded herein but who have also read and critized most of the book in the manuscript stage; to Mrs. Barbara Hunt for her excellent typing; and to the many other friends, colleagues and research students, too numerous to mention individually, who have helped with advice or contributed experimentally to our knowledge of the subject matter of the book. The writing of the book was begun while I was still at Oxford and completed after I joined Imperial Chemical Industries Limited. I should like to record my appreciation both to the Medical Research Council of London, who supported the work carried out at Oxford under the direction of Dr. R. J. P. Williams in the field of inorganic biochemistry, including vitamin B_{12}, and to the senior management of I.C.I.'s Petrochemical and Polymer Laboratory, who have given full support and encouragement to the writing of this book.

Runcorn, Cheshire.   J. M. PRATT
September 1971

CONTENTS

Section 3: Equilibria

Section 4: Reactions

Section 5: Summary

Section 1

Background

1

INTRODUCTION

Vitamin B_{12} or cyanocobalamin was isolated in 1948 in the form of dark red crystals. It is a diamagnetic, six-co-ordinate cobalt(III) complex. The molecule has the formidable empirical formula $C_{63}H_{88}O_{14}N_{14}PCo$; its structure is shown in Figs 1.1 and 1.2. The crystals contain a further 18–25 molecules of water of crystallization per molecule of B_{12}. (N.B. In this book we shall usually omit the word "vitamin" and refer to the compound simply as "B_{12}").

1948 marks the beginning of the study of the chemistry of B_{12} and its derivatives (the cobalt corrinoids), to which contributions have been made by scientists in fields as far apart as microbiology and theoretical chemistry. The theme of this book is the inorganic chemistry, or more specifically the co-ordination chemistry, of the cobalt corrinoids. The aim of this chapter is to put the co-ordination chemistry of B_{12} into historical perspective and to provide references to reviews on other aspects of B_{12} chemistry (Section I). This leads on to a discussion of the aims and scope of the present book (Section II) and the way in which the material is arranged (Section III).

I. THE CHEMISTRY OF B_{12} IN HISTORICAL PERSPECTIVE

There can be few areas that have attracted the attention of a wider range of scientists than the study of B_{12}—from research workers in medicine and agriculture at one end of the spectrum through microbiologists, biochemists, organic chemists and co-ordination chemists to X-ray crystallographers at the other end; even theoretical chemists have been attracted by the problems of describing the electronic structure and interpreting the absorption spectra of B_{12} and its derivatives. It is interesting to observe the ebb and flow of activity in these different fields and to see how development in one area sparks off research in another.

1

The early history of B$_{12}$ belongs entirely to medicine. The disease, now known as pernicious anaemia, was first described in 1821. The next hundred years witnessed a slow but steady increase in our knowledge of the signs of the disease and methods of diagnosis but a total absence of any advance in the treatment of the disease, which remained incurable and was usually fatal. Then

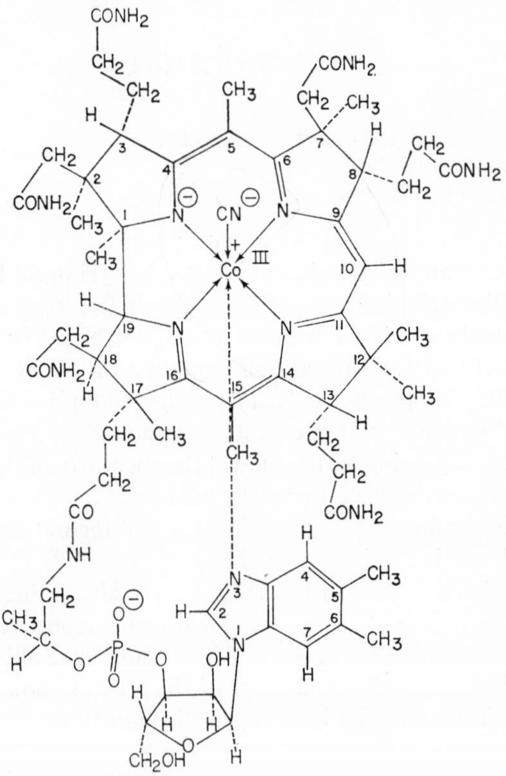

Fig. 1.1. Molecular structure of B$_{12}$. The positive charges of the cobalt(III) ion are balanced by the negative charges on the corrin ring, the cyanide and the phosphate.

in 1920, Whipple in California showed that the regeneration of red blood cells in dogs made anaemic by bleeding was stimulated by a diet containing liver, and in 1926 Minot and Murphy in Boston, Massachusetts reported a remarkable improvement in patients fed a diet of raw liver. This clue started the search for the "liver factor" or "anti-pernicious anaemia factor", which lasted over twenty years. Whipple, Minot and Murphy were awarded the Nobel Prize in Physiology and Medicine in 1934. The race to isolate the factor was very close. The isolation of crystalline vitamin B$_{12}$ was reported independently by two teams in 1948, first by Folkers and his colleagues at Merck Laboratories in the U.S. (Rickes *et al.*, 1948) and then by Smith and Parker at Glaxo Laboratories in the U.K. (Smith, 1948; Smith and Parker, 1948), and in the following year by Ellis, Petrow and Snook at British Drug Houses in the U.K. (Ellis *et al.*, 1949).

1948 can be considered as the date which marks the beginning of the study of the chemistry of vitamin B_{12}. The role of B_{12} and cobalt salts in medicine and agriculture is still being actively investigated, and some of these aspects are

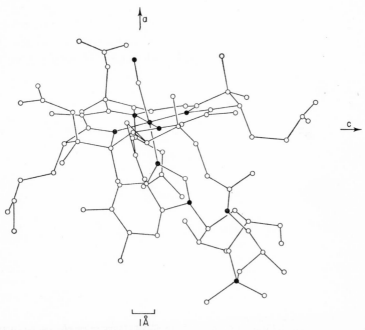

Fig. 1.2. Atomic positions in the molecule of B_{12} viewed parallel with the crystallographic *b*-axis in crystals of wet B_{12}. The solid circles represent cobalt, nitrogen or phosphorus atoms. (From Brink-Shoemaker *et al.*, 1964.)

discussed in Chapter 3. From the chemists' point of view the most interesting developments in this area will be the elucidation of the exact role played by B_{12} in metabolism in man and other animals.

Developments in the fields of biochemistry (including microbiology), organic chemistry, co-ordination chemistry and X-ray crystallography are much more closely linked and have probably been much more dramatic over the last twenty years than those in medicine and agriculture. One can, at the risk of being accused of oversimplification, attempt to pick out the main lines of research within these four related areas and their periods of maximum activity. After the original impetus received from medicine in 1926 the main stimuli have come from the fields of microbiology and biochemistry, in which one can discern four successive and overlapping phases of activity. The first phase ended with the successful isolation of B_{12} in 1948. The second phase (mainly 1948–1955, but still continuing) involved the development of methods for the large-scale production of B_{12} by fermentation techniques through the screening and selection of micro-organisms; see the reviews by Perlman (1959) and by Mervyn and Smith (1964). It soon became clear that B_{12} was only one of a family of closely-related compounds (corrinoids) occurring in nature, and the third phase (with peak activity from 1950 to 1962) may be considered as answering the question "which corrinoids occur in nature"; for fuller details of this phase see the reviews by Kon and Pawełkiewicz (1958), Perlman (1959), Mervyn and Smith (1964) and Wagner (1966). The most extensive work carried

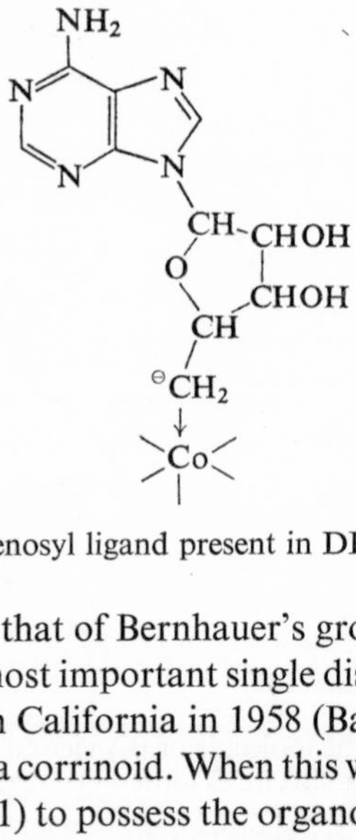

Fig. 1.3. The 5′-deoxyadenosyl ligand present in DBC and other coenzymes.

out under this heading was that of Bernhauer's group at Stuttgart (Bernhauer *et al.*, 1963, 1964), but the most important single discovery was the isolation by Barker and his associates in California in 1958 (Barker *et al.*, 1958) of the so-called "coenzyme" form of a corrinoid. When this was shown by X-ray analysis (Lenhert and Hodgkin, 1961) to possess the organoligand shown in Fig. 1.3, it led directly to a sharp increase in interest in both synthetic work for the preparation of organo-corrinoids and in the co-ordination chemistry of corrinoids in general. Barker's discovery of the coenzyme can also be considered as the start of the fourth phase of activity, that of enzymatic reactions, in which one aims to answer the questions "what reactions do corrinoids catalyse in conjunction with proteins and how". The synthesis of methionine had been shown to require B_{12} in one particular case in 1954, but the spate of work in discovering and studying the enzymatic reactions really got under way in 1958 and is still continuing. In no case has the mechanism of reaction yet been unravelled, but there can be little doubt from the quantity and quality of work being carried out in this field that the situation may soon be changed.

The enzymatic reactions are discussed in Chapter 17; see also the reviews by Weissbach and Dickerman (1965), Barker (1967), Stadtman (1967) and Hogenkamp (1968).

X-ray analysis, carried out by Professor Dorothy Hodgkin and her associates at Oxford, has played a very important part in the development of vitamin B_{12} chemistry. Their work revealed the presence of two structures hitherto unknown in nature, namely the corrin ring which is present in all corrinoids (see Fig. 1.1) and the cobalt–carbon bond which is present in the coenzymes (see Fig. 1.3). The structure of the corrinoids which have been examined in detail also provide a unique insight into hydrogen-bonding, inter- and intramolecular interactions and subtle changes in configuration (e.g. of the corrin ring) in such complex molecules or co-ordination compounds. After the isolation of B_{12} in 1948 the task of elucidating its structure was taken up by both organic chemists and by X-ray crystallographers. The two approaches were complementary. The classical degradative techniques used by the organic chemists provided evidence for the structure of the periphery of the molecule, while X-ray diffraction located the atoms near the cobalt atom in the centre. The structure of the corrin ring was announced by the X-ray crystallographers in 1954 (Brink *et al.*, 1954) and the complete structures of several corrinoids within the next few years. History repeated itself again shortly afterwards. The problem of determining the structure of the coenzyme, isolated by Barker in 1958, was taken up by both organic chemists and by X-ray crystallographers, but it was the latter who established the existence of the cobalt–carbon bond (Lenhert and Hodgkin, 1961). Although work on the X-ray analysis of the corrinoids began in 1948, the hey-day of crystallography (as far as the outside world was concerned) can probably be considered as lasting from 1954 into the late 1960's. Professor Hodgkin's elegant work in applying X-ray diffraction techniques to such complicated molecules was rewarded with the Nobel Prize for Chemistry in 1964. X-ray diffraction will probably be called in again in the future to elucidate the structure of the enzymatically active complexes formed between the corrinoids and proteins and hence provide information on finer points of detail in the mechanism of the enzymatic reactions. Professor Hodgkin has reviewed the work of her group (Hodgkin, 1958, 1964, 1965).

The first phase in the organic chemistry of B_{12} was the determination of the structure, chiefly by classical degradative methods, which began immediately after the isolation of B_{12} in 1948. Most of this work was carried out in the pharmaceutical firms by teams led by Folkers (Merck, U.S.), Smith (Glaxo, U.K.) and Petrow (B.D.H., U.K.) respectively and by Todd and his colleagues at Cambridge. This phase came to an end shortly after 1954, when the structure of B_{12} was finally established by X-ray analysis (see above). For an account of this structural work see the reviews by Folkers and Wolf (1954), Smith (1955), Johnson and Todd (1957) and Bonnett (1963). The isolation of the coenzyme in

1958 again led to work on structural elucidation, which lasted until X-ray analysis in 1961 showed the coenzyme to be an organometallic complex with a cobalt-carbon bond. This in turn led to a great deal of work on the synthesis of organocorrinoids and on the properties and reactions of these compounds, which has continued unabated up to the present and which overlaps with work on the co-ordination chemistry of the corrinoids (see below). The last phase of organic chemistry, beginning in the early 1960's, has as its aim the total synthesis of the corrinoid structure with the correct substituents and stereo-chemistry found in the naturally occurring compounds. Johnson and his co-workers in the U.K. have been interested in the synthesis of corroles and tetradehydrocorrins, which differ from corrinoids in possessing extra double bonds in the periphery of the ring, while the problem of synthesizing the corri-noids themselves has been undertaken by Eschenmoser in Switzerland, Cornforth in the U.K. and Woodward in the U. S. Johnson's work is summarized in his review articles (Harris *et al.*, 1966; Johnson, 1967). Eschenmoser has summarized his earlier work in a review article and a later paper gives refer-ences to work up to and including 1969 (Eschenmoser *et al.*, 1965; Yamada *et al.*, 1969). Woodward gave an account of his work in 1968, but Cornforth's work has so far only been reported in lectures. See also the recent review by Melent'eva, Pekel' and Berezovskii (1969).

The last area of B_{12} chemistry to gain momentum has undoubtedly been that of co-ordination chemistry. Co-ordination chemistry is here taken to mean essentially the properties and reactions of the cobalt atom and the axial ligands and includes the organo-metallic chemistry of the corrinoids, i.e. the chemistry of corrinoids in which one of the axial ligands is an organo-ligand. Although the co-ordination chemistry of the corrinoids has, in fact, been studied ever since the isolation of B_{12} in 1948, the real upsurge in interest can be dated back to 1961 when Lenhert and Hodgkin (1961) showed by X-ray analysis that the coenzyme form of B_{12} contained a cobalt-carbon bond and was therefore the first known naturally occurring organo-metallic compound. This discovery led to an immediate outburst of activity amongst organic chemists in synthe-sizing both the coenzyme itself and a wide range of other organo-corrinoids, which provided co-ordination chemists with a wealth of different unidentate organo-ligands (e.g. CH_3CH_2—, CH_2=CH—, HC≡C—, CH_3CO—, HOOC.CH_2—, etc.) whose properties and reactions could be investigated. It was soon shown that these organocorrinoids were diamagnetic and could be considered as cobalt(III) complexes containing a co-ordinated carbanion (e.g. $CH_3^- \rightarrow Co^{III}$). It also soon became clear that corrinoids which contained an organo-ligand or certain sulphur-bonded ligands (notably SO_3^{2-}) showed pro-perties and reactions (e.g. spectra, formation constants for the binding of other ligands, photochemical reactions) which were very different from those of corrinoids containing the ligands more commonly studied by co-ordination chemists such as H_2O, NH_3, CN^-, NCS^- etc. As will be described in further detail in the final chapter the two main developments in the co-ordination chemistry of B_{12} have been in our knowledge and understanding of (A) organo-metallic compounds containing a σ-bonded carbanion ligand (in contrast to π-bonded ligands such as CO, olefins, acetylenes, cyclopentadienyl, etc.), and (B) the nature of the metal-ligand bond and cis- and trans-effects. The role of organo-corrinoids in enzymatic reactions has provided the stimulus for work under (A), while the existence of a wide range of easily handled corrinoids with different ligands and such different properties has stimulated research under (B). Results achieved with the corrinoids have, in turn, sparked off similar work on other cobalt(III) complexes. Contributions to the co-ordination chemistry of corrinoids have come from many laboratories throughout the world, and much of the work has been done by organic chemists, who have been interested primarily in the organometallic aspects. Of the work on co-ordination chemistry reported in the 1960's particular mention should be made of the contributions from the laboratories of Johnson in the U.K., of Bernhauer and his former colleagues in West Germany and of Hogenkamp in the U.S. The group at Oxford, including Williams and the author, represents the most inorganic wing of those involved in studying the co-ordination chemistry of the corrinoids.

It would probably be true to say that of the four areas of the chemistry of B_{12} delineated in this section (namely biochemistry, organic chemistry, X-ray crystallography and co-ordination chemistry) the greatest developments over the last decade have occurred within the areas of biochemistry and co-ordination chemistry. But, although the biochemistry has been well reviewed several times within the last few years, there has been no adequate review of the co-ordination chemistry. Some aspects of co-ordination chemistry have been included in the reviews by Bernhauer et al. (1963, 1964), Wagner (1966) and Hill et al. (1969) and information relating to the corrinoids has been included in a review on cis- and trans- effects in cobalt(III) complexes by Pratt and Thorp (1969). But there would appear to be a need for a more comprehensive review of the co-ordination chemistry of the corrinoids.

II. AIM AND SCOPE OF THE PRESENT WORK

The scope and treatment of the material in this book, as in any other, is determined mainly by

1. the need to have some unifying theme,
2. the readership it is intended to serve,
3. the existence of other reviews or books on similar topics and, of course,

4. personal preference and prejudice (for which any good writer should be able to find cogent reasons and arguments).

The theme of this book is the co-ordination chemistry of the cobalt corrinoids (vitamin B$_{12}$ and related compounds). It is useful to divide the corrinoid molecule (see Fig. 1.1) into the following four regions:

1. the axial ligands,
2. the cobalt atom,
3. the conjugated corrin chain of the equatorial ligand and
4. the side-chains; the outer ring of carbon atoms could be placed in either (3) or (4).

The co-ordination chemistry of the corrinoids concerns primarily regions (1) and (2). The importance of the corrin ring (region 3) resides mainly in the fact that the absorption spectra of the cobalt corrinoids are due to electronic transitions within the conjugated chain and provide a very sensitive indicator of changes at the cobalt atom due to changes in the valency or in the number and nature of the axial ligands. The few known "organic" reactions of the corrin ring are also of interest for the evidence they provide of *cis*-effects within the complex. As a broad generalization, therefore, one can say that the proportion of the total chemistry which is relevant to co-ordination chemistry falls and that to organic chemistry rises, as we progress from the centre (cobalt and axial ligands) out to the periphery (the side-chains). This will be reflected in the thoroughness with which the chemistry of the different regions is covered in this book.

The co-ordination chemistry of the corrinoids is probably of interest to several different groups of chemists, for example:

1. those already working in the field,
2. biochemists working on the enzymatic reactions of the corrinoids, who may obtain useful clues about the binding of the corrinoids to proteins and the mechanism of enzymatic reactions from studies on simpler systems,
3. biochemists interested in other metal complexes and metal-containing enzymes, in particular the iron porphyrins,
4. co-ordination chemists, working with other cobalt complexes, which often show similarities to the corrinoids,
5. co-ordination chemists in general, who may be interested in the contributions to the theory of the metal-ligand bond, which have come from the study of cobalt(III) corrinoids and
6. organometallic chemists, since the organocorrinoids have probably contributed more than any other group of complexes to filling the gap in our knowledge about the simplest possible type of transition metal organometallic complex, viz. the complex containing a unidentate σ-bonded carbanion.

For readers in groups 4–6 a short chapter has been included, which provides a brief sketch of the role of Vitamin B_{12} in medicine and in nature in general (Chapter 3). The enzymatic reactions, which are catalysed by corrinoids in conjunction with a protein, are summarized in Chapter 17; in no case has the mechanism of reaction yet been completely elucidated. One might think there would also be a case for including a chapter on the theory of transition metal complexes, including crystal field theory: quite the reverse. The main contribution of B_{12} chemistry to co-ordination chemistry has been to overthrow some of our most cherished existing theories and preconceived ideas, such as the importance of crystal field theory in correlating chemical properties, the kinetic inertness of cobalt(III) complexes and the instability of the bond between a transition metal and an alkyl group. The main contributions within the area of the co-ordination chemistry of B_{12} which are of interest and relevance to co-ordination chemists and biochemists outside this area are summarized in the final chapter.

The way in which the chemistry of vitamin B_{12} has been and still is developing, together with the available reviews, has been summarized in the preceding section. The only other book written on the subject is the valuable monograph called simply "Vitamin B_{12}" by E. Lester Smith, which was first published in 1957 and finally revised and brought out as the third edition in 1965; this concentrates mainly on the organic and medical aspects of vitamin B_{12}. It seems that the areas of biochemistry, organic chemistry and X-ray crystallography have been or are being adequately surveyed and reviewed, but that there is a real need to review the co-ordination chemistry of B_{12}. There is also undoubtedly scope for a new monograph on the subject of B_{12}, but to survey the whole field from medicine to X-ray crystallography would probably be too much for any single author and perhaps even too much to include in one book.

The aim of this book is, therefore,

1. to cover fairly thoroughly the co-ordination chemistry of B_{12} (including the relevant areas of X-ray crystallography), i.e. to include all relevant material, to provide comprehensive references and a brief historical background and, where necessary, to discuss points at issue and to make suggestions and
2. to cover rather superficially the areas of organic chemistry and biochemistry, i.e. to provide only brief surveys together with references to reviews on the subject.

III. ARRANGEMENT OF THE MATERIAL

Both the collection and the organization of the information have presented problems. Information which is relevant to the co-ordination chemistry of the corrinoids is scattered through vast numbers of different journals, ranging from journals in the field of medicine and pharmacy to those in physical and theoretical chemistry. The amount of relevant material is also, by the usual standards of co-ordination chemistry, immense. This is, firstly, because the corrinoids are large and complex molecules; secondly, because their important role in medicine and biochemistry has stimulated remarkably detailed studies (particularly by X-ray analysis); and, thirdly, because the ease with which they can be handled and studied (e.g. stability under a wide range of conditions, solubility in water) has encouraged an extensive investigation of their chemistry.

The arrangement of the chapters in this book is as follows. The physical and chemical properties of the corrinoids are described in Chapters 5–18 inclusive. Chapters 2–4 present certain background material which is either essential (Nomenclature, Chapter 2), is intended as interesting reading (B_{12} in Biochemistry, Medicine and Agriculture, Chapter 3) or is related to the chemistry of the corrinoids (Preparation, Purification and Identification, Chapter 4). The organization of material in Chapters 5–18 is rather more complicated. We wish to include information on bond-lengths and bond angles, spectroscopic properties, equilibria and reactions; we have to deal with weak interactions, in particular hydrogen-bonds, as well as strong interactions (covalent or co-ordinate bonds); these interactions may occur at several different sites and even between sites within the corrinoid molecule. The following scheme has been adopted. The electronic (or u.v.-visible) spectra, which have provided the most widely used tool for studying the equilibria and reactions of the corrinoids, are discussed in Chapter 5. The structures and certain other physical properties of the corrinoids (bond-lengths and bond-angles; inter and intra-molecular hydrogen-bonding; steric repulsion and van der Waals interaction between the different parts of the corrinoid molecule; evidence from absorption spectra, nuclear magnetic resonance and infrared spectra for strong electronic interaction extending from the conjugated corrin ring through the cobalt ion to the co-ordinated atoms of the axial ligands) are described in Chapter 6. Some physical properties which provide evidence for the valency of the cobalt ion (e.g. magnetic susceptibility, e.s.r. and n.m.r. data) are also included in Chapter 7.

The remaining material, i.e. the chemical properties, has been roughly arranged according to a twofold classification: first, into equilibria (Chapters 7–10) and reactions (Chapters 11–17) and, secondly, according to the site of the equilibria or reactions (the axial ligands, the cobalt ion, the corrin ring, the side-chains) or the type of reaction. This arrangement provides a fairly logical system for handling the bulk of the material, though some overlap is inevitable and some inconsistencies have been allowed to remain. The equilibria considered in this book and the way in which they are distributed amongst Chapters 7–10 is shown below (where L is an axial ligand, R the corrin ring,

S a side-chain, and M any metal cation). We have treated as equilibria all reactions which involve the binding or loss of Lewis acids or bases which can exist free in aqueous solution, even though some of these reactions have not yet been shown to be reversible (e.g. the binding of cyanide by aquocobalamin and of cobalt by metal-free corrin ligands).

Site	Equilibrium Involved	Chapter	Section
Co	Electrons (i.e. change in valency)	7	—
Co–L	Substitution of one L by another in octahedral Co(III) corrinoids	8	II, IV, V
	Loss of one L to give five-co-ordinate Co(III) corrinoids	8	III
	Substitution and/or loss of L in Co(II) corrinoids	7	III, IV
L	Co-ordinated ligand $\pm$ H$^+$, M	8	IV
R, Co–R	Metal-free corrin $\pm$ H$^+$	9	I
	$\pm$ M (including Co)	9	II
	Co-corrin + H$^+$ (addition to conjugated chain)	9	III
	$-$ H$^+$ (loss from C$_8$)	15	I
S	Side-chains $\pm$ H$^+$	10	I
	$\pm$ M	10	II

The material on reactions has been distributed amongst the chapters as follows:

Site	Reaction	Chapter	Section
(1) Rates of (and qualitative observations on) the above-mentioned equilibrations involving ions and electrons only.			
Co	Electron transfer reactions	11	—
Co–L	Ligand substitution reactions of cobalt(III) complexes	12	II
(2) Simple (i.e. stoichiometric) reactions involving the making or breaking of covalent bonds (including Co–C and Co–S bonds).			
Co, Co–L	Other redox reactions	11	—
	Formation and cleavage of Co–C bonds	13	I, II
	Formation and cleavage of Co–S bonds	13	III
	Photochemical reactions	14	—
R	Reactions of the corrin ring	15	—
S	Reactions of the side-chains	16	—
(3) Catalytic reactions.			
Co–L	Redox reactions	11	VI
	Enzymatic reactions	17	—

The final chapter (Chapter 18) summarizes the main findings which are of general interest to co-ordination chemists or to biochemists and draws together related material which because of the above arrangement is scattered over several chapters. It should be emphasized once again that the detail with which the material of each chapter is treated varies considerably. Those chapters which are of greatest relevance to co-ordination chemistry (Chapters 7, 8, 11–14) together with the chapter on nomenclature (Chapter 2) are treated comprehensively. Some of the other chapters are treated in reasonable detail (Chapters 5, 6, 9, 15), others only superficially (Chapters 3, 4, 10, 16, 17).

2

NOMENCLATURE, ABBREVIATIONS AND CONVENTIONS

The corrinoids are large and complicated molecules and they pose commensurate problems of nomenclature. There are two main difficulties in devising any systematic nomenclature for the corrinoids. Firstly, there are so many different possible types of derivative (involving changes in both the equatorial and axial ligands) that any fully comprehensive and systematic nomenclature is bound to be unwieldy; there will inevitably be a conflict between devising a more systematic but rather unwieldy system and a less systematic but more convenient system. Secondly, the corrinoids have been studied by a wide spectrum of scientists, and a system of nomenclature which is convenient for one group may not be convenient for another. In particular, the present IUPAC–IUB* rules have been drawn up on the basis of treating the corrinoids as organic molecules (i.e. the rules can readily cope with changes in the corrin ring and side-chains), and are therefore less convenient when treating them as co-ordination complexes (i.e. they cannot so readily cope with changes in the number and nature of the axial ligands).

Interest in the co-ordination chemistry of the corrinoids has developed much more recently than interest in the organic chemistry, and many essential features of their co-ordination chemistry have only been established or investigated within the last few years. It is therefore not surprising that rules of nomenclature drawn up to cope with the organic chemistry should prove inadequate to cope with the co-ordination chemistry.

The IUPAC–IUB rules for nomenclature of the corrinoids are presented and discussed in Section I.

The rules for nomenclature which have been devised for use in this book are given and exemplified in Section II. The aim has been twofold:

---

* IUPAC is the International Union of Pure and Applied Chemistry; IUB is the International Union of Biochemistry.

(1) To develop a system of nomenclature which can cope with extensive variation in both (i) the large organic equatorial ligand (the corrin ring and side-chains), and (ii) the axial ligands;

(2) To devise a set of rules which can be applied rigorously and systematically when required, but which can also be simplified and modified to give a more concise nomenclature if and where the context permits.

It is hoped that the type of approach adopted here may perhaps find application in the nomenclature of other groups of co-ordination complexes such as the porphyrins and phthalocyanines, where one has to cope (or probably will have to cope in the future) with extensive variations in two rather different parts of the molecule, viz. the conjugated equatorial ligand and the axial ligands.

Section III contains a brief glossary of some of the more common "trivial" or non-systematic names (i.e. names which do not conform to the IUPAC–IUB rules), which are also used in this book. Section IV lists abbreviations (e.g. for ligands) and conventions in common use throughout the book together with diagrams of other tetradentate ligands such as "salen" which, like the corrin ring, form a square planar or "equatorial" arrangement around the cobalt ion.

I. THE IUPAC–IUB RULES

There are three stages in the development of internationally accepted rules of nomenclature. First, experts in each field are requested to suggest rules for naming the compounds or concepts they are working with. These suggestions or reports are then studied by the Commissions of the International Union of Pure and Applied Chemistry. From these deliberations and with the approval of the Council of IUPAC the so-called tentative rules are published. After about two years, if the tentative rules prove to be satisfactory even with modest revision, they are then declared definitive. This is the third and final stage. However, definitive rules as well as tentative rules may be revised and changed as experience dictates. In the case of the corrinoids the stages have been as follows:

(1). An *ad hoc* Nomenclature Commission met during the First European Symposium on "Vitamin B_{12} and Intrinsic Factor", which was held in Hamburg in 1956, and its recommendations were published in the proceedings of that symposium (Smith, 1957).

(2). The Commission on the Nomenclature of Organic Chemistry of the IUPAC authorized "Tentative Rules for Nomenclature in the Vitamin B_{12} field" in 1957, which were published in 1958 (IUPAC, 1958).

(3). The Commission on the Nomenclature of Biological Chemistry of the IUPAC met in 1959 and the "Definitive Rules for the Nomenclature of Vitamins" were published in 1960 (IUPAC, 1960b).

(4) A round table discussion on nomenclature was held at the Second European Symposium on "Vitamin B_{12} and Intrinsic Factor" in Hamburg in 1961 and several suggestions were made in the light of recent developments (Smith, 1962).

(5) The Definitive Rules mentioned under (3) were revised by a Joint IUPAC–IUB Commission on Biochemical Nomenclature, whose Tentative Rules were published in 1966 (IUPAC–IUB, 1966) and replace the former Definitive Rules.

These Tentative Rules for the nomenclature of corrinoids are as follows:

(1) Compound I should be designated *corrin*. The number 20 is omitted in the corrin nucleus so that the numbering system will correspond to that for the porphyrin nucleus. The generic name for compounds containing the corrin nucleus is *corrinoid*. Pentadehydrocorrin should be designated *corrole*.

(2) Compound II should be designated *cobyrinic acid*. The terminal carboxyl groups or modified carboxyl groups are designated by letters *a* to *g*, as shown in II.

Cobyrinic acid *a, b, c, d, e, g*-hexa-amide, also known as Factor V_{1a}, should be designated *cobyric acid*.

(3) Compound III (R = —OH; R' = —H) should be designated *cobinic acid*. Compound III (R = —NH$_2$; R' = —H) should be designated *cobinamide*.

(4) Compound III (R = —OH; R' = X) should be designated *cobamic acid*. Compound III (R = —NH$_2$; R' = X) should be designated *cobamide*.

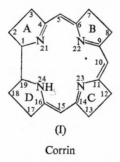

(I)

Corrin

(5) For nucleotides of this series the name of the additional heterocyclic radical, ending in -yl, should be added to the name of the appropriate ion designated in Rules 1–6.

Examples

α-(5,6-dimethylbenzimidazolyl)cobamide cyanide, also known as vitamin B_{12} (Formula IV)

α-(2-methyladenyl)cobamide cyanide, also known as Factor A

α-(5-hydroxybenzimidazolyl)cobamide cyanide, also known as vitamin $B_{12\,III}$

(6) For molecules formed from the ions designated in Rules 1–4, the ligand attached to the metal should be designated by the methods used in inorganic chemistry and not by a prefix which would denote substitution in the organic part of the molecule.

Examples

cobamic acid dichloride

dinitrocobamic acid

α-(5,6-dimethylbenzimidazolyl)aquocobamide, also known as vitamin B_{12b}

(7) When the cobalt atom in compounds I, II or III is replaced by that of another metal, the symbol "co-" should be replaced by the name of the other metal followed by "o" or "i" according to the valence. When the cobalt is replaced by hydrogen, the prefix "hydrogeno" should replace "co".

Examples

ferrobamic acid

nickelibamic acid

hydrogenobamic acid

(8) Other compounds should be designated systematically from the largest of the compounds I–III that is contained in that derivative.

Examples

cobyrinic acid *a,b,c,d,e,g*-hexa-amide *f*-2-hydroxyethylamide 3,8,13,17-tetraethyl-1,2,2,5,7,7,12,12,15,17,18-undecamethylcobalticorrindichloride (for the dichloride of fully decarboxylated cobyrinic acid)

12,1'-carboxycobyrinic acid (for cobyrinic acid in which one of the 12-methyl groups has been replaced by —CH_2COOH)

(9) The compound α-(5,6-dimethylbenzimidazolyl)cobamide cyanide, also known as vitamin B_{12}, may be designated *cyanocobalamin*.

The tautomeric compounds α-(5,6-dimethylbenzimidazolyl)aquocobamide and α-(5,6-dimethylbenzimidazolyl)hydroxocobamide, also known as vitamin B_{12a} or vitamin B_{12b}, may be designated *aquocobalamin* or *hydroxocobalamin*.

The compound α-(5,6-dimethylbenzimidazolyl)cobamide nitrite, also known as vitamin B_{12c}, may be designated *nitritocobalamin*.

Where it is necessary to specify the state of oxidation of the cobalt atom, the oxidation number may be inserted after "cob", *e.g.*

vitamin B_{12}	cyanocob(III)alamin
vitamin B_{12r}	cyanocob(II)alamin
vitamin B_{12s}	cyanocob(I)alamin

(10) The coenzyme forms of the B_{12} vitamins and their analogues, in all of which an organic ligand is attached to the cobalt atom, may also be named according to these rules. For example, the compound known to be concerned in methionine biosynthesis in some systems, in which a methyl group is attached to cobalt, may be designated methylcobalamin or α-(5,6-dimethyl-benzimidazolyl)-*Co*-methylcobamide.

Coenzyme B_{12} may be designated 5'-deoxyadenosylcobalamin or α-(5,6-dimethylbenzimidazolyl)-*Co*-5'-deoxyadenosylcobamide.

The coenzyme form of pseudovitamin B_{12}, active in glutamate metabolism in some systems, may be designated α-(adenyl)-*Co*-5'-deoxyadenosylcobamide.

Notes on formulae (see p. 18)

(1) In formulae II and III, the corrin nucleus is represented as being roughly in the plane of the paper. Bonds joining peripheral substituents to the nucleus are shown by the same conventions as in the steroid series, *viz.*: ⎯⎯ full (heavy) lines, bonds *above* the plane of the ring system; ------ dashed lines, bonds *below* the plane of the ring system.

(2) Formulae II, III and IV represent the true absolute stereochemistry of the structures as determined by the X-ray work of Hodgkin *et al.*

(3) Formula X represents the already known absolute stereochemistry of the ribofuranose unit. For convenience in comparison with IV, formula X is written with the α-substituent at C-1 *above* the plane of the ring system (*i.e.* the reverse of the usual carbohydrate fashion).

Since there are differences between the successive sets of rules which may confuse the reader when reading the literature, the most important ones are here summarized.

Rings A–D have the same lettering in all sets. The numbering of the carbon atoms is the same in all sets of rules except IUPAC's 1958 publication where the numbering begins with C_1 at the present C_{19} and terminates with C_{19} at the present C_{18}. The nitrogen atoms on rings A–D respectively have been designated A–D in Smith (1957), 20–23 in IUPAC's "Tentative Rules for Nomenclature in The Vitamin B_{12} Field" (1958) and 21–24 in all the other Rules.

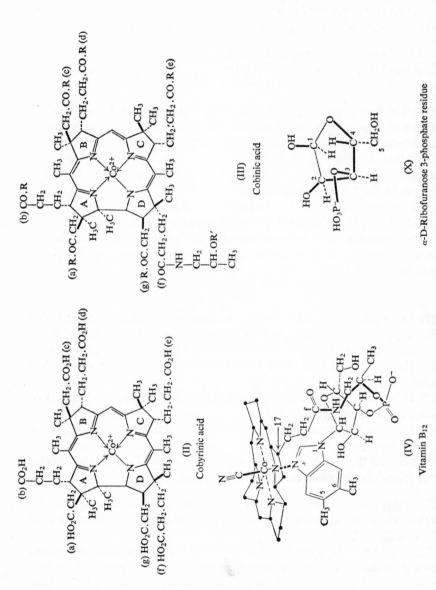

(II)

Cobyrinic acid

(III)

Cobinic acid

(IV)

Vitamin B$_{12}$

(X)

α-D-Ribofuranose 3-phosphate residue

Formula IV is a sketch based on Hodgkin *et al.* Details of substituents on corrin nucleus (except side-chain at C-17) omitted for the sake of clarity.

The number 20 is omitted so that the numbering of the remaining carbon and nitrogen atoms corresponds to that for the porphyrin nucleus, where C_{20} is the *meso*-carbon atom between rings A and D.

The names "cobyric acid" and "corrole" were suggested in Smith, 1962 and adopted in 1966 by IUPAC–IUB and are therefore not met in earlier work. Several differences are found between Smith, 1957 and other rules:

Smith, 1957	All others
Corphyrin	Corrinoid
Corphyrinic acid	Cobyrinic acid
Corphinic acid	Cobinic acid
Corphinamide	Cobinamide

Cobamic acid and cobinamide are the same in all sets.

It should be noted that the methyl group on C_1 is situated below the plane of the diagram and the bond should therefore be represented by a broken line instead of a full line; a full line has been used by mistake in sets 1–3.

Recent research has revealed several inadequacies and inconsistencies in the present IUPAC–IUB Rules, which are discussed below. A more fundamental problem, however, is presented by the conflict between these rules and the IUPAC Rules for the nomenclature of co-ordination compounds (IUPAC, 1960a). In the following discussion the former rules are referred to as "Corr", the latter as "Co-ord". Section 7.2 ("Formulas and Names for Complex Compounds in General") of the Co-ord Rules, which is the most relevant for the purposes of comparing the Corr Rules and the new nomenclature proposed below, can be summarized as follows:

Section 7.21. The central atom (i.e. the metal atom) should be placed after the ligands.
Section 7.22 (and 2.252). The oxidation number of the central atom is indicated by Roman numerals placed in parentheses immediately following the name.
Section 7.23. Names may be supplemented with the prefixes *cis*, *trans* etc.
Section 7.24. Complex anions shall be given the termination -ate. Complex cations and neutral molecules are given no distinguishing termination.
Section 7.25. The order of citation of ligands shall be anionic ligands (in the sequence H^-, O^{2-}, HO^-, other monatomic anions, polyatomic anions, organic anions), then neutral and cationic ligands (in the sequence H_2O, NH_3, other inorganic ligands, organic ligands).

The following examples show some of the differences between the Corr and Co-ord rules. In conflict with Co-ord 7.21 the Corr rules include the name of the metal in the name of the organic equatorial ligand in the form of a prefix. This leads to the confusing situation that when the cobalt is replaced by some other metal the whole name of the organic part must be changed, e.g. *co*bamic acid and *ferro*bamic acid for the cobalt and iron analogues with the same ligand (Corr 7). Corr 9 stipulates, in conflict with Co-ord 7.22, that the Roman numerals which indicate the oxidation state are inserted into the middle of name of the equatorial ligand, e.g. cyanocob(I)alamin; presumably this would lead to forms such as ferrob(I)amic acid. A further illogicality is that there is no cyanide co-ordinated to the cobalt in "cyanocob(I)alamin" (see Chapter 7, Section V). According to Corr 6, "the ligand attached to the metal should be designated by the methods used in inorganic chemistry and not by a prefix which would denote substitution in the organic part of the molecule". However, the following examples (from Corr 9 and 10) show three different methods of specifying the ligands in corrinoid complexes which differ only in the nature of one axial anionic ligand [α-DMB is α-(5,6-dimethylbenzimidazolyl)]:

α-DMB-hydroxocobamide
α-DMB-cobamide cyanide
α-DMB-*Co*-methyl cobamide

It is not at all obvious how they conform to "methods used in inorganic chemistry" or why or when three different methods have to be used. In fact, it is not clear that the axial ligands have to be specified at all; Factor V$_{1a}$, which has been shown by X-ray analysis to possess CN$^-$ and H$_2$O as axial ligands (Hodgkin *et al.*, 1962) "should be designated cobyric acid" (Corr 2).

Further difficulties arise in the nomenclature of compounds whose structure has only recently been established and for which adequate provision had not been made in the Corr rules. The Corr rules can, for example, define the nature of the nucleotide in the side-chain, but there is no method given by which one can indicate whether the heterocyclic base is co-ordinated or not. Reference to Fig. IV of the Corr rules shows that the base is co-ordinated in the case of cyanocobalamin or α-(5,6-dimethylbenzimidazolyl)cobamide cyanide; but in α-(adenyl)-*Co*-5'-deoxyadenosyl-cobamide (example in Corr 10) the base is now known not to be co-ordinated and the cobalt is in fact five-co-ordinate (Hill *et al.*, 1970b). Nor have any rules been made for the naming of the two stereoisomers which are possible when the axial ligands are different.

II. RULES FOR NOMENCLATURE USED IN THIS BOOK

In the light of our present knowledge of the equilibria and reactions shown by the corrinoids, one would wish any system of nomenclature to convey clearly and concisely the following information about the different parts of the molecule:

1. Cobalt
   a. The valency
   b. Whether four-, five- or six-co-ordinate.
2. Axial ligands
   a. Their number (0, 1 or 2), i.e. the same information as in 1b.
   b. Their identity, including those cases where the co-ordinated ligand can
   (i) show ligand isomerism, as in Co—NCS and Co—SCN, (ii) lose a
   proton, as in Co—CH_2COOH, (iii) add a proton, as in 5-deoxyadenosyl,
   the glutathionate anion or adenine in ψ-B_{12}, (iv) co-ordinate further to
   another metal, as in the case of Co—CH=CH_2 which probably forms a
   π-complex with the Ag(I) cation and (v) form a bridged complex, as in the
   derivatives which contain the structures Co(III)—$(CH_2)_4$—Co(III) and
   Co(II)—I—Co(II).
   c. The relative orientation of the two axial ligands (if different).
3. The corrin ring
   a. Possible isomers of the ring due, for example, to stereoisomeric change
   at C_8.
   b. Possible gain (e.g. at C_{10}) or loss (e.g. from C_8) of a proton.
   c. Changes caused by reactions such as substitution at C_{10}.
4. The side-chains
   a. The identity of the side-chains and whether any functional groups are
   dissociated (e.g. —COOH, —OH in the sugar), protonated (e.g.
   —$CONH_2$, the phosphate in the nucleotide, the heterocyclic base), co-
   ordinated to another metal (e.g. the heterocyclic base), alkylated or otherwise modified.
5. The corrinoid complex as a whole.
   a. The identity of ionic salts, in which the corrinoid may be either an
   anion or cation.

The main principles adopted in devising the present set of rules have been

1. To make a clear and consistent separation between the naming of (i) the
axial ligands and (ii) the corrin ring with its side-chains by placing them in a
systematic order.
2. To incorporate as much as possible of the existing IUPAC–IUB rules and
certain common trivial names for the naming of the corrin ring and its side-
chains.
3. To adhere as closely as possible to the IUPAC rules on the nomenclature
of co-ordination compounds, and to treat the corrin ring and its side-chains
as one ligand. The main exception is that the corrin ring is always placed after
the names of the axial ligands, even if the latter are neutral bases.
4. Finally allowance is made for each rule to be simplified or otherwise
modified, as and where the context permits, to give a shorter name. The way

in which each rule can be modified is given in italics and preceded by an asterisk. Explanatory notes are enclosed in brackets.

Proposed Rules for the Nomenclature of Corrinoid Co-ordination Compounds.
Rule 1. The order of citation shall be:

1. Prefixes to denote the relative orientation of the two axial ligands, when they are different.
2. The axial ligands, including ligands which may form part of a side-chain to the corrin ring.
3. The equatorial ligand (the corrin ring together with its substituents and side-chains).
4. The metal.
5. The oxidation number of the metal.

The names under (3) shall be enclosed in square brackets.
(The order prefixes–ligands–metal–valence is in accord with Co-ord sections 7.21, 7.22 and 7.23; the separate and fixed position of the equatorial ligand and its enclosure in square brackets is, of course, not. The use of square brackets is designed to separate the names or suffixes belonging to the axial and equatorial ligands and hence to prevent confusion between, for example, methyl or cyanide as an axial ligand and as a substituent of the corrin ring, e.g.

    dicyano-[cobinamide]-cobalt(III)   (CN as ligand)
    diaquo-[10-cyanocobinamide]-cobalt(III)   (CN as substituent)

A second difference from the Co-ord Rules is the absence of the termination -ate for complex anions (cf. Co-ord. 7.24). This is because the overall charge on the corrinoid is usually determined by the presence of positive or negative charges so far from the cobalt ion (e.g. carboxylates in the side-chains, phosphate in the nucleotide side-chain, protonation of adenine in the 5-deoxyadenosyl ligand) that they have little relevance to the co-ordination chemistry. It seems simplest, therefore, not to use any suffix which indicates the presence of an overall negative charge on a corrinoid complex).

The above order of citation may not be varied, but certain members may be omitted. The prefixes are only required in certain cases (see Rule 5). The name "cobalt" may be omitted when, as in this book, we are dealing only with cobalt complexes, except when the valency is expressed, e.g.

    dicyano-[cobalamin]
    [cobalamin]-cobalt(I)

Amongst cobalt corrinoids the valency may be omitted for cobalt(III) complexes only (see Rule 2). The square brackets may be omitted when the name of the equatorial ligand is a single word (such as cobalamin) and comes either first or last in the name of the whole complex (see Rule 6). The base present in the cobalamins, namely 5,6-dimethylbenzimidazole, is abbreviated to Bzm (Rule 4). These modifications to Rule 1 are used in many of the exemplifications to the rules given below.

(Since all the ligands, including those which form part of a side-chain to the corrin ring, are named explicitly, the co-ordination number of the cobalt (4, 5, or 6) is therefore given by the number of axial ligands specified (0, 1 or 2), e.g.

Methylaquo-[cobinamide]	for the six-co-ordinate form
Methyl-[cobinamide]	for the five-co-ordinate form
[Cobalamin]-cobalt(I)	for four-co-ordinate B_{12s}

The only exception to this rule is that the specification of Bzm as the second axial ligand in the cobalamins may sometimes be omitted (see Rule 3)).

Rule 2. The oxidation number of the metal is indicated by Roman numerals placed in brackets after the metal (in accordance with Co-ord 7.22). Organo-ligands (such as CH_3—, CH_2=CH—, CH_3CO—, $HOOC.CH_2$— etc., but not, of course, CO or RNC) are treated as if the ligand atom carried a negative charge when computing the oxidation number (cf. Co-ord. 7.324), e.g.

methyl-Bzm-[cobalamin]-cobalt(III)

The oxidation number and the "cobalt" may be omitted for cobalt(III) complexes, but are retained for cobalt(I) and cobalt(II) complexes,
e.g. methyl-Bzm-[cobalamin]

[cobalamin]-cobalt(I)

Rule 3. The order of axial ligands. The axial ligands are cited in the order anionic, then neutral and cationic ligands (cf. Co-ord 7.25), with the exception that if one of the ligands is the heterocylic base of a nucleotide side-chain this is named last of all, regardless of charge. Ligands are defined as anionic, neutral or cationic when the charges on the co-ordinated atom and those atoms with which it interacts strongly (i.e. all the atoms and hence all the charges in SO_3^{2-}, the imidazolate anion, $[Fe(CN)_6]^{4-}$, etc., but not in —CH_2COO^-, the 5-deoxy-adenosyl ligand protonated on the adenine ring, etc.,) are negative, zero and positive respectively. Amongst anionic ligands the order is organo-ligands, cyanide, sulphite, hydroxide, halides, other inorganic anions, other organic anions.

(This last order differs from that in Co-ord. 7.25 in placing the organo-ligands, cyanide and sulphite first. This is done to avoid possible confusion from two sources. First, "cyano-methyl" could mean either that there were two ligands (CN^-, CH_3^-) or only one ($NC.CH_2^-$); if the organo-ligand is placed first (methyl- cyano-) no confusion can occur. Secondly, the stereoisomers involving the axial ligands are defined in terms of the position of the first

2

mentioned axial ligand (see Rule 5). If the organo-ligand were placed after the inorganic anion we would have the confusing situation that the u-isomer of, say, a vinylaquo complex reacted with azide ion to give the l-isomer of the azidovinyl complex. Hence it is better to place first those ligands which are least likely to undergo substitution reactions; and the order of general inertness falls in the order organo-ligands > cyanide > sulphite > others).

*The commonly used names such as aquocobalamin and methylcobalamin, in which only one axial ligand is specified, are acceptable in certain circumstances. Since the cobalt ion in aquocobalamin is six-co-ordinate and Bzm is co-ordinated, while the cobalt is five-co-ordinate and Bzm not co-ordinated in certain cobalamins such as isopropylcobalamin, the generic name of "X-cobalamin" (where X is one axial ligand) does not identify the second axial ligand unambiguously. These names must therefore only be used where the nature of the second axial ligand is immaterial or can be assumed from the context.

Rule 4. The axial ligands are named in accordance with the IUPAC Rules for the Nomenclature of Co-ordination Compounds. If one of the ligands is the heterocyclic base of a nucleotide side-chain, then this is indicated by giving the name of the heterocyclic base (neglecting the ribose substituent) and underlining it, e.g.:

cyano-adenine-[adenylcobamide] for ψ-B_{12}
bisimidazole-[cobinamide]
vinylaquo-[cobinamide]
isothiocyanato-(or S-thiocyanato-)-Bzm-[cobalamin]
μ-tetramethylene-bis{Bzm-[cobalamin]}

*5,6-dimethylbenzimidazole, the heterocyclic base present in cobalamins, may be represented as Bzm, i.e.

cyano-Bzm-[cobalamin] for B_{12}

*Where the systematic name of the ligand is cumbersome or confusing it may be replaced in part or in whole by a formula. In the case of the organo-ligands the point of attachment to the cobalt is indicated by a hyphen and the whole formula is enclosed in brackets. Where the usual form of the ligand has been reversibly modified by the loss or gain of a proton, the co-ordination of a metal ion, etc., the ligand may be indicated by giving the name of the usual form followed by sufficient information in brackets to specify the structural modification, e.g.:

$(HOOC.CH_2—)$-Bzm-[cobalamin]
$(^-OOC.CH_2—)$-Bzm-[cobalamin]
cyano-adenine(N_7H^+)-[adenylcobamide] for ψ-B_{12} in acid
vinyl($—CH{=}CH_2 \rightarrow Ag^+$)aquo-[cobinamide]

S-glutathionato(—COOH, —NH$_3^+$)-B̲z̲m̲-[cobalamin]
S-glutathionato(—COO⁻, —NH$_3^+$)-B̲z̲m̲-[cobalamin]
S-glutathionato(—COO⁻, —NH$_2$)-B̲z̲m̲-[cobalamin]
NCS⁻-B̲z̲m̲-[cobalamin] for isothiocyanato-B̲z̲m̲-[cobalamin]

Rule 5. The relative orientation of the axial ligands is denoted by prefixing u- or l- when the first named ligand is in the upper or lower co-ordination site respectively. The upper side is defined as that toward which the acetamide side-chains project or that side from which a viewer will see rings A, B, C, and D form a clockwise sequence (this second definition can include synthetic corri-noids as well as porphyrins and chlorins).

The prefix may be omitted when one of the axial ligands is the heterocyclic base of a nucleotide side-chain, since these bases can apparently only co-ordi-nate in the lower position, i.e. only the u-isomer is known.

Rule 6. Naming the equatorial ligand. The corrin ring together with its sub-stituents and side-chains is named in accordance with the IUPAC–IUB (Corr.) Rules 2–5 and 8 (i.e. we neglect the fact that the Corr. names include the cobalt atom) and the name is enclosed in square brackets. The name "cobalamin" is used for all α-(5,6-dimethylbenzimidazolyl)cobamides (i.e. the name is not restricted to the four cobalamins named in Corr. Rule 9).

Examples:

Cyanoaquo[-cobyric acid] is Factor V$_{1a}$
5-deoxyadenosyl-[adenylcobamide] is AC, the five-co-ordinate coenzyme
    form of vitamin ψ-B$_{12}$
Dicyano[cobalamin]

The square brackets may be omitted when the name of the equatorial ligand is a single word such as cobalamin, cobamide or cobinamide used without any modifications and comes either first or last in the name of the whole complex, e.g.:

Cyanoaquocobinamide
Cobalamin-cobalt(I)
Cyanoaquo-[cobalamin(BzmH⁺)]
Aquo-[cobinamide]-cobalt(II)

* Since the α-glycosidic linkage occurs in all but one of the corrinoid nucleotides so far examined, the prefix α is omitted and all corrinoid nucleotides are assumed to have this linkage unless the prefix β is used.

*5,6-Dimethylbenzimidazole and 5,6-dimethylbenzimidazolyl are abbreviated to Bzm (as already mentioned under Rule 4).

*Where the usual form of the equatorial ligand has been reversibly modified by the loss or gain of a proton, the co-ordination of a metal ion etc. the nature of the equatorial ligand may be indicated by giving the name of the usual form

followed by sufficient information in brackets to specify the structural modification, e.g.:

Cyanoaquo-[cobalamin(BzmH$^+$ or N$_7$H$^+$)] for B$_{12}$ at pH < 0

Cyanoaquo-[cobalamin(BzmAg$^+$ or N$_7$Ag$^+$)]

Cyano-Bzm-[cobalamin(R$_2$POOH)] for B$_{12}$ in which the phosphate residue has been protonated.

Rule 7. Formation of salts. Where the corrinoid carries an overall charge and it is desired to indicate the formation of a particular ionic salt, then the name of the counter-cation or anion is added before or after respectively the unmodified name of the corrinoid complex, e.g.:

aquo-Bzm-[cobalamin]-cobalt(III) chloride or aquocobalamin chloride.

sodium dicyano-[cobalamin]-cobalt(III) or sodium dicyanocobalamin.

μ-iodo-bis{[cobyrinic acid heptamethylester] cobalt(II)} iodide.

Three general points can be made about the application in practice of these (or any) rules for the nomenclature of the corrinoids.

Firstly, there are many cases where the exact structure of the complex is not known; this applies to the structure of both the axial and the equatorial ligands. The problems of establishing the structure are, of course, far greater for the corrinoids than for the simpler complexes usually studied by co-ordination chemists. In addition, the axial ligands may undergo rapid ligand substitution reactions, so that a structure which has been established for the solid state (e.g. NCS$^-$ co-ordinated through S in the cobalamin or CN$^-$ co-ordinated in the lower position in Factor V$_{1a}$) cannot always be assumed to persist in solution. We do not yet know, for example, whether cobalamin-cobalt(II) is five- or six-co-ordinate, whether NO$_2^-$ is co-ordinated through N or O, or what is the relative orientation of the axial ligands in the sulphitocobinamide; nor do we know the position of the different side-chains in many of the corrinoids which contain both amide and carboxylic acid side-chains, or the site of protonation of the corrin ring in strong acid. One could indicate those complexes where the structure has not been established by, for example, prefixing the names with an asterisk; but it seems simpler in practice (i) merely to omit details of the structure (such as the identity of the ligand atom, the relative orientation of the two different axial ligands, the site of protonation of the corrin ring or the letters indicating which side-chains carry carboxylic acid groups), where these are uncertain, (ii) to use the name which corresponds to the simplest or most likely structure or which incorporates the simplest name (e.g. nitro- instead of nitrito-) and (iii) only to point out the uncertainty in structure where this is necessary in order to prevent erroneous conclusions from being drawn.

Secondly, since axial ligand substitution reactions occur so readily, an apparently single compound may in fact be present as a mixture, even in the solid state. Methyl cobinamide, for example, exists as a mixture of the five- and six-co-ordinate complexes (with and without H_2O as the sixth ligand) both in solution and in the solid state; equilibration is very rapid in solution (see Chapter 8, Section II). The cobalamin containing NCS^- appears to be present in solution as a mixture of the isomers co-ordinated through N and S (Thusius, 1968). Most cyanoaquocorrinoids isomerize fairly readily, so that the dissolution of one isomer in water soon leads to an equilibrium mixture of the two isomers (see Chapter 8, Section III). One might indicate the presence of a mixture by some suffix to the name. But here again it is probably simpler in practice merely to omit details which identify one isomer etc. and only to point out the presence of a mixture where this is essential. Corrinoids which contain both amide and carboxylic acid side-chains can obviously exist in a large number of isomeric forms; but these isomers are not readily interconvertible and can be separated by chromatographic techniques.

Thirdly, since we are mainly concerned with the co-ordination chemistry of the corrinoids and since the most commonly used technique for study is spectrophotometry, we are not usually interested in any changes, reversible or irreversible, in those parts of the molecule which do not affect the spectrum beyond 300 nm (i.e. the spectrum due to the corrin ring); such changes include, for example, the protonation of the phosphate or the ionization of the ribose in the nucleotide side-chain, the protonation of adenine in the 5-deoxyadenosyl ligand, and the ionization of the $—NH_3^+$ group in co-ordinated cysteine. In these cases it is obviously simplest to name the complex on the assumption that the "irrelevant" part of the molecule has the structure normally found in neutral solution, i.e. the reversible loss or gain of a proton etc. is neglected when it does not affect the chromophore.

Certain common trivial names and abbreviations such as B_{12a}, B_{12r}, $\psi\text{-}B_{12}$ and DBC are used in this book; they are explained in the next section.

III. TRIVIAL AND NON-SYSTEMATIC NAMES OF CORRINOIDS

It can readily be appreciated that many trivial names have been used in the B_{12} field because there is often a long period between the isolation or preparation of a corrinoid and the elucidation of its structure, during which time a trivial name becomes firmly entrenched (e.g. vitamin B_{12r}, the coenzymes) and also because the trivial name may be much more convenient than the systematic name (e.g. B_{12a}). Many workers in the B_{12} field use trivial names and abbreviations of their own; part of Friedrich's nomenclature has, in fact, been used in the section on stereoisomers involving the axial ligands (see Chapter 8, Section II).

The following is a list of common trivial names which are also used in this book. Those marked with an asterisk(*) are normally prefixed with the word "vitamin"; but this seems unnecessary in the context of this book and the word is therefore omitted. A few additional trivial names which are not used in this book are mentioned in brackets.

Cobalamins: According to the IUPAC-IUB Rules (see Section I) only cyano-, aquo-, hydroxo- and nitrito-cobalamin are accepted: other cobalamins are "trivial". But in the nomenclature proposed for this book (see Section II) the names of all cobalamins are accepted.

*B_{12}. Cyanocobalamin.

*B_{12a}. Aquo- or hydroxo-cobalamin, depending on pH (pK ~8) and other conditions.

(*B_{12b} = B_{12a})

*B_{12c}. Nitro- or nitrito-cobalamin. The identity of the ligand atom has not been established.

*B_{12r}. The cobalt(II) derivative of B_{12a}, which is *probably* five-co-ordinate, existing as Bzm-[cobalamin]-cobalt(II) or aquo-[cobalamin(BzmH$^+$)]-cobalt(II) depending on pH (pK ~2.5).

*B_{12s}. [Cobalamin]-Cobalt(I).

Coenzymes are corrinoids which possess the organo-ligand 5′-deoxyadenosyl. AC, BC and DBC are coenzymes which differ in the nature of the nucleotide side-chain and hence also in the equilibrium between five- and six-co-ordinate complexes; AC, for example, is present mainly as the five-co-ordinate complex.

AC.   5′-deoxyadenosyl-[adenylcobamide].
BC.   5′-deoxyadenosyl-benz-[benzimidazolylcobamide].
DBC. 5′-deoxyadenosyl-Bzm-[cobalamin].

According to the IUPAC–IUB Rules their names are:

AC.   α-(adenyl)-*Co*-5′-deoxyadenosylcobamide.
BC.   α-(benzimidazolyl)-*Co*-5′-deoxyadenosylcobamide.
DBC. α-(5,6-dimethylbenzimidazolyl)-*Co*-5′-deoxyadenosylcobamide.
DBC   is also known as "cobalamin coenzyme" or "coenzyme B_{12}".

*ψ-B_{12}. Cyano-adenine-[adenylcobamide].

Factor B. Cyanoaquo-[cobinamide] (in either or both isomeric forms).

Factor V_{1a}. Cyanoaquo-[cobyric acid] (in either or both isomeric forms).

Lactam (or dehydrovitamin B_{12}) is the derivative of B_{12} in which a lactam ring has been fused onto ring B by the elimination of the hydrogen atom at C_8 and a hydrogen atom of the amide side-chain at c, as shown in Fig. 2.1. Its systematic name is cyano-Bzm-[8-amino-(5,6-dimethylbenzimidazolyl)cobamic acid abdeg-pentamide c-lactam].

Lactone. The lactone analogue of the above-mentioned lactam.

Chlorolactam (or chlorodehydrovitamin B_{12}). The lactam in which the hydrogen at C_{10} in the corrin ring has been substituted by chlorine, i.e. cyano-Bzm-[8-amino-10-chloro-(5,6-dimethyl-benzimidazolyl)cobamic acid abdeg-pentamide c-lactam].

Hexacarboxylic acid is 1-cyanochloro-[8-aminocobyrinic acid-c-lactam], i.e. the corrinoid part contains the lactam ring as in the previous examples, but all the other side-chains (a, b, d–g) terminate in carboxylic acid groups.

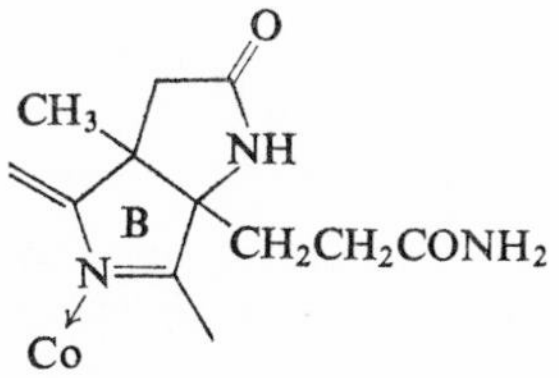

Fig. 2.1. Partial structure of dehydrovitamin B_{12} showing the lactam ring fused onto ring B.

IV. ABBREVIATIONS AND CONVENTIONS

The following abbreviations for well-known ligands have been used: tu, thiourea; py, pyridine; aden, adenine; imid, imidazole; benz, benzimidazole.

"Bzm" is the heterocyclic base present in the nucleotide side-chain of the cobalamins, viz. 5,6-dimethylbenzimidazole (see diagram of formula IV in Section I). The author has in the past often used the abbreviation "Bz", but this is clearly undesirable as it is commonly used in organic chemistry to signify benzyl or benzoyl.

There are several other tetradentate ligands which form a square planar or "equatorial" arrangement around the cobalt as in the corrinoids, the coordination sphere being completed by the presence of two unidentate "axial" ligands. The structures of some of these ligands are shown in Fig. 2.2; certain other ligands of this type are mentioned in the text. A similar equatorial arrangement is formed by two DMG ligands which are joined by symmetrical hydrogen-bonds (see Fig. 2.2). These ligands are abbreviated as follows:

DMG, dimethylglyoximato-
Salen, N,N′-ethylenebis(salicylideneiminato)-
BAE, N,N′-ethylenebis(acetylacetonemonoximeiminato)-

The bisdimethylglyoximatocobalt complexes are sometimes called "cobaloximes".

The axial ligands are labelled X, Y and Z according to the following convention. X is the ligand in whose properties we are most interested, e.g. its structure

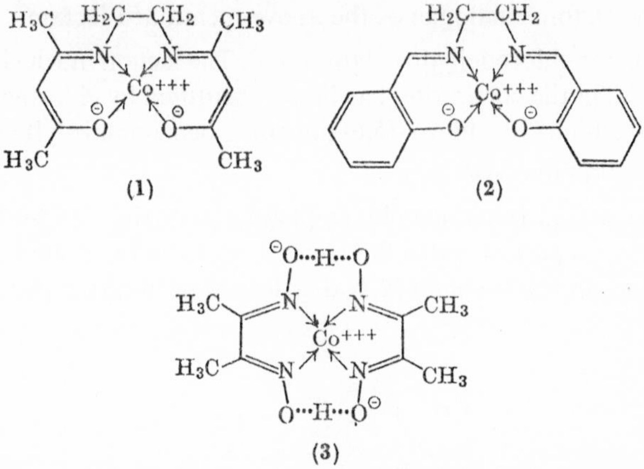

Fig. 2.2. The "equatorial" ligands in (1) BAE, (2) salen and (3) bis-DMG complexes; the co-ordination sphere is completed by two unidentate "axial" ligands.

as shown by X-ray analysis, its fate during photolysis, its effect on the absorption spectrum of the corrin ring, on the stretching frequency of cyanide co-ordinated in the trans-position or on the rates and equilibria of ligand substitution in the trans-position. For ground-state effects Y is the "probe", e.g. CN^-, when we study the dependence of the CN stretching frequency on the nature of X. For thermodynamic and kinetic effects Y and Z are the ligands involved in the equilibrium or reaction and Y is the common denominator, if any, in the set of equilibria or reactions under investigation. The axial ligands may also be designated by other letters as follows:

L, any ligand, which one does not wish to specify as X, Y or Z.
S, a solvent molecule which can be co-ordinated.
B, a nitrogeneous base.
R, any organo-ligand.
RS^-, a thiolate anion, e.g. thioglycollate $^-OOC.CH_2.S^-$
X_s, any ligand co-ordinated through a sulphur atom.

The term "organo-ligand", as used here, includes all ligands co-ordinated through a negatively charged carbon atom, except cyanide (CN^-); for the purposes of distributing the charge in organo-corrinoids the cobalt ion is considered as trivalent. The term "organo-ligand" includes ligands in which the carbon atom may be involved in a triple bond (e.g. ethinyl $HC{\equiv}C—$), a double bond (e.g. vinyl $CH_2{=}CH—$, phenyl $C_6H_5—$, acetyl $CH_3CO—$) or only single bonds (e.g. alkyl and substituted alkyl ligands). The term "carbanion" includes organo-ligands and cyanide. Neutral molecules such as CO and RNC are not included in either term.

The terms "formation constant" and "equilibrium constant" are used almost synonymously. The constants are defined in the appropriate part of the text.

In most cases where equilibria or reactions are written down only the axial ligands are given and the charge on the complex is neglected, e.g.:

$$[NC—Co—OH_2] + CN^- = [NC—Co—CN] + H_2O$$

Equilibria may also be shown schematically, e.g.:

$$\begin{array}{ccc} \text{X} & & \text{X} \\ | & & | \\ \text{Co} \quad + \quad H_3O^+ \quad \rightleftharpoons & & \text{Co} \\ | & & | \quad | \\ \text{Bzm} & & {}^+\text{HBzm} \quad OH_2 \end{array}$$

where the rectangle represents the corrin ring together with the four equatorial co-ordination positions and the nucleotide side-chain is attached at the left-hand end.

3

B₁₂ IN BIOCHEMISTRY, MEDICINE AND AGRICULTURE

Because of the great interest and importance of B_{12} in medicine and agriculture, a very brief outline of these and related topics is presented in this chapter. Much of the general information has been gleaned from the monograph by Smith (1965) and from review articles (references given in the relevant paragraphs), although certain points have been simplified and certain personal interpretations added—without, one hopes, any distortion of the truth.

Vitamin B_{12}, like other vitamins, is required by humans and other animals in small amounts to perform (with or without further structural modification) some catalytic role, but it cannot be synthesized by the organism and must therefore be obtained from the diet. It is, however, the only vitamin which contains a metal, i.e. which is a co-ordination compound. It is also the largest of the vitamins and apparently the only one which requires a special mechanism for absorption into the body from the gut. Oddly enough, it is mainly or wholly an artefact. Vitamin B_{12} is—officially—cyanocobalamin, yet the corrinoid present in animal tissues is almost exclusively in the form of 5-deoxyadenosylcobalamin. The organo-ligand of the latter is, however, readily split off by the action of light, acid or cyanide during the process of isolation and purification. A much wider range of corrinoids is found amongst microorganisms, which differ from the cobalamins in the nature of the side-chains. For further information on these analogues see the reviews by Mervyn and Smith (1964) and by Wagner (1966) and Chapter nine of Smith's monograph (Smith, 1965); the analogues which possess a nucleotide side-chain are mentioned in the section on the co-ordination of heterocyclic bases (Chapter 8, Section IV, F). The overwhelming majority of naturally occurring corrinoids contain the organo-ligand 5-deoxyadenosyl (for structure see Fig. 1.3), though certain corrinoids containing a methyl ligand have been found both in animals and in microorganisms (Lindstrand, 1964; Irion and Ljungdahl, 1968), and there is some evidence for the occurrence of a carboxymethyl-corrinoid (Co—CH₂COOH) (Ljungdahl et al., 1965). Corrinoids have also been isolated which do not contain an organo-ligand, but it is usually very difficult to establish whether or not this is due to the removal of an

32

organo-ligand during isolation. Growing cultures of bacteria reduce vitamin B_{12} to B_{12r}, the cobalt(II) complex (Scott *et al.*, 1964), and it is very likely that any corrinoid which does not contain an organo-ligand will be present *in vivo* as a reduced complex because of the reducing power of cellular material.

As far as we know at present, vitamin B_{12} is required by all members of the animal kingdom together with certain bacteria and algae. Corrinoids are not required by green plants or fungi, though they may be found in plants as a result of bacterial activity, e.g. in the root nodules which contain nitrogen-fixing bacteria. Corrinoids, are, however, synthesized only by microorganisms (certain bacteria, moulds, blue-green, brown and red algae, but not green algae). It would appear that the genes and enzymes required for some particular step in the biosynthesis of corrinoids have been lost at some early point in the course of evolution between microorganisms and animals; it would be interesting to know what chemical reaction this is. It also appears that animals have lost the ability to utilize any corrinoids other than the cobalamins (B_{12}, B_{12a} and DBC), which are selectively absorbed from the mixture of corrinoids provided by microbial synthesis.

Corrinoids are probably synthesized by bacteria in the lower gut, and hence in the faeces, of all animals including man, but the most intensive synthesis occurs in the fore-stomach of ruminants (cattle, sheep, etc.). Corrinoids are also present in abundance in sewage. It is ironic that the intestinal synthesis of B_{12} does not occur in the stomach, which is relatively sterile because of its acidity, but further on in the lower gut, from where it cannot be absorbed. The ruminants can, of course, absorb from the stomach the B_{12} synthesized in the fore-stomach. Most vertebrates must therefore obtain their supply of B_{12} in other ways such as (1) eating other animal food, (2) eating their faeces (a fairly common practice, usually referred to euphemistically as coprophagy) and (3) perhaps from soil, contaminated water, etc.

A number of steps have now been identified in the biosynthetic pathway leading to the corrinoid coenzymes. It has been shown by the use of isotopically labelled compounds that the synthesis of the corrin ring, like that of the porphyrin ring, proceeds by the route involving glycine, Δ-aminolaevulic acid and porphobilinogen (see Fig. 3.1) and that the methyl group on C_1 in the corrin ring corresponds to the methine carbon atom between rings A and D in the porphyrin ring. One methyl group on C_{12} in the corrin ring arises from the decarboxylation of the acetic acid side-chain of the porphobilinogen unit. The other six methyl groups of the corrin ring originate from methionine. It is the presence and position of these methyl groups which really distinguish the corrin and porphyrin structures. The C_1 atom in the corrin ring is forced to remain tetrahedral because of the methyl group and thereby breaks the conjugated system of double bonds at the point between rings A and D. The presence of the other methyl groups on the β atoms of the rings fixes the corrin ring in a state which corresponds to a reduced porphyrin. It is not yet known whether the cobalt atom is normally introduced before or after the corrin structure has been formed by closure of the ring to form the cyclic ligand. But

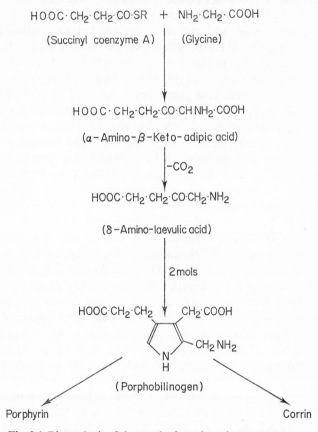

Fig. 3.1. Biosynthesis of the porphyrin and corrin structures.

certain metal-free corrinoids have been isolated from photosynthetic bacteria which will incorporate cobalt, but not Fe(III), Mn(II) or Ni(II), ions to give cobalt corrinoids (Toohey, 1965, 1966). The first cobalt corrinoid to which the biosynthetic pathway can be traced back is some derivative (i.e. axial ligands not known) of cobyrinic acid, in which all the side-chains a–g are carboxylic acids. The structure of the corrinoid coenzymes is then developed by reactions of three types:

1. The successive conversion of the carboxylic acids in side-chains a–e and g into amides.
2. The successive condensation onto the carboxylic acid of side-chain f of aminopropanol, phosphate, ribose and 5,6-dimethylbenziminazole or some other heterocyclic base to form the nucleotide side-chain.
3. The formation of the ligand 5-deoxyadenosyl (or possibly the methyl ligand in some cases).

The large number of naturally occurring corrinoids arises

(i) because of variations in the nature of the heterocyclic base in the side-chain and
(ii) because these three groups of reactions apparently occur independently.

For a summary of the evidence on the biosynthetic pathway and of the compounds isolated see the reviews by Mervyn and Smith (1964) and by Wagner (1966).

By contrast very little is known about the degradation of corrinoids by living organisms. B_{12} is excreted by animals both in urine (i.e. unchanged by metabolic processes within the body) and of course in faeces (as the product of microbial synthesis in the gut). It seems that cultures of many microorganisms will reversibly reduce B_{12} to B_{12r} but that very few will irreversibly degrade corrinoids (Helgeland et al., 1961; Scott et al., 1964). The first stage in the degradation of corrinoids is the formation of "stable yellow corrinoids", which are discussed in Chapter 15, Section II. There is little doubt that corrinoids are remarkably stable under natural conditions with the exception that the 5-deoxyadenosyl ligand may be split off by the action of light etc. B_{12} can be detected in the soil, in pond-water and even in sea-water.

The fate of B_{12} in animals can be considered under the headings of

(1) absorption from the gut,
(2) transport,
(3) storage and
(4) enzymatic reactions.

In each stage B_{12} is tightly bound to a protein; free, unbound B_{12} hardly ever occurs inside cells or organisms except immediately after injection. This is not surprising since the presence of numerous amide side-chains makes the corrinoids similar to proteins in their tendency to form hydrogen-bonds (this is discussed in Chapter 6, Section II). In absorption we have to transfer molecules of B_{12} (B_{12a} or DBC) from the gut, where they are present in complexes firmly attached to proteins, through the wall of the intestine into the blood. Although some B_{12} may be absorbed independently, most of the absorption is accomplished by the action of two proteins named "Intrinsic Factor" (I.F.) and "Releasing Factor" (R.F.). I.F. is secreted into the gastric juice by the gastric mucosa and is apparently able to compete successfully with all other B_{12}-binding proteins (the only exception so far known is a protein from a certain tape-worm). I.F. from hog pylorus has recently been isolated and purified; it is a glyco-protein with a molecular weight of about 50,000 which binds B_{12} about twelve times as strongly as ψ-B_{12} (the analogue with adenine in the nucleotide side-chain) (Ellenbogen and Highley, 1967; Highley *et al.*, 1967). In the next step the B_{12}–I.F. complex is adsorbed by the wall of the intestine. However, since I.F. is apparently not able to pass through the intestinal wall into the blood, the B_{12} must first be released from its thermodynamically stable complex with I.F. This is achieved by the action of R.F. which breaks down the B_{12}–I.F. complex catalytically. We can now see why B_{12}, alone of all the vitamins, requires such a special mechanism for its absorption. Vitamin B_{12} is carried in the blood principally in the form of a complex with one of the α-globulins and apparently in the form of *methyl*–cobalamin. All animal tissues contain some B_{12}, but in man and most other animals the main storage organ is the liver, where most or all of it is present in the form of 5-deoxyadenosylcobalamin (DBC) bound to proteins or polypeptides. For further information on these topics see the review by Ellenbogen and Highley (1963).

A considerable number of B_{12}-dependent reactions have been identified and studied in microorganisms. These are discussed in Chapter 17. The reactions can be classified into two groups: (A) reactions which involve the transfer of a methyl group (to give methionine, acetic acid, methane, even the methylmercuric ion) and which probably involve the intermediate formation of a methylcorrinoid (i.e. with methyl on the cobalt) and (B) reactions which involve a hydride transfer (and often lead to the isomerization of a carbon chain) and which depend on the presence of a 5-deoxyadenosylcorrinoid. In each case the catalyst is the complex (or "holo-enzyme") formed from a corrinoid (acting as the "coenzyme") together with a protein (or "apoenzyme"). The same corrinoid may, in fact, act as the coenzyme for several different reactions by complexing with different apoenzymes, as DBC does for the various isomerase reactions. So far only two B_{12}-dependent reactions have been identified in mammals, viz. the methylation of homocysteine to give methionine and the isomerization of L-methylmalonyl-CoA to succinyl-CoA. For recent summaries of our knowledge of the function of B_{12} in man and other mammals see Mahoney and Rosenberg (1970) and Silber and Moldow (1970).

The ruminants (cattle, sheep, goats) deserve a paragraph to themselves. These animals possess a rumen or fore-stomach in which the vegetable matter is broken down by the action of a mass of microorganisms. The real "food" of these animals is therefore the product of fermentation in the rumen; it has in fact been shown that ruminants deprived of their rumen microflora die of starvation! This "food" contains an unusually high concentration of propionic acid and ruminants are more dependent than other animals on propionic acid as a source of energy. Corrinoids play an important role at two points in the metabolism of ruminants—in addition to those common to other animals. Firstly, the microorganisms present in the rumen include many species which require corrinoids, but of these many can synthesize the corrinoids themselves. The rumen microorganisms can therefore be maintained in a healthy state by the provision of a supply of simple cobalt salts and the B_{12} synthesized in the rumen can be absorbed by the animal from the stomach. But the majority of the corrinoids required and synthesized by these microorganisms are not cobalamins (such as B_{12}) but analogues with purines in the nucleotide side-chain. Secondly, propionic acid is metabolized within the animal by carboxylation to methylmalonic acid, followed by isomerization to succinic acid, which then enters the tricarboxylic acid cycle; the isomerization step is dependent on B_{12}, or rather on the coenzyme form 5-deoxyadenosylcobalamin. These isomerase reactions are discussed in Chapter 17. A deficiency of cobalt in the diet of sheep and cattle leads to progressive wasting and causes the milk-flow to cease and abortion to be common. This disease is observed in certain parts of the world where the soil is deficient in cobalt or contains cobalt in a form in which it is not available to plants (and hence to animals) and is known by a variety of names, such as pining in Scotland, coast disease in Australia, bush disease in New Zealand, nakuruitis in East Africa. It was traced to a deficiency of cobalt by Australian workers in 1935, but the connection with B_{12} has only recently been established. It can be cured by providing a supply of simple cobalt salts (the daily dose is ~2 mg/100 kg of live weight). The cobalt is usually added to the feed or the drinking water, mixed with fertilizer for application to the soil or simply sprayed onto the soil in the form of the soluble cobalt sulphate or chloride. Where, however, the animals range over an extensive area or are tended infrequently, it is usual to introduce into the rumen a pellet of rather insoluble cobalt oxide, which slowly releases its cobalt over a period of up to one year (Latteur, 1962).

We can now understand more clearly the role of B_{12} in medicine, the role of B_{12} and cobalt salts in animal nutrition and the methods used for the industrial preparation of B_{12}.

Vitamin B_{12} is associated in man with the disease called "pernicious anaemia", which almost invariably proved fatal before methods of treatment were discovered. The disease is caused by failure of the stomach to secrete hydrochloric acid and the protein called intrinsic factor and hence by the failure—amongst other things—to absorb B_{12}. Tests show that the blood contains a lower concentration of B_{12} and fewer but larger red blood cells than normal. The B_{12} deficiency affects the production of red and white blood cells in the bone marrow. Although their nuclear development has been retarded, the red blood cells function normally, but have a reduced life-span; hence the anaemia. In man prolonged B_{12} deficiency leads to neurological disorders. The symptoms of pernicious anaemia include tiredness, sore tongue and, if the central nervous system is affected, there may be loss of sensation in the legs and hands and difficulty in walking. The disease is treated by monthly intramuscular injections of B_{12} or B_{12a}. The reported B_{12} requirement for humans is amazingly low; about 1 μg per day or less than 1 mg per year. It should be mentioned that some, but not all, of the effects of pernicious anaemia can be counteracted by an increased intake of folic acid; the complex relationship between B_{12} and folic acid in metabolism is not yet understood.

Although anaemia can be produced experimentally in other animals by feeding on a B_{12}-deficient diet, these anaemias have little in common with pernicious anaemia in man (Stokstad, 1968).

The most important outlet for commercially produced B_{12} is not in medicine but as an additive to feedstuffs for pigs and poultry. A deficiency of B_{12} retards growth and causes failure in the hatching of eggs. With the increased use of feedstuffs of purely vegetable origin there has been an increasing need for the addition of B_{12} to their diet. The situation with cattle and other ruminants is different and has already been discussed.

Not only do animal feedstuffs represent the most important use of B_{12} but the lines of research leading up to this application also provided the clues for the means of large-scale production of B_{12}. Attempts during the second world war to raise pigs and poultry on purely vegetable rations revealed the need for some "animal protein factor" (or A.P.F.), which was also found to be present in dung and droppings. This suggested the possibility of producing APF commercially by some fermentation process using microorganisms. In 1948, not only was crystalline B_{12} isolated from liver, but APF was shown to be identical with B_{12} and it was also shown that B_{12} was actually produced by the existing fermentation process for the production of the antibiotic grisein from *Streptomyces griseus*. This opened the way to the large-scale production of B_{12} very shortly after its isolation and, of course, on a scale which would have been quite impossible if animal liver had remained the sole source. B_{12} was initially produced as a by-product of fermentations (mainly of species of *Streptomyces*) which produced antibiotics (such as streptomycin, aureomycin and neomycin). As the demand for B_{12} grew, fermentation processes were developed to produce B_{12} as the primary product. The microorganisms most commonly used now are species of the genera *Streptomyces* and *Propionibacter* together with

Bacillus megatherium and *Nocardia rugosa*. For medicinal use B_{12} is obtained in pure, crystalline form; but for animal feedstuffs partially purified concentrates are generally used. For further information on the industrial production of B_{12} see the reviews by Perlman (1959) and by Mervyn and Smith (1964).

It is interesting to see in retrospect how several different lines of research, which for a long time appeared to have nothing in common, have converged on B_{12}; for example, the search for the anti-pernicious anaemia factor in liver, the animal protein factor and the cause of pining in ruminants. Studies on the metabolism of microorganisms have revealed several B_{12}-dependent enzymatic reactions. The most recently discovered role of B_{12} concerns the more sinister area of mercury pollution, whereby mercury compounds are methylated to give the methylmercury cation CH_3Hg^+ and dimethylmercury $(CH_3)_2Hg$ by a B_{12}-dependent reaction. These B_{12}-dependent reactions of microorganisms are discussed in Chapter 17. Doubtless many more such reactions remain to be discovered. The most interesting developments will be the elucidation of the more important B_{12}-dependent pathways in the metabolism of humans and other animals.

4

THE PREPARATION AND IDENTIFICATION OF COBALT CORRINOIDS

This section aims only to provide a brief introduction to the methods used in the preparation and identification of cobalt corrinoids and is limited mainly to those which have played a significant role in the development of the co-ordination chemistry of the corrinoids. For experimental details see the references given in the sections mentioned below.

The vast bulk of our knowledge of the co-ordination chemistry of the corrinoids has come from the study of the cobalamins and cobinamides. The importance of the cobinamides lies in the fact that they are the most easily prepared corrinoids which do not possess a heterocyclic base which can co-ordinate to the cobalt; they therefore provide the opportunity of studying the properties of ligands other than Bzm in the position *trans*- to CN^-, CH_3^- etc. Since the substitution of axial ligands occurs very rapidly in the corrinoids (with the exception of the organo-ligands and in some cases ligands such as CN^- and SO_3^{2-}) many corrinoids are prepared and studied only in solution; the aquo- complexes such as aquocobalamin, cyanoaquocobinamide and methylaquocobinamide are most frequently used for these experiments in solution.

Most of the corrinoids which have been isolated as solids contain either one cyanide or one organo-ligand. The monocyanide is the usual form in which a corrinoid is isolated, when interest centres on obtaining corrinoids in which the side-chains have been modified, either synthetically (see Chapter 16) or biosynthetically (see Chapter 8, Section IV.E); this is because of the widespread use of organic solvents containing HCN in the chromatographic step in the isolation procedure together with the high formation constant for the binding of CN^- in the position trans to Bzm, H_2O or HO^- (see Table 8.7). A very large number of different organo-ligands have been placed on the cobalt in organo-cobalamins and cobinamides, but few with other modified corrin ligands (see Chapter 13, Section I). Other corrinoids which have been isolated as solids include cobalamins where X is NCS^-, $NCSe^-$ and NO_2^- (all used in X-ray crystallographic work; see Chapter 5, Section II and Chapter 6, Section I).

The main starting material for synthetic work is cyanocobalamin (B_{12} itself), which has long been available commercially; aquocobalamin (B_{12a}), methylcobalamin and 5-deoxyadenosylcobalamin (DBC) are now also available commercially. The main routes for the synthesis of solid corrinoids of interest to co-ordination chemists are shown in the following scheme:

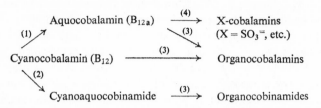

(1) Catalytic hydrogenation, followed by aerial oxidation (see Chapter 11)
(2) Treatment with concentrated HCl at 65° for 5 min or with $Ce(OH)_3$ and KCN in neutral solution at 95° for 10–20 min (see Chapter 16).
(3) Reduction to the cobalt(I) corrinoid using BH_4^-, Cr(II) or zinc and ammonium chloride, followed by alkylation with, for example, methyl iodide (see Chapter 13, Section I).
(4) Addition of ligand (e.g. SO_3^{2-}) in solution.

The aim of purification is to separate the corrinoids from inorganic and organic purities and to separate the corrinoids from each other. The first is usually accomplished by extracting the corrinoids from aqueous solution into a phenol-chloroform mixture and then displacing the corrinoids back into pure water by the addition of acetone to the organic phase (for further details see Chapter 6, Section II). The second is accomplished by the use of some chromatographic technique; the methods most commonly used now in research laboratories are paper and thin-layer chromatography and ion-exchange cellulose columns. Electrophoresis is often useful for separating mixtures of compounds which differ in, for example, the number of carboxylic acid side-chains.

The corrinoids are usually obtained in the solid state by one of two methods. Where the axial ligand is stable towards substitution and no excess reagent is required (e.g. organocorrinoids, cyanoaquocobinamide) the aqueous solution may be freeze-dried, i.e. the solution frozen at the temperature of liquid nitrogen and the ice removed by sublimation under vacuum; this reduces the occurrence of any side-reactions, but produces a non-crystalline solid. Where crystalline material is required, as in X-ray crystallographic work, or where the formation constant for the binding of the ligand is rather low and excess ligand must be present in solution, an organic solvent such as acetone is allowed to diffuse through the solution to induce slow crystallization.

Most of the standard techniques used in organic and co-ordination chemistry for establishing the structure of a new compound or proving that two compounds are identical (e.g. chemical analysis, melting point, n.m.r. and i.r. spectra) are of little use when applied to such complex molecules as the corrinoids. Paper and thin-layer chromatography are used to establish the identity of two corrinoids. The structure of a corrinoid is, in the ultimate analysis, established by reference to one of the compounds whose structure has been established by X-ray analysis through either reactions or equilibria. As regards side-chains a–e and g it is usually easy to establish their number and nature (e.g. the number of carboxylic acid side-chains can be determined by pH titration or from electrophoresis) but difficult to establish their positions without recourse to X-ray analysis. The structure of side-chain f differs from the others (and contains the nucleotide, if present) and can usually be established by degradation and synthesis. The methods which have been used to identify the products of reaction at C_8 and C_{10} in the corrin ring are described in Chapter 15, Section I.

The main points in identifying the axial ligands are the following:

(1) The absorption spectrum at wavelengths longer than 300 nm is almost always due to π-π^* transitions within the conjugated corrin chain and is very sensitive to changes in the valency of the cobalt, and in the number and nature of the axial ligands, but rather insensitive to changes in the side-chains; changes involving the conjugated chain itself (such as chlorination at C_{10}) also affect the spectrum, but these need not concern us here. Close similarities in spectra can therefore be used as evidence for the identity of the axial ligands; for example, the cobalamins in acid show the same spectra as the cobinamides, which shows that Bzm cannot be co-ordinated under these conditions. For further discussion of the absorption spectra see Chapter 5, Section I.

(2) Bzm absorbs below 300 nm. The position of the absorption bands can show whether the base is protonated (band at 284 nm) or free or co-ordinated to the cobalt (both 288 nm), while the degree of resolution of the bands can sometimes distinguish between the latter two (see Chapter 5, Section I). Bzm is, for example, not co-ordinated to the cobalt in cobalamin-cobalt(I). Similar information could, in principle, be obtained from the absorption spectra of most other nucleotide bases, but none have yet been examined in any detail.

(3) Where the axial ligand is a Lewis base, which can exist free in aqueous solution, its identity can be established from the stoichiometry of the reaction or equilibrium. In this way we can start with the known cyano-cobalamin and establish the identity of the following cobalamins (axial ligands only given):

[NC—CN] $\leftarrow$ [Bzm—CN] $\rightarrow$ [Bzm—OH$_2$] $\rightarrow$ [Bzm—OH], [Bzm—N$_3$] etc.

The formation constants are tabulated in Chapter 8, Table 8.7.

(4) In the case of the organocorrinoids, where the axial ligand cannot exist free in aqueous solution, the presence of an organo-ligand is assumed on the basis of evidence such as analogies to 5-deoxyadenosylcobalamin (DBC) in methods of synthesis, absorption spectra and sensitivity to light. This problem is discussed in more detail in Chapter 13, Section I.

(5) The nature of the ligand atom (where more than one donor atom is present) has been established by X-ray analysis (NCS$^-$ and NCSe$^-$ in the cobalamins in the solid state), infra-red spectra (SO$_3^{2-}$ in the solid cobalamin), similarities in the absorption spectra (glycine through N, cysteine through S in the cobalamins in solution) and comparison of the formation constants (histidine probably through the iminazole N in the cobalamin in solution), but there are still certain unresolved problems (e.g. NO$_2^-$ and NCS$^-$ in the cobalamins in solution). For a fuller discussion see Chapter 8, Section IV.C.

(6) The most direct method of establishing the relative orientation of two different axial ligands (e.g. CN$^-$ and H$_2$O) is by X-ray analysis, but other less direct methods are possible (see Chapter 8, Section II).

(7) The existence of five-co-ordinate cobalt(III) corrinoids (usually organo-corrinoids) or conversely the absence of a co-ordinated H$_2$O or other solvent molecule can only finally and conclusively be established by X-ray analysis. But strong evidence for this structure is provided by the observation of well-defined equilibria, which can only be explained on this basis, together with the existence of other organo-cobalt(III) complexes, where five-co-ordination has been established by X-ray analysis. These presumed five-co-ordinate cobalt(III) corrinoids are discussed in Chapter 8, Section III.

Section 2

Structure and Physical Properties

5

ELECTRONIC SPECTRA

Absorption spectroscopy has played such an important role in the study of cobalt corrinoids that it deserves a chapter to itself. In addition, the corrinoids are of interest to theoretical chemists because they provide a wealth of experimental data on the effects of changes in the axial ligands, the valency of the cobalt, the substituents in the corrin ring and even the metal on properties such as the energies and oscillator and rotational strengths of the electronic transitions, which are amenable to theoretical calculations. The cobalt corrinoids, in fact, provide a unique example of a ligand whose electronic structure can be profoundly altered by the nature of the ligands attached to the metal (see, for example, the spectra shown in Figs 5.1, 5.3 and 5.4); in this respect they differ strikingly from complexes such as the iron porphyrins and the phthalocyanines.

All corrinoids are highly coloured, varying from yellow or brown (e.g. methylcobinamide, B_{12r}) through red (e.g. B_{12}) to purple or violet (e.g. dicyanocobalamin), and sometimes even greenish (B_{12s}) or blue (e.g. the analogue of dicyanocobalamin in which C_{10} carries a chlorine atom). This wide variation in spectra, which makes different corrinoids readily distinguishable, together with the high extinction coefficients, which enable experiments to be carried out with very small amounts of material, provides the main reason why absorption spectroscopy has played such an important role in the chemistry of B_{12}. It has provided a general technique, e.g. for studying reactions and equilibria, for determining concentrations and for aiding structural elucidation, and a probe for the *cis*-effect of the axial ligands. Relatively few results have yet been obtained with newer techniques such as CD or ORD, though it appears that CD spectra are even more sensitive to changes in ligands, temperature etc. than the absorption spectra and may provide a more sensitive tool for certain purposes (see below).

The aim of this chapter is, therefore, to provide a brief introduction to the results of absorption spectroscopy and of related physical techniques depending on electronic transitions such as optical rotatory dispersion (ORD), circular dichroism (CD), magnetic circular dichroism (MCD) and fluorescence or emission spectroscopy.

Examples of the effect on the spectra of changes in the axial ligands, the substituents in the corrin ring, the side-chains, temperature, solvent etc. are given in Section I together with the conclusions which can be drawn about the nature of the electronic interaction between the axial ligands and the corrin ring. Experimental evidence and theoretical calculations relating to the assignment of the different electronic transitions (π–π^*, d–d, charge transfer) are discussed in Section II. References to work on the CD, ORD, MCD and fluorescence spectra of corrinoids are given in Section III.

This chapter is concerned mainly with the spectra of cobalt(III) corrinoids, in which the corrin ring retains six double bonds and of certain metal-free corrinoids. For the spectra of cobalt(II) and cobalt(I) corrinoids see Chapter 7, of additional metal-free corrinoids see Chapter 9, Section I, and of cobalt(III) corrinoids in strong acid, where the corrin ring is probably protonated, see Chapter 9, Section III. Information on the spectra of other cobalt(III) corrinoids not mentioned in this chapter may be obtained from the references in Tables 8.7 and 13.3; in many cases only the wavelength of the γ-band (the most intense band in the near ultraviolet) is given.

I. TRENDS IN THE ABSORPTION SPECTRA OF COBALT(III) CORRINOIDS

As will be shown in Section II the major bands observed in the absorption spectra of cobalt(III) corrinoids beyond 300 nm correspond to π–π^* transitions within the corrin ring. The number, position and intensities of these bands are surprisingly variable. They are very sensitive to changes in the number and nature of the axial ligands, apparently rather less sensitive to changes in the nature of substituents in the conjugated chain (though this may be due merely to the small range of substituents so far studied) and only slightly affected by changes in the side-chains, in the solvent and in temperature (except, of course, where this causes a change in the nature of the axial ligands). Wavelengths and extinction coefficients are most frequently quoted for the γ-band, less frequently for the $\alpha\beta$ bands, and only rarely for other bands. Most of our information on spectra relates to the cobalamins. Our picture is therefore far from complete, but the main features have probably been established.

Since cobalt corrinoids usually crystallize with a large and variable amount of water of crystallization, the extinction coefficients cannot be determined directly from the observed optical density and the weight of the sample. The ultimate standard of reference is B_{12}, which can be obtained pure and crystalline with a known number of molecules of water of crystallization under given conditions (see Chapter 7, Section III,C). The usual reference standard is, however, the γ-band of dicyanocobalamin or some other dicyanide; it is assumed that the spectra of dicyano-cobalamin and cobinamide and perhaps other dicyanides are virtually identical above 300 nm. This is a useful working standard since B_{12} can be converted directly into dicyanocobalamin in solution (by the action of excess cyanide), the γ-band of the dicyanide is the most intense band of all the cobalt corrinoids, and a dicyanide can be prepared in one or at most a few steps from all other cobalt corrinoids (by the action of excess cyanide and, if necessary, light etc.). Although there is some variation in the reported extinction coefficients due to uncertainties in the molecular weight, three laboratories have obtained virtually identical values for the molar extinction coefficient of the γ-band (367–368 nm) of dicyanocobalamin, viz. 3.08×10^4 (Friedrich, 1964), 3.04×10^4 (Barker et al., 1960a) and 3.04×10^4 (Hill, J. A. et al., 1964); cf. also dicyano-[8-aminocobyrinic acid-c-lactam] $\log_{10}\epsilon$ 4.48, i.e. $\epsilon\sim3.02 \times 10^4$ (Bonnett et al., 1957b). Values for the wavelengths and extinction coefficients of B_{12} include:

λ_γ	ϵ_γ	λ_α	ϵ_α	Reference
361	2.78×10^4	—	—	Barker et al., 1960a
362	2.96×10^4	552	0.96×10^4	George et al., 1960
360.5	2.75×10^4	547	0.83×10^4	Hill, J. A. et al., 1964
361	2.81×10^4	550	0.87×10^4	Friedrich, 1964

Differences of up to 2 and 5 nm in the wavelengths reported for the γ and $\alpha\beta$ bands respectively are fairly common and must be borne in mind when comparing wavelengths.

Figure 5.1 shows the spectra of cobalamins (Y = Bzm) containing the ligands cyanide, ethinyl (HC≡C—), vinyl (CH$_2$=CH—) and methyl. The spectrum of the naturally occurring 5-deoxyadenosylcobalamin or DBC is similar to that of methylcobalamin (see, for example, Hill, J. A. et al., 1964). The bands below 300 nm are due mainly to transitions within the co-ordinated Bzm (see Chapter 8, Section IV,C) and will not be considered here. Cyanocobalamin has a "typical" spectrum with an intense γ-band at 360.5 nm. Variation of the ligand in the above order produces an increasingly "atypical" spectrum, characterized by the occurrence of the γ-band at longer wavelength (~370 nm) with considerably reduced intensity and the appearance of other bands of comparable or greater intensity in the 300–350 nm region (Pratt and Thorp, 1966). The pattern of changes shown in the figure suggests that we are justified in assigning a common origin to the first band below 400 nm in each spectrum and calling this the γ-band. Atypical spectra can be produced by several ligands other than these organo-ligands. Table 5.1 shows how the wavelength of the γ-band depends on the nature of various ligands; all the spectra

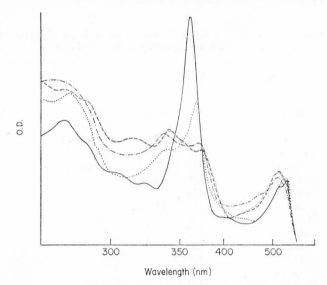

Wavelength (nm)

Fig. 5.1. Absorption spectra of cobalamins containing the ligands cyanide (———), ethinyl (·······), vinyl (—·—·—) and methyl (————). From Hill *et al.* (1965a).

where the wavelength of the γ-band is 364 nm or greater are rather atypical; see, for example, (Pratt and Thorp, 1966). This shows that the more electronegative ligand atoms (N, O, Cl, Br and C in CN⁻) all move the γ-band to shorter wavelengths, the less electronegative ligand atoms (S, Se, I and C in organo-ligands) to longer wavelengths. As will be discussed further in Chapter 6, Section III, these spectroscopic data provide a very useful probe for the *cis*-effect of the axial ligands. It has been pointed out (Pratt and Thorp, 1966, 1969; Firth *et al.*, 1968d, 1969) that both the general order of ligand atoms (N, O, Cl, Br and C in CN⁻ < S, Se, I and C in organo-ligands) and the specific order of carbanions (CN⁻ < ethinyl < vinyl < ethyl) indicate that the most important property of the axial ligand which determines its influence on the rest of the complex is the amount of negative charge donated via the σ-bond to the cobalt, which also shows a positive correlation with its position in the nephelauxetic, but not in the spectrochemical, series.

The cyano-corrinoids ($Y = CN^-$) are the only other series for which a reasonable amount of spectroscopic information is available; see, in particular George *et al.* (1960) and Firth *et al.* (1968d). A detailed study has been made of the effect of changing the axial ligand (HO^-, Bzm, and a range of carbanions) on

(i) the energies and relative intensities of all the absorption bands (not merely the α, β and γ bands) beyond 300 nm and
(ii) the cyanide stretching frequency in the infrared (Firth *et al.*, 1968d).

Table 5.1. *Effect of the axial ligand X on the wavelength of the γ-band in the cobalamins ($Y = Bzm$), tabulated according to the ligand atom*

	X	λ(nm)		X	λ(nm)
C	CH_3NC	360	S	NCS^{-a}	357
	NC^-	360.5		SO_3^{2-}	364
	$HC\equiv C-$	367		Thiourea	366
	$CH_2=CH-$	372		$S_2O_3^{2-}$	367
	$CH_3.CH_2-$	~375		Cysteine (RS^-)	370
N	NH_3	356	Se	$NCSe^-$	371
	NO_2^{-a}	356			
	NCO^-	357	Halides	Cl^-	352
	N_3^-	358		Br^-	353
	Imidazole	358		I^-	371
	Pyridine	360			
O	H_2O	350			
	$CH_3CO_2^-$	352			
	$C_6H_5O^-$	355.5			
	HO^-	357			

[a] Donor atom not known with certainty, though NCS^- is co-ordinated through S in the solid state. Data taken from Firth *et al.* (1969) except for $C_6H_5O^-$ (Hill *et al.*, 1970b).

The results are tabulated in Table 5.2 and shown graphically in Fig. 5.2. The Table and the figure show, firstly, that all the absorption bands move in the same direction on changing the ligand, though not at the same rate, and, secondly, that there is a good correlation between the cyanide stretching frequency and the wavelength of the absorption bands, i.e. between the ground-state *trans*-effect of the axial ligand and its *cis*-effect (see also Chapter 6, Section III). Thirdly, the table emphasizes how the intensities of the DE and δ bands rise while those of the α, β and γ bands fall from $X = CN^-$ downwards.

A much more limited amount of spectroscopic data is available for aquo-corrinoids ($Y = H_2O$). However, when the second axial ligand is a polarizable group such as SO_3^{2-} or an organo-ligand, the supposedly six-co-ordinate aquo

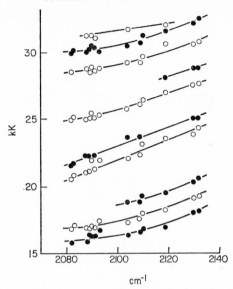

Fig. 5.2. Correlation between the stretching frequency of co-ordinated CN⁻ and the energies of the various transitions in the u.v.-visible spectra of a series of cyanocorrinoids; for the nature of the second axial ligand see the original paper. From Firth *et al.* (1968d).

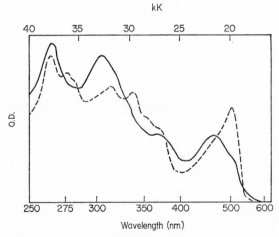

Fig. 5.3. Absorption spectrum of methylcobinamide in ethanol at +20° (———) and −180° (– – – –). From Firth *et al.* (1968a).

complex may in fact be the corresponding five-co-ordinate complex or a mixture of the five- and six-co-ordinate complexes (see Chapter 8, Section III). Figure 5.3 shows the absorption spectrum of "methyl-cobinamide" at +20° and −180° in ethanol, where it is present as a mixture containing 90 and 20%

Table 5.2. *U.v.-visible and i.r. spectra of cyanocorrinoids*[a]

Each u.v.-visible entry lists: wavelength (nm), molar extinction coefficient (×10⁻³), relative absorbance.

Axial ligand (X)	U.v.-visible absorption spectra				γ				β	α	I.r. spectra (cm⁻¹)
H₂O			323, 30.96, 1.37		354, 28.25, 2.66	387, 25.84, 0.33	407, 24.57, 0.32	(470), (21.28), 0.75	496, 20.16, 1.00	526, 20.16, 1.01	
HO⁻		309, 32.36, 1.32	(325), 30.77, 1.36	(345), 28.99, 1.69	361, 27.70, 2.49	(397), 25.19, 0.42	416, 24.04, 0.53	(490), 20.41, 0.73	520, 19.23, 1.00	552, 18.12, 1.08	2130
Bzm		306, 32.68, 1.03	323, 30.96, 0.98	(345), 28.99, 1.63	360, 27.78, 3.42	397, 25.19, 0.51	(408), (24.51), 0.49	(484), (20.66), 0.68	518, 19.31, 1.00	549, 18.21, 1.15	2132
NC⁻	(310), (32.26), 0.98	315, 31.75, 1.00	(325), (30.77), 0.70	(354), (28.25), 1.50	369, 27.10, 3.27		422, 23.70, 0.30	(512), (19.53), 0.61	545, 18.35, 1.00	586, 17.06, 1.24	2119
HC≡C—		319, 31.35, 0.98	336, 29.76, 1.04		377, 26.53, 2.40		(430), (23.36), 0.43	(515), (19.42), 0.53	554, 18.05, 1.00	593, 16.86, 1.121	2110
—SO₃.CH₂—		325, 30.77, 1.52	(341), (29.33), 1.40		381, 26.25, 2.43	(420), (23.81), 0.72	(445), (22.47), 0.58	(530), (18.87), 0.77	565, 17.70, 1.00	(599), (16.69), 0.82	~2109
CF₃.CH₂—	(314), (31.85), 1.05	327, 30.58, 1.29	340, 29.41, 1.10		386, 25.91, 2.34	(421), (23.75), 0.63	(452), (22.12), 0.42	(530), (18.87), 0.53	574, 17.42, 1.00	609, 16.42, 0.97	~2104
—OOC.CH₂—	(318), (31.45), 1.63	327, 30.58, 1.70	(345), (28.99), 1.44		391, 25.58, 2.23		(455), (21.98), 0.68		584, 17.12, 1.00	(612), (16.34), 0.91	2090

Compound									
CH₂=CH—		331	(346)	393		(454)	572	(596)	2093
		30.21	(28.90)	25.45		(22.03)	17.48	(16.78)	
		1.34	1.22	1.89		0.43	1.00	0.97	
5'-Deoxy-adenosyl	(320)	329	(348)	396	447	468	588	(620)	2091
	(31.25)	30.40	(28.74)	25.25	22.37	21.37	17.01	(16.39)	
		1.84	1.61	1.84	0.64	0.63	1.00	0.85	
CH₂OH.CH₂—		330	(350)	397	451	472	589	(610)	2089
		30.30	(28.57)	25.19	22.17	21.29	16.98	(16.39)	
		1.97	1.75	1.73	0.65	0.65	1.00	0.92	
CH₃—	(319)	332	(346)	398	447	473	588	(627)	2088
	(31.35)	30.12	(28.90)	25.13	22.37	21.14	17.01	(15.95)	
	1.68	1.70	1.62	1.73	0.58	0.58	1.00	0.75	
CH₃.CH₂—		333	(349)	399	462	484	593	(631)	2082
		30.03	(28.65)	25.06	21.65	20.66	16.86	(15.85)	
		2.07	1.94	1.56	0.67	0.72	1.00	0.72	
CH₃.CH₂.CH₂—		331		396	459	480	585		2083
		30.21		25.25	21.79	20.83	17.09		
		2.24		1.67	0.73	0.75	1.00		

[a] For each compound the top lines gives the wavelength in nm, the second line the energy in kK, and the bottom line the optical density relative to the optical density of the β-band (values in parentheses denote shoulders). From Firth et al. (1968d).

of the six-co-ordinate methylaquocobinamide respectively. The spectrum of the six-co-ordinate methylaquocobinamide shows α and β bands at 529 nm (shoulder) and 503 nm (Firth et al., 1968a) and is obviously not so very different from that of the six-co-ordinate methylcobalamin (cf. Figs 5.1 and 5.3). The five-co-ordinate vinyl-, methyl-, ethyl-, isopropyl- and sulphitocobinamides, on the other hand, are all yellow in colour and the first band in their absorption spectra occurs in the 440–460 nm region (Firth et al., 1968a); their spectra are, therefore, very different from those of the six-co-ordinate

Table 5.3. *Comparison of the effect of the axial ligand X on the wavelength of the γ-band (in nm) in three series of corrinoids ($Y = H_2O$, Bzm, CN^-)*

X	$Y = H_2O$	$Y = Bzm^a$	$Y = CN^-$
H_2O	348^f	350	355^e
NH_3	348.5^g	356	362^e
HO^-		357	362^e
Imidazole	351^g	358	362^e
N_3^-		358	363^e
Pyridine		360	363^e
CH_3NC		360	368^e
CN^-	353^b	360.5	368^e
SO_3^{2-}	351^b	364	372^d
$HC\equiv C-$	355^h	367	377^c
Cysteinate (RS^-)		370	377^d
$CH_2=CH-$	363^b	372	393^c
CH_3-	369^b	$\sim374^h$	398^c
CH_3CH_2-	$\sim373^b$ (shoulder)	~375	399^c

[a] Data taken from Table 5.1 except for $X = CH_3$.
[b] Firth et al., 1968a; [c] Firth et al., 1968d; [d] Firth et al., 1969; [e] George et al., 1960; [f] Hayward et al., 1965; [g] Hayward et al., 1971; [h] Hill, J. A. et al., 1964.

complexes and caution must be exercised when discussing the spectra of corrinoids in which one axial ligand is a very polarizable ligand and the second is supposedly a solvent molecule.

Table 5.3 compares the effect of varying one axial ligand (X) in the three series where $Y = H_2O$, Bzm and CN^-. We can also keep X constant and see the effect of varying Y by comparing data across the rows. Comparison of the equilibrium constants listed in Table 8.8 suggests that the "ethinylaquo" complex is truly six-co-ordinate. If we exclude the sulphitoaquo complex, very similar ligand orders are observed in each case. As a broad generalization we can say that the greater the *sum* of the donor strengths of the two axial ligands, the longer the wavelength of the γ-band. Sulphite has the ability to co-ordinate through either S or O; although it is almost certainly co-ordinated through S both in the stable form of the cobalamin and when Y is CN^-, there is evidence for an unstable O-bonded cobalamin (Firth *et al.*, 1969) and the anomalously short wavelength of the sulphitoaquo complex may indicate co-ordination through O in this complex as well.

If we now compare the effect of varying both axial ligands on the extinction coefficient of the γ-band, which provides some measure of how "typical" or "atypical" the spectrum is, we find a very different correlation (see Table 5.4). It appears that the extinction coefficient of the γ-band falls (i.e. the spectrum becomes more atypical) as the *difference* in the donor strength of the two axial ligand increases. The highest extinction co-efficients are found when both axial ligands are identical (H_2O or CN^-), the lowest when one is H_2O and the

Table 5.4. *Comparison of the effect of the axial ligand on the molar extinction coefficient of the γ-band ($\times 10^{-4}$ M^{-1} cm^{-1}). Wavelength (in nm) given in parentheses*[a]

	H_2O	Bzm	CN^-
H_2O	2.8 (348)	2.62 (350)	2.4 (353)
CN^-	2.4 (353)	2.75 (360.5)	3.04 (367)
HC≡C—	1.7 (355)	1.8 (367)	2.28 (373)
CH_2=CH—	⩾1.0 (363)[b]	1.3 (372)	~1.4 (393)[c]
CH_3	~1.3 (369)[b]	1.16 (374)	~1.3 (398)[c]

[a] Data from Hill *et al.* (1965a) with the following corrections:

[b] Original data referred to mixtures of five- and six-co-ordinate complexes. Tabulated wavelengths are those of the pure six-co-ordinate complexes (Firth *et al.*, 1968a); the extinction coefficient of the methyl complex has been calculated from data in Firth *et al.* (1968a).

[c] Original wavelengths superseded by more recent data (Firth *et al.*, 1968d); extinction co-efficients are probably still comparable.

other an alkyl ligand. Figure 5.1 showed how, when the unchanged ligand is Bzm (i.e. a ligand of relatively low donor strength), the anomaly increases as the donor strength of the second axial ligand increases in the order $CN^- \ldots CH_3$. The opposite effect is shown in Fig. 5.4, namely that when the unchanged ligand is ethinyl (a much better donor), then the anomaly decreases as the donor strength of the second ligand increases in the order $H_2O < $ Bzm $< CN^-$.

We can also examine the effect of inverting the two axial ligands by comparing the spectra of l- and u-isomers; for a discussion of l- and u-isomers involving the relative orientation of the axial ligands see Chapter 8, Section II. Friedrich and co-workers have reported the spectra of several pairs of isomers of cyanoaquocorrinoids (Friedrich, 1966b; Friedrich *et al.*, 1967). Figure 5.5 shows the spectra of two such isomers; some other data are given in Chapter 8, Section II. As can be seen from Fig. 5.5 and Table 5.4, the cyanoaquo complexes are slightly "atypical" (prominent shoulder ~320 nm, rather low γ-band,

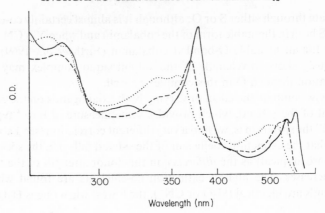

Fig. 5.4. Absorption spectra of ethinylcobalamin in 1 N H$_2$SO$_4$ ($\cdots\cdots$), 1 N NaOH (––––) and 1 N NaOH and 0.5 N KCN (———), where the second axial ligand is H$_2$O, Bzm and CN$^-$ respectively. From Hill *et al.* (1965a).

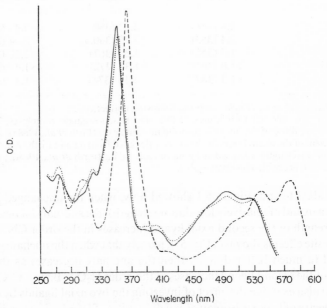

Fig. 5.5. Absorption spectra of the 1-(———) and u-($\cdots\cdots$) isomers of the cyanoaquo complex of a tetracarboxylic acid derivative in 0.04 M sodium acetate, and of the corresponding dicyano complexes, which are identical (––––). From Friedrich *et al.* (1967).

β-band higher than α-band). The differences between the isomers are obviously very small compared to the differences discussed in previous paragraphs. This suggests (Firth *et al.*, 1968c) that the corrin ring is sensitive to the difference in donor strength between the two axial ligands but, although it lacks any plane of symmetry, is nevertheless insensitive to the sign of this difference, as shown by the similar spectra of the two isomers. Much larger differences in spectra are observed between the l- and u-isomers of methyl- and ethyl-corrinoids (see Table 8.3); but these differences in spectra may be due primarily to differences in the relative proportions of five- and six-co-ordinate species.

We can summarize the above results on the effect of the axial ligands on the spectra of six-co-ordinate cobalt(III) corrinoids in the following generalizations:

1. The nature of the axial ligands has a marked effect on both the energies and intensities of the absorption bands.
2. The most relevant property of the ligand is its σ-donor strength.
3. The γ-band moves to increasingly longer wavelengths (and other bands show comparable movements) as the *sum* of the donor strengths of the two axial ligands increases.
4. The intensity of the γ-band falls (and other bands also show changes in intensity) as the *difference* between the donor strengths of the two axial ligands increases, without regard to their relative orientation.

The evidence for these generalizations comes mainly from the study of complexes containing carbanions. It is to be hoped that future work will show how far they are valid when applied to a wider range of ligands. There is, for example, something unusual about HO^-; hydroxocobalamin has a low γ-band with a very prominent shoulder on the high-energy side (Hill *et al.*, 1962), while dihydroxocobinamide has an even more anomalous spectrum in the γ-band region (Hayward *et al.*, 1971).

The absorption spectra can provide evidence for steric as well as electronic effects in the metal-ligand bond. Compare the wavelengths (in nm) of the γ-band in cobalamins with the following ligands: H_2O, 350; pyridine, 360; α-picoline, 356; β-picoline, 361; γ-picoline, 361; imidazole, 358; benzimidazole, 354 (Hill *et al.*, 1962). It is clear that the shift in wavelength on replacing H_2O by a nitrogeneous base is least for just those two ligands where considerable steric hindrance is expected, viz. α-picoline and benzimidazole.

Table 5.5 shows the effect of substituents in the corrin ring. It is interesting that the substitution of hydrogen by either chlorine or bromine moves all the bands to longer wavelength, but that the $\alpha\beta$ bands (and the 458 nm band in the last two complexes) are affected far more than the higher-energy bands. This must obviously be related to differences in the electron density at C_{10} in the excited states corresponding to the various transitions. Corrinoids carrying the substituents NH_2 and NO_2 at C_{10} have also been reported (Wagner, 1965), but their structure cannot be regarded as established (see Chapter 15, Section I). Comparison of the spectra of synthetic cobalt corrinoids, in which one can

3

Table 5.5. *Effect of substituents at C_{10} on the absorption spectra*

Compound	Axial ligands	Subst. at C_{10}	λ (nm)							Reference
						γ	β		α	
Lactam	Bzm, CN^-	H				359	517		548	Bonnett *et al.*, 1957a
		Cl				365	548		580	
Cobalamin	Bzm, CN^-	H				361	520		550	Wagner, 1965
		Br				363	550		575	
Cobalamin	CN^-, CN^-	H				367	540		580	Wagner and Bernhauer, 1964
		Cl				369	561		602	
		H				367	550		580	Wagner, 1965
		Br				370	561		602	
Lactam	CN^-, CN^-	H				366	541		581	Bonnett *et al.*, 1957a
		Cl				369	568		609	
		H				367	541		581	Wagner and Bernhauer, 1964
		Cl				369	565		616	
Cobalamin	Bzm, CH_3	H	278	343		377		525		Johnson *et al.*, 1963a
		Cl	283	347				548		Dolphin *et al.*, 1964a
Cobalamin	Bzm, 5-deoxyadenosyl	H	262	342				518		
		Cl	262	347				543		Wagner and Bernhauer, 1964
Cobalamin, (pHI)	(H_2O), CH_3	H	276	340	303		458	525		
		Cl	278	345	306		481	543		
Cobalamin (pHI)	(H_2O), 5-deoxyadenosyl	H	263		304		458			
		Cl	266		306		474			

replace the hydrogen at C_{15} by CH_3 or CN, shows similar small changes in wavelength and differences between the $\alpha\beta$ and γ bands (Briat and Djerassi, 1969).

In contrast to the effects of changes in the axial ligands or substituents of the conjugated ring, changes in the side-chains or even in the outer ring of carbon atoms have very little effect on the spectrum. Compare, for example, the wavelengths (in nm) of the bands in dicyanide complexes containing the following equatorial ligands:

	γ	β	α	Reference
Cobalamin	367	540	580	Wagner and Bernhauer, 1964
Lactam	366	541	581	Bonnett et al., 1957a
Lactone	365	544–5	584–6	
Pentacarboxylic acid	365	540	579–80	Bonnett et al. 1957b
Hexacarboxylic acid	363	537	576–7	

The effects of changing the temperature or the solvent have also been studied with a wide range of cobalt(III) corrinoids (Firth et al., 1967a, 1968a). Lowering the temperature causes a sharpening of all the absorption bands; two examples are given in Fig. 5.6 in the next section. Change of temperature or solvent may cause a marked change in spectrum through changing the number or nature of the axial ligands, in particular through displacing the equilibrium between five- and six-co-ordinate complexes (see Chapter 8, Section III). But where no change in the axial ligands occurs, only very small changes in the spectrum are observed, e.g. $\leqslant 2$ nm for the γ-band of B_{12} or dicyanocobinamide.

Reflection spectra have been measured of several corrinoids in the solid state (Hill, J. A. et al., 1964; Firth et al., 1968a). Varying the water vapour pressure, and hence the water content of the solid, may cause large changes in the spectrum; drying tends to convert aquocobalamin and cyanoaquocobinamide into the corresponding hydroxo complexes and six-co-ordinate organo-cobalamins and cobinamides into the five-co-ordinate complexes. Where no such changes occur, there is a good correspondence between the wavelengths observed for the reflection spectrum of the solid and the absorption spectrum of the solution both for six-co-ordinate corrinoids such as B_{12} (Hill, J. A. et al., 1964) and five-co-ordinate complexes such as ethylcobinamide (Firth et al., 1968a).

II. NATURE AND THEORY OF THE ELECTRONIC TRANSITIONS

As mentioned in the previous section, lowering the temperature sharpens all the bands in the absorption spectra and makes them easier to resolve. Figure 5.6 shows the spectra of a "typical" red corrinoid, viz. dicyanocobinamide, and an "atypical" red corrinoid, viz. methyl-cobalamin, at −180°; for the characteristics of typical and atypical spectra see the previous section. The spectrum of the dicyanide is particularly well resolved and reveals a very large number of bands. The question to be discussed here is: what are the origins of these transitions? As will be shown below, we now have a reasonable understanding of the nature of the transitions observed in "typical" spectra, but not of those in "atypical" spectra.

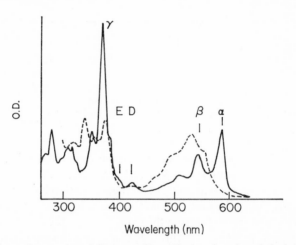

Fig. 5.6. Absorption spectra of dicyanocobinamide (——) and methylcobalamin (----) in ethanol at −180°; letters refer to the bands of the dicyanide. From Firth *et al.* (1967a).

The cobalt corrinoids may be expected to show absorption spectra due to transitions of the following limiting types:

(A) d–d transitions of the cobalt ion,
(B) internal transitions of the equatorial corrin ligand,
(C) internal transitions of the axial ligands (e.g. the absorption spectrum of Bzm in the 260–300 nm region),
(D) charge transfer transitions from the corrin ring to cobalt or vice versa and
(E) charge transfer transitions from an axial ligand to cobalt or vice versa.

In addition, transitions of types A–C may be spin-allowed or spin-forbidden. One expects that the intensities of these different bands will vary by several orders of magnitude, decreasing in the general order: spin-allowed π–π* ~ charge transfer ≫ spin-allowed d–d > spin-forbidden π–π* and spin-forbidden d–d. Some transitions may therefore be obscured by others; the very weak d–d transitions, for example, are probably buried under the intense π–π* transitions (see below).

The main bands in the absorption spectra of cobalt(III) corrinoids above

300 nm are due to π–π* transitions within the corrin ring; the evidence for this assignment is given in the next paragraph. The Bzm present in the cobalamins absorbs in the 260–300 nm region (compare, for example, Fig. 5.6 with Fig. 5.1); for wavelengths and references see Chapter 8, Section IV,C. Very few bands have yet been reported which can be assigned to charge transfer, d–d or spin-forbidden π–π* transitions; these are mentioned at the end of this section.

A. π–π* TRANSITIONS OF THE CORRIN RING

The availability of metal-free corrinoids allows one to identify the internal transitions of the corrin ligand. Several naturally occurring and synthetic

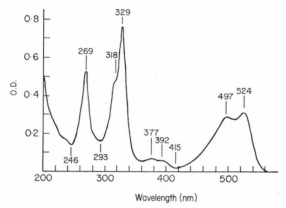

Fig. 5.7. Absorption spectrum of one of Toohey's red metal-free corrinoids from *Chromatium*, 2.55×10^{-5} M in water. From Toohey (1965).

forms have been studied (see Chapter 9, Section I). The naturally occurring forms can all exist in a red and one or more yellow forms depending on the pH and other factors. It appears that in the red form both N_{21} and N_{22} are protonated. The absorption spectrum of one of these red metal-free corrinoids is shown in Fig. 5.7. Comparison with the spectrum of dicyanocobinamide (see Fig. 5.6) shows that all the main bands in the dicyanide (α, β, D, E, γ with shoulder, δ-bands) are present in the metal-free compound; the relative intensities are very similar in both cases except that the δ-band is less intense in the dicyanide, while the energies are all slightly lower in the dicyanide. All these transitions can therefore be ascribed to π–π* transitions within the corrin ring. n–π* transitions from a lone pair on one of the corrin nitrogen atoms (e.g. N_{20} or N_{23}) can be excluded because they would be shifted to much higher energy on co-ordination to the cobalt ion, which would lead to differences between the two spectra. Spin-forbidden π–π* transitions can apparently also be excluded since the addition of ethyl iodide, which is known to enhance the intensity of singlet-triplet transitions, produces no change in the intensity of bands in cobalt(III) corrinoids (Day, 1967b). The main bands in the spectra of the red metal-free corrinoids and of the typical red cobalt(III) corrinoids above 300 nm can therefore be assigned to spin-allowed $\pi-\pi^*$ transitions within the corrin ring. The next question is: how many different electronic transitions are there or, conversely, which bands represent vibrational bands of the same electronic transitions?

All bands in the absorption spectra which represent a vibrational progression of the same electronic transition can be expected to show fairly constant energy differences, a fairly regular distribution of intensities and similarities in, for example, the polarization of the transition or the sign of the circular dichroism. Conversely, bands belonging to different electronic transitions will probably show some differences. With the benefit of hindsight we can group the bands observed in the spectra of typical red corrinoids into the following four regions:

1. The $\alpha\beta$ bands. A series of low to medium intensity bands in the 420–600 nm region. The lowest and next lowest in energy are termed the α and β bands respectively.
2. D and E bands. Two bands of low intensity in the 390–420 nm region.
3. γ-band. The most intense band in the 350–370 nm region, usually accompanied by a shoulder on the high-energy side and perhaps other bands as well.
4. δ-bands. Bands of low to medium intensity in the 300–330 nm region.

The $\alpha\beta\gamma\delta$ nomenclature was adopted from the porphyrin field because of similarities in the spectra of metal porphyrins and cobalt corrinoids (Hill et al., 1962), The low-intensity bands near 400 nm were subsequently named D and E when it was realized that they were distinct from both the $\alpha\beta$ and γ systems (Firth et al., 1967a). A different nomenclature has been used by some authors. One hopes that a more logical system of nomenclature may soon be devised, which would also be applicable to the spectra of atypical corrinoids. Perhaps it would be simplest to name the electronic transitions α, β, γ and δ in order of increasing energy and the individual absorption bands by adding a subscript to denote the vibrational component; in dicyanocobinamide, for example, the present α, β, D, E and γ bands would then (neglecting uncertainties in the numbering of the vibrational components) become α_0, α_1, β_0, β_1 and γ_0 respectively.

Eckert and Kuhn (1960) were the first to look for differences in the polarization of the transitions corresponding to the different bands. They prepared a film of polyvinyl alcohol containing B_{12}, stretched the film in order to induce some orientation of the molecules (they argued that the C_5-C_{15} axis of the corrinoid molecules would tend to align itself parallel to the axis of stretch) and compared the absorption spectra parallel and normal to the axis of stretch; a slight dichroism was observed. The $\alpha\beta$ (or A in their nomenclature) and δ (or C) bands showed greatest optical density parallel to this axis, the D and E (or B') and γ (or B) bands normal to the axis. Thomson determined the polarization ratios of the excitation spectrum of fluorescence in the case of the metal-free red corrin; the cobalt corrinoids, unfortunately, do not fluoresce (Thomson, 1969). The polarization ratios of excitation (relative to emission at 16.7 kK or 600 nm) varied from positive ($\sim50\%$) in the region of the $\alpha\beta$ bands, through zero or slightly negative in the region of the D and E bands, to negative for the γ-band and back to positive again for the δ-bands. The transitions of the $\alpha\beta$ and δ bands are therefore polarized parallel to one another (and to the emitting transition), the γ-band is polarized perpendicular to this direction and the D and E bands are of mixed polarization with the major component in the same direction as the γ-band. Thomson's results on the metal-free red corrin are therefore in excellent agreement with Eckert and Kuhn's data on B_{12} and serve to distinguish four different electron transitions in the region above 300 nm, viz. $\alpha\beta$, DE, γ, and δ.

Thomson has also reported the CD spectrum of the metal-free red corrin, which shows a relatively simple pattern; the values of ($\epsilon_L - \epsilon_R$) are slightly negative in the $\alpha\beta$ region, virtually zero for D and E, strongly positive for the γ-band and strongly negative for the δ-band (Thomson, 1969). Comparison of the polarization ratios of the excitation spectrum of fluorescence with the signs of the rotational strengths in the CD spectrum showed that the relative signs of the latter are determined by the directions of the electric dipole transitions. The CD and MCD spectra of cobalt-containing corrinoids, however, are much more complex. One often observes additional changes of sign in the $\alpha\beta$ region, particularly around 490 nm, and a complicated structure in the γ-band region (Legrand and Viennet, 1962; Briat and Djerassi, 1969; Firth et al., 1967a). Furthermore, the D and E bands which have virtually no rotational strength in the metal-free corrinoid, become the most intense bands in the CD spectra of the cobalt corrinoids. It has been suggested that some of the anomalies observed in the number and rotational strengths of the bands in the CD spectra of cobalt corrinoids may be caused by the presence of or mixing with the d–d transitions of the metal (Firth et al., 1967a).

The large number of bands observed in the spectra of cobalt corrinoids above 300 nm (or 33.3 kK) must therefore be ascribed to the vibrational components of these four electronic transitions. In the spectrum of dicyano-cobinamide at $-180°$ (see Fig. 5.6) the first four bands starting from the low-energy end of the spectrum are separated by intervals of 1.30 ± 0.05 kK and can be ascribed to vibrational components of the same electronic transition, the (0–0) band being the most intense (Day, 1967b); the α and β bands are therefore the (0–0) and (0–1) components respectively. In the case of the metal-free red corrin Thomson concludes that the D and E bands are the vibrational components of the next higher transition with the possibility that the (0–0) band is not seen (Thomson, 1969); the same may be true for dicyanocobinamide. It appears from Fig. 5.6 that the intense γ-band may be the second or (0–1) component of a vibrational progression belonging to the third electronic transition. The δ-band can also be resolved into four components at $-180°$, but the separations are smaller ($\sim$0.7 kK) than for the $\alpha\beta$ system and the (0–1) band is the most intense (Day, 1967b). These vibrational progressions observed in the absorption spectra correspond to vibrational levels in the electronically excited state and are probably related to a stretching frequency of the corrin ring (Day, 1967b; Thomson, 1969). Thomson (1969) has listed the energy separations between the vibrational components in both absorption and emission spectra of red and yellow metal-free corrins.

Using the above assignments, Day (1967b) has calculated the oscillator strengths of the four lowest electronic transitions of dicyano-cobinamide as follows: $\alpha\beta$ 0.13, DE 0.01, γ 0.27, δ 0.13. Calculations were also made for some of the transitions in methylcobalamin.

The first theoretical calculations on the energy levels and hence on the energies of the transitions in the absorption spectra were made by Kuhn (1959) and Kuhn *et al.* (1965) using the one-dimensional free electron model. Molecular orbital calculations have subsequently been made by Offenhartz (1965), Veillard and Pullman (1965), Schrauzer (1966), Day (1967a,b) and Johansen and Ingraham (1969).

The corrinoids, like the cyanines, contain a conjugated chain with an odd number of atoms. The corrin chain contains 13 atoms (4 nitrogen and 9 carbon) and 14 π-electrons; the seven lowest energy orbitals of the π-electron systems are therefore filled. The lowest energy transition observed in the absorption spectrum ($\alpha\beta$ bands) is obviously from the highest occupied to the lowest unoccupied orbital, i.e. $7 \to 8$. There is general agreement that the next two observed transitions in the typical red corrinoids (DE, γ) correspond to $6 \to 8$ and $7 \to 9$, though with strong interaction (see below). There is, however, no general agreement as to the nature of the next transition (δ bands) (Schrauzer, 1966; Day, 1967b; Johansen and Ingraham, 1969). Day has pointed out the importance of configuration interaction between the one-electron energy levels, in particular its effect on the second and third transitions. The two transitions ($6 \to 8$) and ($7 \to 9$) can interact to give a higher-energy in-phase and a lower-energy out-of-phase linear combination, the extent of interaction decreasing as the negative charge on the nitrogen atoms (and hence the donor power of the axial ligands) increases. He suggests that this change in the degree of interaction could explain the striking difference between, say, dicyanocobinamide and methylcobalamin (see Fig. 5.6) in the relative intensities of the bands in the γ-region and the equally striking variation in the rotational strength and even in the sign observed in the CD spectra (see, for example, Firth et al., 1967a), but admits that the spectrum of methylcobalamin cannot yet be fully explained (Day, 1967b). This emphasizes the need for further experimental data, which would allow us to determine the number of different electronic transitions and to assign the observed bands in the absorption spectra of atypical complexes such as methylcobalamin.

In conclusion, one can say that there is good experimental evidence for the number of electronic transitions and for the assignment of the observed bands and a reasonable theoretical understanding in the case of typical red cobalt(III) corrinoids (and metal-free red corrinoids). There is, however, no such firm experimental or theoretical basis for the spectra of "atypical" red cobalt corrinoids (such as methylcobalamin), let alone yellow cobalt corrinoids such as methylcobinamide or cobalt(II) corrinoids.

B. CHARGE TRANSFER BANDS

One might expect to observe transitions due to charge transfer in either direction between the cobalt and the axial ligands or between the cobalt and the corrin ring, depending on the valency of the cobalt and the nature of the axial ligands and substituents in the corrin ring. Since charge transfer transitions, unlike d–d transitions, usually have high intensities ($\log \epsilon \geqslant 3$), they will probably be observable in the absorption spectra, though it may be difficult to identify them as such.

Only one transition assignable to charge transfer from an axial ligand to cobalt has been identified so far. Comparison of the spectra of phenolato- and hydroxo-cobalamin shows that the former contains an additional intense band at 468 nm, which is superimposed on the normal pattern of α, β and γ bands (Hill et al., 1970b). Subtracting out the absorption spectrum due to π–π^* transitions (assumed to be the same as that of hydroxocobalamin) leaves a very broad band with a maximum at 455 nm (molar $\epsilon \sim 7 \times 10^3$ M^{-1} cm^{-1}), which is assigned to charge transfer from the phenolate anion to the cobalt (see Fig. 5.8). Similar charge transfer bands are observed in phenolate complexes of other reducible metal ions (see references in Hill et al., 1970b).

One would also expect to observe charge transfer bands above 300 nm with polarizable and reducing ligands such as I^-, $S_2O_3^{2-}$, RS^- etc.; cf. the wavelengths of the transitions due to transfer of an electron from the iodide to the cobalt in $[Co(NH_3)_5I]^{2+}$ $\lambda = 383$ nm ($\log \epsilon = 3.43$) and 286 nm (4.24) (Linhard and Weigl, 1957) and $[Co(CN)_5I]^{3-}$ 330 nm (3.47) (Adamson et al., 1969). But it will be difficult to distinguish such a transition due to charge transfer from the axial ligand to the cobalt from π–π^* transitions or charge transfer transitions from the cobalt to the corrin ring. For example, cobalamins with "atypical" spectra showing several intense bands in the 300–380 nm region are produced by all polarizable axial ligands, both those such as CH_3^- which are not expected to give rise to a charge transfer transition from the axial ligand at such low energies (since the electron pair of the ligand is held in the cobalt-carbon bond) and by those such as iodide, which almost certainly will.

Nor is there any direct evidence for charge transfer between the cobalt and the corrin ring, though one would expect the spectra of cobalt(I) corrinoids (see Chapter 7, Section V) to contain transitions due to electron transfer from the cobalt to the corrin ring. Could some of the bands in the 300–380 nm region of

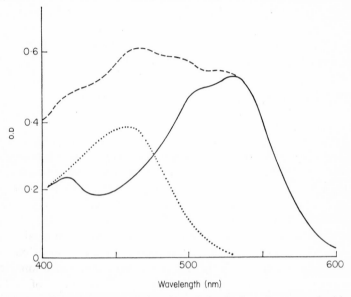

Fig. 5.8. Absorption spectrum of phenolatocobalamin (– – – –) compared with that of hydroxocobalamin (——); the difference (·····) is attributed to a charge transfer band from phenolate to cobalt. From Pratt (unpublished work).

cobalt(III) corrinoids with polarizable ligands be due to charge transfer from the cobalt to the ring?

C. SPIN-ALLOWED d–d TRANSITIONS

The ligand field strength of the corrin ring is not known; but one might expect that the five nitrogen atoms in the cobalamins would exert a ligand field comparable to that of the five nitrogens in the pentammine complexes. The following examples show the range of wavelengths (with molar extinction coefficients in parentheses) observed for the first spin-allowed d–d transition in the pentammine complexes $[Co^{III}(NH_3)_5X]$: CN^-, 440.5 nm

(56 M^{-1} cm^{-1}) (Siebert, 1964); NH$_3$, 475 (55); H$_2$O, 490 (47); N$_3^-$, 520 (265); Cl$^-$, 533 (49); I$^-$, 580 (80) (Candlin et al., 1964; Linhard and Weigl, 1957). The first d–d transitions in the cobalamins are therefore likely to be buried under the much more intense bands of the $\alpha\beta$ system. The d–d transitions might be more readily detected by other techniques such as CD spectroscopy; but, although some of the anomalies observed in the CD spectra of cobalt corrinoids have been ascribed to the influence of d–d transitions (Firth et al., 1967a) (see also Section I), no direct evidence as to their position has yet been reported.

D. SPIN-FORBIDDEN BANDS AT LOW ENERGY

All the transitions considered above are spin-allowed, i.e. singlet–singlet in the case of the diamagnetic cobalt(III) corrinoids. Analogous spin-forbidden transitions (in this case singlet–triplet) will occur at much lower energies and with reduced intensity. Compare, for example, the wavelength and molar extinction coefficient of the spin-forbidden d–d transitions of the following pentammine complexes [Co^{III}(NH$_3$)$_5$X] with the values for the spin-allowed transitions given in the previous paragraph: NH$_3$, ~746 nm (0.6) and ~580 (0.9); Cl$^-$, 877 (0.6) and 657 (0.8); I$^-$, 936 (68) and 725 (43) (Linhard and Weigl, 1957). It is difficult to predict the wavelengths and intensities of the spin-forbidden analogues of the $\alpha\beta$, DE, γ and other π–π^* bands. The presence of a heavy atom, in particular iodine, enhances the intensity of spin-forbidden transitions; this is clearly shown by comparing the relative intensities of the spin-allowed and forbidden transitions for the complexes with NH$_3$, Cl$^-$ and I$^-$.

Transitions have been observed at wavelengths longer than the $\alpha\beta$ bands both in the solid state and in solution. Hodgkin and co-workers noted that all the crystalline cobalamins which they examined were highly pleochroic, the following colours being observed: CN$^-$, red and colourless; NO$_2^-$, red and pale blue; NCS$^-$ and NCSe$^-$, red and deep green (Hodgkin et al., 1957). Blue indicates the occurrence of a transition at the low-energy end of the visible region, green a transition at each end of the visible. The red colour is clearly due to the $\alpha\beta$ bands; the blue and green colours are therefore probably due to transitions with a different polarization and are probably not the spin-forbidden $\alpha\beta$ bands. Absorption bands of low intensity have also been observed for cobalamins in solution (Pratt and Thorp, 1966); they are particularly noticeable (molar ϵ ~500 M^{-1} cm^{-1}) with the ligands I$^-$ (λ_{max} ~740 nm), NCSe$^-$ (~730 nm) and S$_2$O$_3^{2-}$ (~680 nm) (Pratt and Thorp, unpublished results). There is clearly insufficient evidence for assigning the bands as either π–π^* or d–d transitions. One hopes that further study will be made of these low-energy transitions. Identification and study of the spin-forbidden d–d bands might be the only way to obtain information on the position of the corrin ligand in the spectrochemical and nephelauxetic series.

III. OTHER SPECTROSCOPIC TECHNIQUES

A. OPTICAL ROTATION

B_{12} and all other naturally occurring corrinoids are optically active. For references to reported values of specific rotations see Bonnett (1963).

B. ORD SPECTRA

Eichhorn (1961) has reported the ORD spectra of a few cobalt corrinoids.

C. CIRCULAR DICHROISM (CD) AND MAGNETIC CIRCULAR DICHROISM (MCD) SPECTRA

CD spectra of cobalt corrinoids were first measured by Legrand and Viennet (1962). Since then Firth *et al.* (1967a) have studied a much wider range of complexes (see also Hill *et al.*, 1965a). Friedrich (1966b) and co-workers (Friedrich *et al.*, 1967) have compared the l- and u-isomers of several cyanoaquocorrinoids; their data are given in Table 8.3. Thomson (1969) has studied metal-free red and yellow corrinoids. Babior and Li (1969) have used CD to study the binding of B_{12a} and DBC to an enzyme. Briat and Djerassi (1968, 1969) have reported the MCD spectra of several synthetic cobalt, nickel and zinc corrinoids as well as the CD and MCD spectra of dicyano-[cobyrinic acid heptamethyl ester]–cobalt(III). The main results can be summarized as follows. There is a reasonable correlation between the wavelengths of the bands in absorption and in CD spectra for some complexes, but the CD spectra often show additional bands and other anomalies, which might be due to the presence of d–d transitions and to the mixing of these with the $\pi-\pi^*$ transitions (Firth *et al.*, 1967a). The most prominent bands in the CD spectra are usually the D and E bands, which are amongst the least prominent bands in the absorption spectra. The CD spectra appear to be even more sensitive than the absorption spectra to the nature of the axial ligands (Firth *et al.*, 1967a), but comparison of the l- and u-isomers shows that inversion of the axial ligands has only a minor effect (Friedrich, 1966b; Friedrich *et al.*, 1967). Most surprisingly, the signs of all the bands in the CD spectra of cyano-, dicyano- and methyl-cobalamin appear to undergo an inversion on cooling to $-180°$; the cause of this inversion is not known, but it could be associated with some change in the conformation of the corrin ring (Firth *et al.*, 1967a) (see also Chapter 6, Section I). A great deal more work must clearly be done before we can claim to understand the CD spectra of the corrinoids.

D. EMISSION SPECTRA

As already mentioned in Section II above, Thomson has studied the fluorescence of metal-free red and yellow corrinoids. He could not, however, detect any fluorescence in cyano- or dicyano-cobalamin (wavelength of exciting radiation not stated, but probably >300 nm) or any long-lived emission (i.e. phosphorescence) in either these complexes or in the red or yellow metal-free corrinoids down to the limit of detection of the apparatus at 14 kK (~700 nm) (Thomson, 1969). B_{12} will, however, fluoresce when excited with light of wavelength ~275 nm; the fluorescence maximum occurs at ~305 nm and can be attributed to Bzm (Duggan *et al.*, 1957). Metal-free and cobalt(III) corrinoids are, of course, photochemically active (see Chapter 14).

6

STRUCTURE AND BONDING

The aim of this chapter is to present some of the information relating to the details of structure (especially of the cobalt co-ordination sphere and of the conjugated corrin ring) and of the types of bond or interaction, both intra- and inter-molecular (covalent, hydrogen-bond, van der Waals interaction), which are observed in the corrinoids. This forms an essential introduction to the subsequent chapters which deal with the making and breaking of covalent or co-ordinate bonds.

Much of our information comes from X-ray crystallography. As Professor Hodgkin said in 1958 (Hodgkin, 1958): "If one looks closely at the positions of the atoms found within each molecule in each crystal, they provide remarkable illustrations of the interplay of the different factors controlling them, chemical, stereochemical, conformational, intermolecular—all the various forces of attraction and repulsion". Our knowledge has increased considerably since then and evidence from diffraction methods (X-ray and neutron) has been supplemented by spectroscopic techniques (mainly u.v.-visible absorption spectra, but also infrared, nuclear magnetic resonance and electron spin resonance spectra) as well as by chemical observations.

In addition to elucidating the framework of covalent and co-ordinate bonds, X-ray crystallography has shown the occurrence of both inter- and intra-molecular hydrogen-bonds, the existence of several sites of strong steric repulsion and the formation of clathrates within the hydrogen-bonded lattice involving the side-chains. Physical and chemical studies have provided evidence for additional examples in each of these categories. No positive evidence has yet been obtained for the occurrence of any significant interaction of the charge-transfer or donor-acceptor type involving either the corrin ring or a heterocyclic base, though iodine appears to form a weak adduct with aquocobalamin which may be of this type (see Section II).

From the point of view of co-ordination chemistry and biochemistry the most important features of the structure and bonding of the corrinoids can best be thrown into relief by dividing the three-dimensional structures of the corrinoids into three layers as follows:

1. An inner core of atoms, comprising the conjugated corrin ring, the cobalt ion and the donor atoms (and occasionally further atoms) of the axial ligands. These atoms show strong electronic interaction, and contain several reactive sites. Reactions may occur at either of the axial co-ordination positions of the cobalt (ligand substitution, oxidation, reduction, etc.) and at C_8 or C_{10} in the corrin ring (see Chapter 15).

2. An outer layer comprising the nitrogen and oxygen atoms of the amide and nucleotide side-chains, which form inter- and intra-molecular hydrogen-bonds. These side-chains do not appear to undergo any reactions of interest, but play a very important role in, for example, determining the solubility properties of the corrinoids and in the binding of other molecules such as proteins.

3. An intermediate layer, comprising the carbon atoms of the outer ring of the corrin ligand and of the side-chains. With the exception of C_8 (included in the core) these atoms do not undergo reactions under mild conditions, but may exert a subtle influence on the structure and reactivity of the core through steric hindrance and the provision of a hydrophobic region.

The material has been arranged as follows. The structure of the corrin ring and the cobalt co-ordination sphere is described in Section I (mainly X-ray data). The formation of intermolecular hydrogen-bonds and their effects on the chemical and physical properties of the corrinoids are discussed in Section II; direct evidence is provided by X-ray crystallography and indirect evidence comes from properties such as solubility in protic solvents and the formation of adducts with proteins. Examples of weak intramolecular attraction (hydrogen-bonds, van der Waals forces) and repulsion (steric hindrance) are mentioned in Section I where these are relevant to the structure and properties of the corrin ring or the axial ligands. This chapter does not include other structural details such as the bond-lengths and bond-angles in the side-chains or in the 5-deoxyadenosyl ligand or the position and direction of the hydrogen-bonds, for which reference should be made to the original papers. The evidence (mainly spectroscopic) for the existence of strong electronic interaction between the axial ligands and the corrin ring, i.e. ground-state *cis*- and *trans*-effects, is discussed in Section III.

One gets the impression that the corrinoids are remarkably flexible (not only the side-chains, but also the corrin chain) and that effects may readily be transmitted from one part of the molecule to another (either by electronic interaction between the axial ligands, the cobalt ion and the conjugated corrin chain, by steric repulsion or by attraction through the formation of hydrogen-bonds). What relevance, if any, this may have for the biochemical function of the corrinoids remains to be seen.

I. STRUCTURE OF THE CORRIN RING AND THE COBALT CO-ORDINATION SPHERE

The cobalt corrinoids differ from most types of complex studied by co-ordination chemists in the large amount of distortion, steric repulsion and flexibility observed within the complex. No X-ray analysis has yet been carried out on a metal-free corrinoid. But one would expect that the planarity of the conjugated chain would be disrupted by the single bond between rings A and D, the saturated carbon atoms on the outer ring and the large number of substituents. Further distortion of the bond-lengths and bond-angles will occur in the cobalt corrinoids as a result of the compromise between the differing requirements of the cobalt ion (e.g. the octahedral co-ordination of the cobalt(III) ion) and of the metal-free corrin ligand. The distortion is further compounded by steric repulsion or by the formation of intramolecular hydrogen-bonds between different parts of the molecule. Comparison of the structures of different corrinoids emphasizes the remarkable flexibility of the corrinoids, not only in the conformation of the side-chains but also in the conformation of the corrin ring and of the cobalt co-ordination sphere. The relevant information is presented in the above order, viz. the corrin ring, the cobalt co-ordination sphere, steric repulsion and steric hindrance, intramolecular hydrogen-bonds.

The numbering of the atoms in the corrin chain is shown in Fig. 6.1. Early doubts as to whether the chain contained five or six double bonds (see the discussion in Hodgkin (1965)) have finally been settled by a neutron diffraction study of a derivative of B$_{12}$ in which the hydrogen atoms have been located and the existence of a conjugated chain of six double bonds extending from N21 round to N24 has been established (Moore et al., 1967). Since the chain contains an odd number of atoms (thirteen), it is analogous to a cyanine dye and not to a polyene (see Chapter 5, Section II). There are two points of interest in the structure of the conjugated chain:

1. the degree of buckling or deviation from planarity and
2. the alternation of bond-lengths.

Comparison of the structures which have been determined by X-ray analysis shows a surprising variation in the degree and kind of deviation from non-planarity of the corrin ring. Hodgkin (1964) and Lenhert (1968) have pointed out that these corrinoids can be classified into three groups on the basis of the type of deviation from planarity of the corrin ring and the degree of pucker in the five-membered pyrroline rings as follows:

(A) [1,8,8,13,13-pentamethyl-5-cyano-corrin]-nickel(II) chloride;
(B) the hexacarboxylic acid and cobyric acid;
(C) wet and dry cyanocobalamin and 5-deoxyadenosylcobalamin, i.e. all the three cobalamin structures yet determined.

Examples of each type of buckling of the corrin ring are shown in Fig. 6.2. Non-planarity is, of course, the natural consequence of the presence of

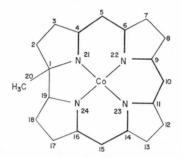

Fig. 6.1. Diagram to show the numbering of the carbon and nitrogen atoms and the extent of the conjugated chain (thick line) in the cobalt corrinoids. Axial ligands and substituents have been omitted, except for CH_3 20.

saturated carbon atoms at C_1 and C_{19} and the differing requirements of the metal ion and the metal-free corrin ligand. Lenhert also emphasizes the importance of minimizing the repulsion between the substituents on the outer ring and suggests that the main reason for the difference between the conformation of the corrin ring in groups A and B lies in the difference in the size and position of these substituents, while the greater distortion around C_5 and C_6 in group C is due mainly to contact with the benziminazole present in the cobalamins (Lenhert, 1968).

The unusually large values found for the C1–C19–C18 bond-angle of a formally tetrahedral carbon atom in different corrinoids, viz. 120° (Hodgkin et al., 1962), 121° (Lenhert, 1968), 122.5° (Hodgkin et al., 1959), 127° (Brink-Shoemaker et al., 1964) and even 129° (Dunitz and Myer, 1965), are probably also caused by the need to reduce repulsion between C18 and C20. The absence of free rotation of the methyl groups about the C–C bond, revealed by neutron diffraction of a derivative of B_{12} (Moore et al., 1967) is probably another indication of extensive overcrowding in the corrinoid molecule.

Table 6.1 lists the experimentally observed bond-lengths in the conjugated corrin ring in cobalt(III) corrinoids and in a square planar nickel(II) corrinoid together with the theoretically calculated bond-lengths for a conjugated system of six double bonds covering thirteen atoms. The calculated bond-lengths show how in a conjugated chain containing an odd number of atoms the difference between double and single bonds is observed at either end of the chain

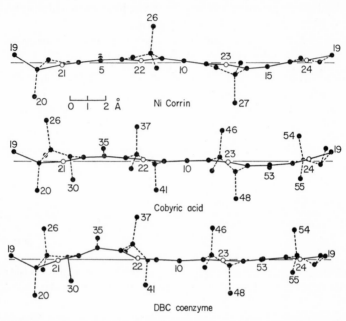

Fig. 6.2. The three types of buckling observed in the corrin ring, shown by cylindrical projections of a nickel(II) corrinoid, cobyric acid and DBC. The molecules are shown as they would be seen when viewed from the metal atom outwards, the atoms being projected onto a cylinder of radius 2.8 Å. The vertical displacement of each atom corresponds to the distance from the least-squares plane of the four nitrogen atoms which are shown as open circles. From Lenhert (1968).

but is eliminated near the centre. In spite of the high error and the deviations from planarity due to buckling, some of the corrinoid complexes do show the expected pattern of bond-lengths, in particular the nickel(II) corrinoid and cobyric acid.

Certain equilibria, which may involve changes in the conformation of the corrin ring, have been shown to occur in several cobalt(III) corrinoids. Studies on the variation of circular dichroism (CD) with temperature revealed that the CD spectra of methyl-, cyano- and dicyano-cobalamin in a methanol-ethanol glass apparently underwent an inversion on cooling from room temperature to −180°, even though the absorption spectra showed no change except for an

Table 6.1. *Bond-lengths (in Å) in the conjugated corrin chain*

	Theory Hodgkin (1965)	Nickel(II) corrinoid Hodgkin (1967)	Hexacarbo-xylic acid Hodgkin et al. (1959)	Cobyric acid Hodgkin (1965)	Wet B$_{12}$ Brink-Shoemaker et al., (1964)	Dry B$_{12}$ Hodgkin et al., (1962)	DBC Lenhert (1968)
N21–C4	1.29	1.28	1.28	1.34	1.39	1.26	1.32
C4–C5	1.44	1.45	1.48	1.47	1.33	1.49	1.39
C5–C6	1.36	1.35	1.30	1.37	1.50	1.42	1.49
C6–N22	1.37	1.40	1.45	1.36	1.30	1.36	1.39
N22–C9	1.32	1.39	1.23	1.38	1.37	1.37	1.41
C9–C10	1.39	1.37	1.39	1.39	1.60	1.41	1.41
C10–C11	1.39	1.39	1.34	1.43	1.28	1.39	1.41
C11–N23	1.32	1.40	1.50	1.33	1.32	1.35	1.31
N23–C14	1.37	1.39	1.41	1.42	1.52	1.44	1.37
C14–C15	1.36	1.33	1.32	1.39	1.37	1.35	1.31
C15–C16	1.44	1.44	1.48	1.44	1.48	1.43	1.49
C16–N24	1.29	1.28	1.33	1.29	1.32	1.41	1.21
E.s.d.			0.07 (C–C) 0.09 (C–N)		Prob. 0.06	0.07	0.06

increase in the sharpness of the bands; the changes in CD correspond to an equilibrium between forms differing in enthalpy (ΔH) by about 2–3 kcal/mole (Firth *et al.*, 1967a). Temperature-jump studies have also shown the existence of a relaxation with an "immeasurably fast time constant" ($\tau^{-1} \leqslant 3 \times 10^{-6}$ sec^{-1} or $k \geqslant 2 \times 10^5$ sec^{-1}) in thiocyanatocobalamin and certain other unspecified cobalamins (Thusius, 1968).

A very different and far slower type of equilibration has been reported to occur in strongly acid media (70% $HClO_4$ at room temperature) between a variety of corrinoids and so-called "iso-corrinoids" (Bernhauer *et al.*, 1968; Friedrich and Moskophidis, 1968). It has been suggested that the methyl group on C_1 and the hydrogen atom on C_{19} have a *cis*-conformation in the iso-corrinoids in contrast to the *trans*-conformation in the natural corrinoids (Bernhauer *et al.*, 1968), but there is no direct evidence for this yet.

The bond-angles and bond-lengths involving cobalt are given in Table 6.2. Lenhert points out that the Co–N bond-lengths are similar to those found for cobalt(III)-ammonia complexes (1.96–1.99 Å) (Lenhert, 1968). The bond-angles in the plane are determined by the structure of the corrin ring; the absence of the bridging carbon atom between rings A and D causes the angle N24–Co–N21 to be less than 90°, while the opposite angle is correspondingly increased. The four corrin nitrogen atoms also show a slight tetrahedral distortion in all compounds studied; N22 and N24 tend to be slightly above, N21 and N23 slightly below the least-squares plane of the four nitrogen atoms (see also Fig. 6.2). It appears that the planar and axial cobalt-ligand bond-lengths are all longer in dry B_{12} than in wet B_{12}; this may, however, be spurious since the bond-lengths in the next sphere (i.e. the C–N in cyanide, the two N–C bonds in Bzm, the N–C bonds in corrin) are almost all longer in wet B_{12}. Lenhert does, however, consider that the cobalt-nitrogen bond-lengths (both to corrin and to Bzm) are significantly longer in DBC than in either form of B_{12} or in the hexacarboxylic acid (Lenhert, 1968). This is an example of the strong *cis*- and *trans*-effect of the organo-ligand, which is related to its strong σ-donor power. For further evidence on the *cis*- and *trans*-effects of the axial ligands, see, in particular, Chapter 6, Section III, Chapter 8, Section V and Chapter 18.

The cobalt-nitrogen bond-lengths are presumably longer in the reduced corrinoids, in particular the four-co-ordinate cobalt(I) corrinoids. It would be interesting to know what effect this has on the buckling of the corrin ring and on the stereochemistry of the cobalt ion. It is conceivable that the cobalt(I) ion would be too large to be accommodated in the plane of the corrin nitrogen atoms and might be displaced above or below the plane. E.s.r. studies indicate that cobalamin-cobalt(II) has a higher symmetry ($g_{\perp} = 2.33$, $g_{11} = g_3 = 2.004$, therefore axial symmetry) than cobinamide-cobalt(II) ($g_1 = 2.60$, $g_2 = 2.2$, $g_3 = 2.006$); see Cockle *et al.* (1969) and Section III.

Table 6.2. *Bond-lengths and bond-angles in the cobalt co-ordination sphere*

		Hexacarbo-xylic acid Hodgkin et al., (1959)	Dry B$_{12}$ Hodgkin et al., (1962)	Wet B$_{12}$ Brink-Shoemaker et al., (1964)	DBC Lenhert (1968)
		Bond-lengths (Å)			
In plane	Co–N21	1.90	1.86	1.80	1.92
	Co–N22	1.96	1.90	1.92	1.91
	Co–N23	1.78	1.91	1.86	1.97
	Co–N24	1.87	1.95	1.87	1.98
	Average	1.88	1.91	1.86	1.95
To upper ligand	Co–Cl	2.41	—	—	—
	Co–CN	—	2.02	1.92	—
	Co–CH$_2$R	—	—	—	2.05
To lower ligand	Co–CN	1.96	—	—	—
	Co–N (Bzm)	—	2.07	1.97	2.23
E.s.d.		0.04	≤0.07	0.06	0.03
		Bond-angles			
In plane	N21–Co–N22	92.5	91.5	89	91
	N22–Co–N23	95	94.1	96	98
	N23–Co–N24	89.5	94	92	90
	N24–Co–N21	83	80.5	84	81
Upper ligand	X–Co–N21	88	89	87	
	X–Co–N22	88	87	87	
	X–Co–N23	91	90	91	89
	X–Co–N24	90	87	89	93
Lower ligand	Y–Co–N21	91	94	96	92
	Y–Co–N22	90	90	88	88
	Y–Co–N23	90	88	87	
	Y–Co–N24	91	97	97	

The large values of the Bzm–Co–N21 and Bzm–Co–N24 bond-angles (see Table 6.2) show that the plane of the Bzm is tilted away from rings A and D; this is shown very clearly in Fig. 6.4. (see below). Both this tilting, which is due to contact with CH_3 20, and a further tilting due to contact with the corrin ring are discussed in more detail below.

Several other bond-angles involving the axial ligands are of interest. The Co–CN group is, as expected, linear in all the corrinoids so far studied (Hodgkin *et al.*, 1959, 1962; Hodgkin, 1965; Brink-Shoemaker *et al.*, 1964; Moore *et al.*, 1967; Nockolds *et al.*, 1967). The Co–CH_2–R bond-angle in DBC has the surprisingly high value of 125° (Lenhert, 1968), which is far greater than the value normally observed for a tetrahedral carbon atom or even a trigonal carbon atom (120°). Similar wide bond-angles have, however, also been found in the two other organo-cobalt(III) complexes which have been examined by X-ray analysis, viz. $[(NC)_5Co–CF_2CF_2H]^{3-}$, where the Co–$C_\alpha$–$C_\beta$ bond-angle is 120° (Mason and Russell, 1965), and a bis-DMG complex possessing the axial ligands pyridine and $CH_3OOC–CH_2$–Co, where the Co–C_α–C_β bond-angle is 115° (Lenhert, personal communication) (see also (Lenhert, 1967)). Obviously the need to maximize the overlap with the relevant hydridized orbital of the cobalt and to minimize various repulsions (in particular between the electron pairs in the C–C and C–H bonds on the one hand and the non-bonded electron pairs of cobalt and nitrogen on the other) brings about a very considerable rehybridization of the normal sp^3-hybridized orbitals of the saturated carbon atom when it forms a σ-bond to the cobalt. Such unusual stereochemistry and hydridization might be expected to lead to unusual chemical properties. This carbon atom (C'_5) is, in fact, known to be involved in enzymatic reactions (see Chapter 17). By contrast, the Co–Se–CN bond-angle in selenocyanatocobalamin is approximately 90° and the $SeCN^-$ ligand is linear (Brink *et al.*, 1954).

The relative orientations of the different parts of the molecule and the contacts between them can best be visualized by reference to Figs 6.3–5. The first two figures show the molecules of cobyric acid (one of the very simplest corrinoids) and DBC (the most complex yet studied) as viewed roughly along the C_5–C_{15} axis, i.e. "from the side". The third shows DBC viewed from the top. These figures demonstrate how the plane of the cobalt and the corrin ring is surrounded by amide side-chains and methyl substituents which project above and below the plane approximately at the four corners of a square. Bulky ligands such as Bzm and 5'-deoxyadenosyl must, therefore, align themselves between the pyrroline rings (as seen in Fig. 6.5). The methyl group on C_1 is, however, situated close enough to the central axis to cause distortion of the bond-angles of ligands in the lower co-ordination position (see below).

Three main sites of steric repulsion can be identified. Firstly, there is bound to be repulsion between the bonding and non-bonding electron pairs on the co-ordinated nitrogen atoms of the corrin ring and those on the co-ordinated atoms (and even β atoms) of the axial ligands and also between these and the electrons of the cobalt ion. The interest lies in the effect of this steric hindrance on the ground-state, thermodynamic and kinetic properties of the ligand. It

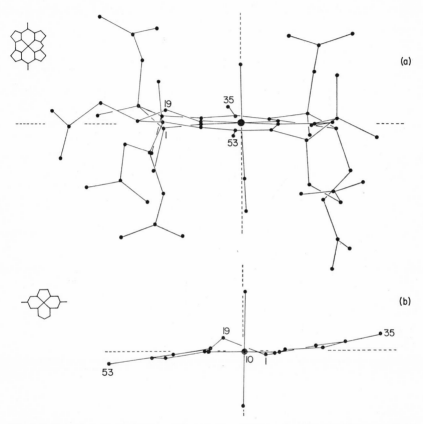

Fig. 6.3. Cobyric acid. Projection of the atomic positions along lines in the plane (least-squares plane passing through cobalt and the four inner nitrogen atoms) parallel (a) and perpendicular (b) to the projection of C1–C19. Part of the structure only is shown in (b). From Hodgkin (1965).

has already been mentioned that the large value found for the Co–CH$_2$–R bond-angle in DBC (125°) can be ascribed in part to repulsion between the β carbon atom (or the bonding electron pair on the co-ordinated atom) and one of the corrin nitrogen atoms. Why then is the Co–Se–CN bond-angle ~90° (Brink *et al.*, 1954); is it simply that the longer Co–Se bond reduces the repulsion or is there some additional attraction between the CN group and the

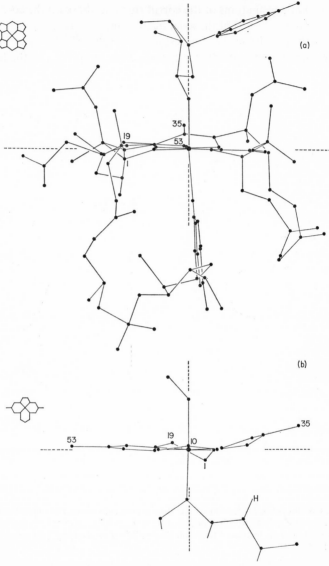

Fig. 6.4. 5-deoxyadenosylcobalamin (DBC). Projection of the atomic positions along lines in the plane (least-squares plane passing through cobalt and the four inner nitrogen atoms) parallel (a) and perpendicular (b) to the projection of C1–C19. Part of the structure only is shown in (b). From Hodgkin (1965).

π-electrons of the corrin ring? The proton magnetic resonance spectrum of iso-propylcobinamide shows that the two methyl groups of the ligand (doublets at 10.70 and 10.94 τ, each corresponding to three protons) are non-equivalent, which suggests the absence of free rotation of the ligand around the Co–C bond (Hill *et al.*, Unpublished results). Absorption spectra also provide evidence for steric hindrance: compare the wavelengths (in nm in parentheses) for the γ-band of the cobalamins with the following ligands: H_2O (350); pyridine (360), α-picoline (356), β-picolinne (361), γ-picoline (361); imidazole

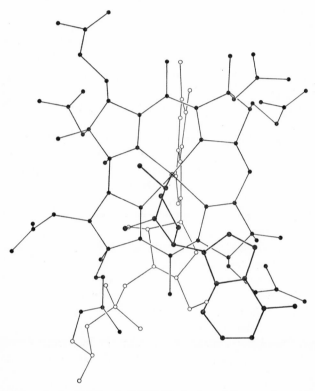

Fig. 6.5. 5-deoxyadenosylcobalamin (DBC). Projection of the atomic positions onto the least-squares plane passing through cobalt and the four inner nitrogen atoms. From Hodgkin (1965).

(358), histidine (357), benziminazole (354) (Hill *et al.*, 1962). It is clear that the shift in wavelength on replacing H_2O by a nitrogenous base is much less for just those two ligands where considerable steric hindrance is expected, viz. α-picoline and benziminazole. No formation constants have yet been reported for any series of ligands where one might be able to see the effects of steric hindrance in reducing the formation constant. But the increased kinetic lability towards mercury(II) ions of the isopropyl ligand over ethyl and n-propyl has been ascribed to electronic changes combined with a weakening of the Co–C bond by steric repulsion between the β atoms in the ligand and between them and the corrin ring (Hill *et al.*, 1970a) (see also Chapter 13, Section II). As can be seen from Fig. 6.2, the nitrogen atoms N22 and N24 tend to project above the plane, while N21 and N23 tend to project below the plane. This will still further increase the barrier to free rotation about the cobalt-ligand bond and lead to a preferred orientation of ligands such as pyridine or selenocyanate.

The second common site of steric repulsion is the methyl group C20, which projects down from C1 (see Fig. 6.1) and is close enough to the cobalt-ligand axis to interact with ligands in the lower axial position. Even the cyanide is pushed away from the normal by contact with CH_3 20 in cobyric acid (Fig. 6.3) and apparently in the hexacarboxylic acid (Hodgkin, 1964), though the deviation is hardly detectable from the bond-angles listed in Table 6.2. In all the cobalamins the plane of the Bzm is quite noticeably tilted away from the normal by contact with CH_3 20; see the bond-angles listed in Table 6.2, which show that Bzm is pushed away from N21 and N24. Lenhert calculates that this departure from octahedral symmetry in DBC increases the distance between C20 and the co-ordinated nitrogen atoms of Bzm from 2.98 Å to the observed value of 3.19 Å (Lenhert, 1968). This contact between Bzm and CH_3 20 can also be detected by proton magnetic resonance, since the shielding effect of Bzm causes a large shift in the position of the methyl resonance (Hill *et al.*, 1968a). Hodgkin has pointed out (Hodgkin, 1964) that the presence of the CH_3 20 may hinder access to the lower co-ordination site and reduce the stability of ligands in this position. The relative stability of the u- and l-isomers is discussed in Chapter 8, Section II. There is virtually no difference in the relative stability of the two isomers containing CN^- and H_2O; but the relative stability of the u-isomer (i.e. the isomer with the organo-ligand in the upper co-ordination position) appears to increase in the order $CN^- < CH_3^- < CH_3CH_2^-$, i.e. with increasing size of ligand, in agreement with Hodgkin's suggestion.

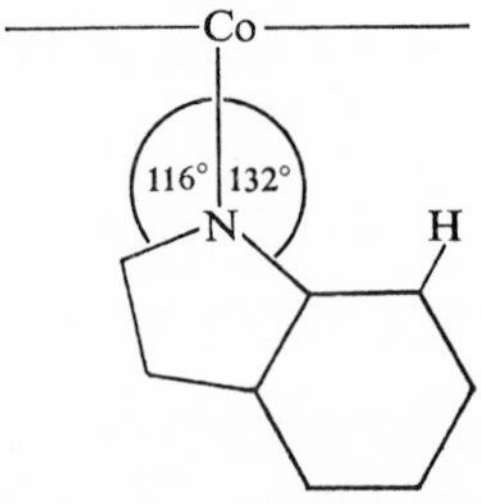

The co-ordinated Bzm is distorted yet further by contact between the hydrogen atom indicated in the figure above and the corrin ring between C5 and C6. This third site of repulsion, which is common to all corrinoids containing Bzm leads both to increased buckling of the corrin ring in the region of C5–C6 (see Fig. 6.2) and to an asymmetrical co-ordination of Bzm. In dry B_{12}, for example, one observes the bond-angles given in the figure above. Since the corrin ring is very unevenly buckled the degree of steric hindrance between the ring and a large co-ordinated base such as Bzm will depend critically on the exact point of contact; one would expect, therefore, to see differences (in, for example, formation constants) between the upper and lower axial positions and between free bases and bases bound in the nucleotide side-chain (and hence restricted in their possible conformations). No data have yet been obtained in which one might observe such effects. It would be interesting to find the limits of steric hindrance which can be tolerated in the lower axial position; can a quinoline derivative, for instance, remain co-ordinated?

A few additional points can be made about the organo-ligand present in DBC. The oxygen atom of the five-membered ribose ring appears to be in contact with the corrin ring between C14 and C15, but this has no obvious effect on the buckling of the latter (Lenhert, 1968). Free rotation of the bulky ligand about the Co–C bond would be hindered by interaction between this oxygen atom and the upward-projecting methylene groups of the acetamide side-chains on rings A and B and the methyl substituents on rings C and D (Lenhert, 1968) (see Fig. 6.4). Hodgkin has also emphasized that the hydrophobic character of these four saturated carbon atoms may influence reactions at the upper co-ordination site (Hodgkin, 1964).

Distortion may also be caused by the formation of intramolecular hydrogen-bonds. The H_2O co-ordinated in the upper axial position of cobyric acid is hydrogen-bonded to the acetamide side-chain on ring B (see Fig. 6.6). This displaces the co-ordinated oxygen atom and affects the pucker in the corrin ring (Hodgkin, 1965). This acetamide side-chain provides a very good example of variable conformation. It also forms an intramolecular hydrogen-bond to the co-ordinated cyanide in dry B_{12}, but in this case the C7–C37 bond is rotated in the opposite sense from that observed in cobyric acid; in wet B_{12} and in DBC, on the other hand, the acetamide turns outwards to form intermolecular hydrogen-bonds (Hodgkin, 1964). For further information on intra- as well as inter-molecular hydrogen-bonding and on the conformations adopted by the side-chains see the papers giving the results of X-ray analysis (Hodgkin et al., 1959, 1962; Brink-Shoemaker et al., 1964; Lenhert, 1968), and the discussions in Hodgkin (1964, 1965, 1967).

Intramolecular hydrogen-bonding may affect the thermodynamic and kinetic properties of the corrinoids, in particular the ionization constants of acids and bases in the side-chains and the formation constants for the binding of axial ligands. Neutron diffraction has shown, for example, that in the derivative of B_{12} in which side-chain c has been hydrolysed to the carboxylic acid, it is the phosphate group which carries a proton while the carboxylate is dissociated (Moore *et al.*, 1967). This apparent reversal of ionization constants can probably be ascribed to stabilization of the phosphoric acid and carboxylate anion forms by favourable hydrogen-bonds. The presence of this neighbouring carboxylate group catalyses the hydrolysis of the nucleotide side-chain (Bernhauer *et al.*, 1966). The ionization constant of carboxylic acid side-chains and the relative stability of stereo-isomers involving different axial ligands (CN^- and H_2O) are also affected by hydrogen-bonding between the side-chain and the co-ordinated H_2O (see Chapter 8, Section II). Other possible effects of hydrogen-bonding on the formation constants for the binding of axial ligands are discussed in Chapter 8, Section V,G.

Very little information concerning the corrin ring or the cobalt co-ordination sphere has been obtained by the use of infrared spectroscopy. The infrared spectra of cobalamins (see, for example, the spectra of cyano-, hydroxo-, methyl- and 5-deoxyadenosyl-cobalamin in Hogenkamp *et al.* (1965)) show a very large number of bands in the region up to 1800 and from 2800 to 3600 cm^{-1}, in which it is virtually impossible to assign frequencies with any certainty. It has been suggested that a weak band at 348 cm^{-1} in methylcobalamin can be assigned to the Co–C stretching vibration (Hogenkamp *et al.*, 1965), but this cannot be regarded as proven. However, a few ligands such as CN^-, which absorb in the "window" between 1800 and 2800 cm^{-1}, are easily seen. The presence of cyanide in B_{12} was in fact detected by infra-red spectroscopy, and the dependence of this stretching frequency on the nature of the axial ligand in the *trans*-position has been studied (see Section III). Some evidence for the vibrational frequencies of the conjugated corrin chain in the electronic ground-state and excited states can be obtained from the vibrational overtones of the electronic transitions (see Chapter 5, Section II).

II. INTERMOLECULAR HYDROGEN-BONDS

The various structures of corrinoids which have been determined by X-ray analysis provide an instructive picture of the role of hydrogen-bonding in such complex molecules. The hydrogen-bonded network of cobyric acid is shown in Fig. 6.6. See also the structures of the hexacarboxylic acid (Hodgkin *et al.*, 1959), the dry and wet forms of B_{12} (Hodgkin *et al.*, 1962; Brink-Shoemaker *et al.*, 1964), and DBC (Lenhert, 1968); the first crystallizes with two molecules of water and one of acetone, the last three with approximately 17, 18 and 22 molecules of water per cobalt respectively. In these structures hydrogen-bonds may be formed inter- and intra-molecularly, directly between two corrinoid molecules or via a bridging water molecule and between water molecules. As Hodgkin and her co-workers (1959) point out when discussing the structure of the hexacarboxylic acid, "so many stereochemical conditions have to be met that it is almost surprising to find that all but one of the groups capable of forming hydrogen-bonds are in fact in positions to do so"; the odd man out appears to be the carboxyl oxygen of one of the acetamide side-chains.

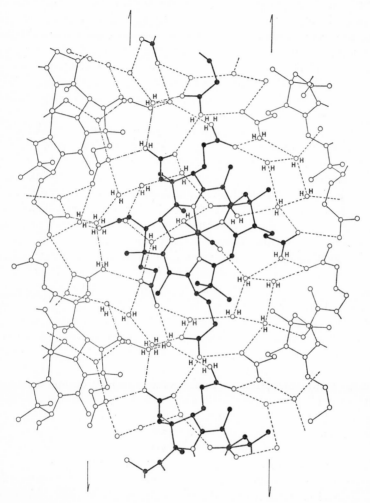

Fig. 6.6. The crystal structure of cobyric acid projected along the crystallographic a-axis. From Hodgkin (1965).

The ease with which the hydrogen-bonded network of the solid corrinoids can be rearranged allows considerable freedom of movement to small molecules. The number of molecules of water of crystallization, for example, varies with the water vapour pressure. As mentioned above, cyanocobalamin contains approximately 18 or 22 molecules of water per cobalt when in contact with dry air or with the mother liquor respectively; it can apparently be dried completely by heating under reduced pressure (Smith, 1965). Even reactions involving the making and breaking of co-ordinate bonds may occur in the solid state and can be studied by examining the reflection spectra of the solids. For example, the drying of aquocobalamin, vinylaquocobinamide and DBC in the solid state leads to the formation of hydroxocobalamin, the five-co-ordinate vinylcobinamide and the five-co-ordinate 5-deoxyadenosylcobalamin respectively (Firth *et al.*, 1968a), while grinding together organocobalamins and KCN in the solid state produces the organocyano complexes (Firth *et al.*, 1968d). The movement of ions is obviously facilitated by the large amount of water of crystallization.

The formation of intermolecular hydrogen-bonds appears to have several other important consequences. It determines the solubility properties of the corrinoids and the formation of adducts with other hydrogen-bonding molecules, including proteins; and hence also the use of extraction into phenolic solvents and precipitation as phenol adducts as methods of purification. It cannot, of course, be proved unambiguously that these chemical and physical properties are due primarily to the formation of hydrogen-bonds; but, as will be shown below, the evidence is fairly conclusive.

Cyanocobalamin and most other corrinoids with amide, carboxylic acid and nucleotide side-chains are soluble in water, the lower alcohols, fatty acids (such as glacial acetic acid), amides (such as acetamide and dimethylformamide), phenols and dimethylsulphoxide; they are insoluble in hydrocarbons, ether, dry acetone, dry pyridine and other non-polar solvents (Bonnett, 1963; Smith, 1965). They also dissolve in strong acids such as concentrated sulphuric acid and liquid HF (see Chapter 9, Section III). The solubility of B_{12} in water at room temperature is reported to be about 1.2% or 8×10^{-3} M (Havemeyer and Higuchi, 1960; Smith, 1965). Higher solubilities may be found with other corrinoids and in other solvents; for example, several cobalamins dissolve to the extent of $2.5-5 \times 10^{-2}$ M in trifluoroacetic acid (Hill *et al.*, 1965a). Partition coefficients have been reported for certain corrinoids between water and, for example, benzyl alcohol (Smith *et al.*, 1952a) and solutions of various phenols (Friedrich and Bernhauer, 1954). Corrinoids are, in fact, usually purified by shaking the aqueous solution with a solution of phenol in chloroform, whereby the corrinoid is extracted into the organic phase, leaving the inorganic impurities behind in the aqueous phase. If a donor solvent, such as ether, is then added to the organic phase, the corrinoid can be displaced back into the aqueous phase by shaking with (pure) water (Friedrich and Bernhauer, 1954). Friedrich and Bernhauer also studied the partition of several corrinoids between water and either solutions of phenols in trichloroethylene or fused phenols. They suggested that the ability of phenols to extract corrinoids was due to the formation of hydrogen-bonds (Friedrich and Bernhauer, 1954).

There can, in fact, be little doubt about the role of hydrogen-bond formation in determining the solubilities and partition coefficients of corrinoids.

There is also plenty of evidence for the role of hydrogen-bonds in the formation of adducts between corrinoids and molecules ranging from carboxylic acids to proteins. Particular interest attaches to the mode of binding of corrinoids to polypeptides and proteins, since the latter play such an important role in the absorption, transport, storage and enzymatic activity of the corrinoids. Greenberg *et al.* (1957) were among the first to point out, even if only indirectly, the importance of hydrogen-bonds. They found that the absorption of B_{12} from the gut was enhanced by the addition of carbohydrates such as D-mannitol, L-sorbose and D-xylose (but not sucrose or several other sugars). Since Intrinsic Factor, the protein required to mediate the absorption of B_{12} from the gut, was known to contain a high proportion of carbohydrates they suggested that "the carbohydrate portion of intrinsic factor may play the major part in effecting B_{12} absorption", presumably by binding through the formation of hydrogen-bonds. In his review in 1963, Bonnett concluded that "it is likely that hydrogen-bonding between the protein molecule and the peripheral amide and alcohol groups is important as a secondary binding process"; secondary, that is, to binding through co-ordination by the cobalt of some functional group of the protein (Bonnett, 1963). With our more recent knowledge of the factors which determine the magnitude of the formation constants for the binding of axial ligands it has been possible to show (Hill *et al.*, 1970b) that the formation constants at pH 7 for the displacement of H_2O in aquocobalamin or of Bzm in B_{12} and DBC by any amino-acid functional group will be less than 1 (litre/mol). The formation of a co-ordinate bond clearly cannot be the primary cause of the firm binding between corrinoid and proteins or polypeptides. Furthermore, the corrinoid structure scarcely provides any opportunity for the formation of any covalent bond with a protein. One can therefore conclude that the binding of corrinoids to proteins and polypeptides is due primarily to the formation of hydrogen-bonds between the two partners. There are several cases where spectroscopic and other studies have provided some evidence about the nature of the axial ligand in the adduct; see, for example, the complex of aquocobalamin with a polypeptide where the presence of the γ-band at 350 nm suggests that no co-ordination has occurred (Hedbom, 1960, 1961), complexes of B_{12} with a polypeptide (Heathcote and Mooney, 1958) and with proteins (Wijmenga *et al.*, 1954; Gregory and Holdsworth, 1955) and complexes of B_{12}, DBC and other cobalamins with the protein ethanolamine deaminase (Babior *et al.*, 1969; Babior and Li, 1969).

Yurkevich and co-workers have reported the isolation of crystalline adducts of B_{12} and B_{12a} with phenol, resorcinol and pyrogallol; the only adduct, whose composition has been reported, contained three molecules of resorcinol per molecule of B_{12} (Yurkevich *et al.*, 1966, 1969). The presence of the phenolic component in the B_{12} adducts did not affect the cyanide stretching frequency in the solid state (Yurkevich et al., 1966) or the wavelength of the γ-band in the absorption spectrum of the solution, though it did cause slight changes in the relative optical densities of the different absorption bands (Yurkevich et al., 1965, 1966). They concluded that Bzm had been displaced from co-ordination by the phenol (Yurkevich et al., 1966). But this conclusion seems untenable in the light of the very low formation constant for the co-ordination of the phenoxide ion (see Table 8.7) and clearly cannot explain the presence of three resorcinol molecules in the adduct. Again the only reasonable conclusion seems to be the formation of an adduct through hydrogen-bonding (Hill et al., 1970b). Greater changes in the absorption spectrum are found for B_{12a} in the presence of phenols (Yurkevich et al., 1966), but these are difficult to reconcile with more recent work and may be due to the presence of the products of some irreversible reaction (Hill et al., In press). Yurkevich and co-workers found that the absorption spectrum of B_{12} was also altered slightly by the presence of imidazole or the amino-acids histidine, lysine and tyrosine and concluded that the cyanide had been displaced (Yurkevich et al., 1965); here again it seems most likely, in the light of more recent evidence on the magnitude of formation constants, that the amino-acids interact with some part of the corrinoid molecule through the formation of hydrogen-bonds (Hill et al., 1970b). Havemeyer and Higuchi (1960) also mention the formation of complexes between B_{12} and sugars, sugar alcohols, phenolic compounds, carboxylic acids, amines, amides and diols, but give no experimental details.

Some thermodynamic data has been obtained for the interaction of B_{12} with solids such as ion-exchange resins and talc. Samsonov et al. (1965), for example, studied the adsorption of B_{12} by certain sulphonated resins; they showed that the magnitude of the equilibrium constants for adsorption was determined mainly by a large increase in entropy and concluded that this was due to the formation of a large number of weak bonds (i.e. hydrogen-bonds) between the corrinoid and the stationary phase. On the other hand, the adsorption of B_{12} onto talc, which was stronger than for any other adsorbent examined (starch and cellulose derivatives, magnesium aluminosilicate), is determined mainly by a favourable enthalpy change (Moriguchi and Kaneniwa, 1969).

The presence of a hydrogen-bonded network also allows the incorporation, through the formation of a clathrate structure, of other molecules which do not form strong hydrogen-bonds themselves; for a review of clathrate compounds see Jeffrey and McMullan (1967). X-ray analysis of the hexacarboxylic acid revealed the presence of a molecule of acetone in a hole in the crystal structure near C_{13} on ring C in which it appears to have some freedom of movement (Hodgkin et al., 1959). It has also been suggested (Hill et al., 1970b) that in the solid complexes obtained from the reaction of triphenylphosphine with B_{12} and DBC (Yurkevich *et al.*, 1969) the phosphine may be held in the form of some clathrate structure (see also Chapter 8, Section IV,H).

Finally, one should mention that the addition of iodine increases the partition coefficient for the extraction of B_{12a} from water into benzyl alcohol (Smith *et al.*, 1952a). This could be due to some equilibrium between B_{12a} and I_2 (? charge transfer interaction with Bzm or the corrin ring or clathrate formation involving the side-chains), but the experimental data do not completely exclude the occurrence of some irreversible reaction.

III. ELECTRONIC INTERACTION BETWEEN THE AXIAL LIGANDS, THE COBALT AND THE CORRIN RING

Several lines of evidence (from X-ray diffraction, infrared, u.v.-visible and proton magnetic resonance spectra) indicate that a change in one of the axial ligands can have a marked effect on the physical properties of the other axial ligand and of the equatorial corrin ring, i.e. that there is a strong electronic interaction between the conjugated corrin ring, the cobalt ion and the donor atoms (and in many cases probably additional atoms) of the axial ligands. The effects of one ligand upon the properties of other ligands in the *cis*- and *trans*-positions are termed *cis*- and *trans*-effects respectively. These effects can be divided (Pratt and Thorp, 1969) into

(1) ground-state effects (basically, the effect of changing one ligand on the physical properties of the other ligands),
(2) thermodynamic effects (effects on equilibrium constants for the addition, loss or substitution of another ligand) and
(3) kinetic effects (effects on the rates of addition, loss or substitution).

In this section we deal with ground-state effects, i.e. the effects on physical properties; for reasons given below we shall include the effects on electronic transitions of the corrin ring, even though this is not a property of the ground-state of the molecule only. Thermodynamic effects are discussed in Chapter 8, Section V, kinetic effects in Chapter 12, Section II, and all the information on *cis*- and *trans*-effects is summarized in Chapter 18.

A. X-RAY DATA (COBALT-LIGAND BOND-LENGTHS)

It has already been mentioned that the Co–N bond-lengths are significantly longer in DBC than in B_{12} (see Table 6.2), i.e. that the substitution of CN^- by the organo-ligand 5'-deoxyadenosyl leads to an increase in the cobalt-ligand bond-lengths in both the *cis*- and *trans*-positions.

B. INFRARED SPECTRA (STRETCHING FREQUENCY OF CO-ORDINATED CN⁻)

Firth *et al.* (1968d) have studied the effect of varying one axial ligand on the stretching frequency of CN^- co-ordinated in the second axial position. Their results are shown in Table 6.3. It is clear that as the axial ligand becomes a better donor (i.e. $HO^- < CN^- < CH_3^-$, etc.), so the stretching frequency falls towards the value for free ionic cyanide (2079 cm⁻¹). A very similar effect has been observed in the pentacyanocobalt(III) complexes $[Co^{III}(CN)_5X]$ (Halpern and Maher, 1965). It is unusual for the force constant of a ligand to

Table 6.3. *Effect of the axial ligand X on the stretching frequency of CN⁻ co-ordinated in the* trans-*position in cobalamins and cobinamides*

Ligand X	ν_{CN} (cm⁻¹)
Bzm	2132
HO⁻	2130
NC⁻	2119
HC≡C—	2110
⁻SO₃.CH₂—	~2109
CF₃.CH₂—	~2104
CH₂=CH—	2093
5′-deoxyadenosyl	2091
⁻OOC.CH₂—	2090
HOCH₂.CH₂—	2089
CH₃—	2088
CH₃.CH₂.CH₂—	2083
CH₂.CH₂—	2082
(Ionic CN⁻	2079)

From Firth *et al.* (1968d).

increase on co-ordination, as occurs with cyanide; this peculiarity of cyanide has been discussed by Purcell (1967). These results provide direct evidence for a strong ground-state *trans*-effect of the axial ligand.

C. ABSORPTION SPECTRA (π–π* TRANSITIONS OF THE CORRIN RING)

The u.v.-visible spectra of the corrinoids have been discussed in Chapter 5; only the most important conclusions will be mentioned here. The absorption bands at wavelengths longer than 300 nm are due almost entirely to π–π* transitions within the corrin ring and their energies and intensities are very sensitive to changes in the axial ligands. Furthermore, spectra have been reported for a very wide range of axial ligands. The absorption spectra, therefore, provide a good probe for the *cis*-effect of the axial ligand. Even though the wavelength of an absorption band represents the difference in energy between the ground-state of the molecule and an electronically excited state, we are justified in treating the spectra as a measure of the ground-state *cis*-effect because the changes in spectra form a regular pattern and there is a good correlation between the effect of changing the axial ligand both on the stretching frequency of cyanide co-ordinated in the *trans*-position, mentioned in the previous section, and on the energies of the absorption bands (see Table 5.2 and Fig. 5.2).

It was shown in Chapter 5, Section I that the most important property of the axial ligand is its σ-donor strength, and that as the donor strength of the ligand increases so the $\alpha\beta$ and γ-bands move to longer wavelength; this agrees with theoretical calculations, which show that both bands should move to longer wavelength as the electron density on the co-ordinated nitrogen atoms of the corrin ring is increased by electron donation from the axial ligands. The data of Table 5.1 show that ligands with the more electronegative donor atoms (N, O, Cl, Br and C in CN^-) tend to move the γ-band to shorter wavelength and those with the less electronegative donor atoms (S, Se, I and C in the organo-ligands) to longer wavelengths, while amongst the carbanions we find the order $CN^- < HC{\equiv}C^- < CH_2{=}CH^- < CH_3CH_2^-$.

D. PROTON MAGNETIC RESONANCE SPECTRA (C_{10}-H)

A more limited amount of data is available for the effect of the axial ligands on the p.m.r. of the hydrogen atom on C_{10}, the bridge carbon atom between rings B and C, and this is given in Table 6.4. The results show that for the six-co-ordinate corrinoids the τ-value increases as the axial ligand becomes a better donor, the following orders being observed:

when $Y = H_2O$: $H_2O < CN^- < $ methyl $\leqslant$ vinyl
when $Y = Bzm$: $H_2O < HO^- < $ vinyl $<$ methyl $=$ ethyl
when $Y = CN^-$: $H_2O < CN^- < $ methyl

In the five-co-ordinate cobinamides, on the other hand, it seems as though the reverse order obtains, i.e. vinyl $\geqslant$ methyl $\geqslant$ ethyl $=$ isopropyl, though the experimental error is too large to be certain. The τ-value of the p.m.r. of C_{10}-H shows a positive correlation with the energy of the absorption bands, especially the $\alpha\beta$ bands (Hill *et al.*, 1968a; Firth *et al.*, 1968a). This suggests that both of these physical techniques reflect the same type of change in the corrin ring, i.e. the change in electron density on the co-ordinated nitrogens and hence in the corrin ring, even though the transitions monitored by the two techniques involve energies of totally different magnitudes. Proton magnetic resonance therefore provides another probe for the ground-state *cis*-effect of the axial ligands.

Table 6.4. *Effect of the axial ligands on the proton magnetic resonance of $C_{10}-H$ of the corrin ring*

Compound	Solvent	Axial ligands	τ-value	References
		(1) Six-co-ordinate cobalt(III) corrinoids		
Aquocobalamin	TFA	H_2O-OH_2 (or ? CF_3CO_2)	3.29	Hill *et al.* (1965b)
Cyanoaquocobinamide (see below)		H_2O-CN^-	~3.5	
Vinylcobinamide	D_2O and CD_3OD	H_2O-Vinyl	$3.60-3.70^a$	Firth *et al.* (1968a)
Methylcobinamide	D_2O and CD_3OD	H_2O-Methyl	$3.45-3.65^a$	
Aquocobalamin	D_2O	$Bzm-OH_2$	3.72	Hill *et al.* (1965b)
Hydroxocobalamin	D_2O	$Bzm-OH^-$	3.92	
Vinylcobalamin	D_2O	$Bzm-$Vinyl	4.05	Hill *et al.* (1968a)
Methylcobalamin	D_2O	$Bzm-$Methyl	4.12	
Ethylcobalamin	D_2O	$Bzm-$Ethyl	4.12^a	
Cyanoaquocobinamide	D_2O (0° to +95°)	$NC-OH_2$	$\begin{cases} 3.47-3.49 \\ 3.53-3.55 \end{cases}$	Firth *et al.* (1968a)
	CD_3OD (−50° to +30°)	$NC-OH_2$	$\begin{cases} 3.51-3.46 \\ 3.54 \end{cases}$	
Cyanocobalamin	TFA	$\begin{cases} NC-OH_2 \\ (or \\ NC-CF_3CO_2^-) \end{cases}$	$\begin{cases} 3.45 \\ 3.45 \\ 3.5 \end{cases}$	Hill *et al.* (1965b)
Hexacarboxylic acid	TFA			Bonnett and Redman (1965)
Dicyanocobinamide	TFA			
	D_2O (0° to +95°)	$NC-CN^-$	$4.14-4.20$	Firth *et al.* (1968a)
	CD_3OD (−50° to +30°)	$NC-CN^-$	$4.18-4.20$	
Dicyanocobalamin	d-DMSO	$NC-CN^-$	4.35	
	d-DMSO	$NC-CN^-$	4.3	Hill *et al.* (1965a)
Methylcyanocobalamin	d-DMSO	$NC-$Methyl	4.5	
		(2) Five-co-ordinate cobalt(III) corrinoids		
Vinylcobinamide	D_2O and CD_3OD	Vinyl	$3.10-3.20^a$	Firth *et al.* (1968a)
Methylcobinamide	D_2O and CD_3OD	Methyl	$3.0-3.15^a$	
Ethylcobinamide	D_2O	Ethyl	3.04	
Isopropylcobinamide	D_2O	Isopropyl	3.03	

^{a} Extrapolated values, taking into account the presence of both five- and six-co-ordinate species.

Some τ-values (error $\pm 0.03\tau$) have also been reported (Hill *et al.*, 1965b, 1968a) for the hydrogen atoms and methyl groups of co-ordinated Bzm in cobalamins with the following axial ligands:

H on C_2: H_2O (2.75) < HO$^-$ (2.88) = vinyl (2.88) < methyl (3.03)

H on C_4: H_2O (3.47) < HO$^-$ (3.52) < vinyl (3.58) < methyl (3.71)

H on C_7: H_2O (3.54) > HO$^-$ (3.25) > methyl (2.80) $\geqslant$ vinyl (2.77)

CH$_3$ on C_5 and C_6: H_2O (7.68, 7.73) $\leqslant$ vinyl (7.71) $\leqslant$ HO$^-$ (7.73) < methyl (7.80)

(N.B. Data for ethylcobalamin have been omitted since no allowance was made in the original paper for the presence of a mixture of five- and six-co-ordinate complexes.) The similarity between this ligand order and those obtained above suggests that these changes also reflect the ground-state *trans*-effect of the axial ligand.

The p.m.r. of the co-ordinated methyl ligand is also very dependent on the nature of the trans-ligand. Compare the following τ-values in D_2O and CD_3OD: trans to Bzm 10.14 (Hill *et al.*, 1968a), trans to H_2O 10.4–10.6 (Firth *et al.*, 1968a), five-co-ordinate 10.0–10.1 (Firth *et al.*, 1968a). But no conclusions can be drawn from such limited data.

E. ELECTRON SPIN RESONANCE SPECTROSCOPY

E.s.r. measurements have been made on a variety of cobalt(II) corrinoids, prepared either by the addition of potential ligands to solutions of cobalamin- or cobinamide-cobalt(II) or by the reduction of certain naturally occurring analogues which contain bases other than Bzm in the nucleotide side-chain (Bayston *et al.*, 1969; Cockle *et al.*, 1969; Schrauzer and Lee, 1968). The products show a wide and interesting variation in the cobalt coupling constant (see Table 6.5), but no really significant variation in *g*-values or, where observable, in the nitrogen coupling constants (for experimental values see the references in Table 6.5). These results cannot, however, be considered as strictly quantitative in all cases. The main reason for uncertainty lies in our lack of knowledge of the number of the axial ligands, their formation constants and rates of substitution under the experimental conditions, compounded by discrepancies between the results of different groups. We do not, in particular, know whether the quoted results refer to one species only or represent the mean of two or more species in rapid equilibrium (on the time-scale of e.s.r. transitions). The only direct evidence bearing on the number of axial ligands is that the observation of three and five lines in the superhyperfine structure means the presence of one or two co-ordinated nitrogen atoms respectively in the axial positions. It is very difficult, however, to determine the number of co-ordinated solvent molecules or cyanides, or to decide whether Bzm has been replaced by, for example, imidazole.

The spectrum of cobalamin-cobalt(II) is that of a molecule with axial symmetry ($g_\perp = g_1 \sim g_2 > g_3 = g_{11}$); the cobalt hyperfine structure and the nitrogen superhyperfine structure (three lines, indicating interaction with only one nitrogen) are well resolved for g_{11} but not for $g_\perp$. The spectrum is consistent with a low-spin d^7 complex in which the unpaired electron occupies the d_{z^2} orbital (along the X–Co–Y axis) and interacts with the nitrogen of Bzm (Cockle et al., 1969; Schrauzer and Lee, 1968). The e.s.r. spectra of cobinamide-cobalt(II) and of cobalamin-cobalt(II) at pH 0, where Bzm has been displaced from coordination and protonated, indicate a much lower symmetry ($g_1 \neq g_2 \neq g_3$) and an increase in the cobalt coupling constants (see Table 6.5); there is no superhyperfine structure observable due to interaction with the four nitrogen atoms of the corrin ring and there is, of course, no Bzm in the axial position (Cockle et al., 1969). The e.s.r. spectrum of bispyridine-[cobinamide]-cobalt(II) also gives three g-values; the cobalt hyperfine structure associated with g_3 is well resolved and further split by interaction with the two co-ordinated nitrogen atoms (Cockle et al., 1969). All other cobalt(II) corrinoids so far reported appear to give two g-values, i.e. to show axial symmetry.

E.s.r. studies have also been carried out on a slightly different type of corrinoid. Bayston et al. (1969) have shown that cobalt(II) corrinoids will reversibly pick up O_2 at low temperature to give mononuclear, paramagnetic complexes and that a range of ligands can be co-ordinated in the second axial positions (the O_2 adduct of cobalamin-cobalt(II) has subsequently been observed by other workers (Cockle et al., 1970a; Schrauzer and Lee, 1970)). It appears from their data that the cobalt hyperfine structure can be resolved for $g_\perp$ as well as for g_{11}. Since the cobalt coupling constant is very much reduced on oxygenation (see last column of Table 6.5) and the superhyperfine structure due to interaction with a nitrogeneous base in the other axial position completely disappears, they conclude that the oxygenated product is best represented as a cobalt(III) complex with a superoxide ligand (O_2^-), i.e.

$$Co^{II} + O_2 \;\rightleftharpoons\; Co^{III}O_2^-$$

The cobalt coupling constants found for both the normal and the oxygenated cobalt(II) corrinoids are listed in Table 6.5. If we assume that the reported values correspond to one species only (which is unlikely to be completely true in all cases) and that with the exception of the phosphine complex (see below) all the non-oxygenated cobalt(II) complexes are five-co-ordinate and contain the ligands listed in the first column, then the coupling constants can be seen to show a definite pattern. For the simple cobalt(II) corrinoids the coupling constants fall as the axial ligand is varied in the order: H_2O, MeOH, DMF $\geqslant$ PPh_3 $>$ NCS^- $>$ adenine and derivatives $\geqslant$ isoquinoline, pyridine $\geqslant$ benziminazoles including Bzm $>$ RNC $>$ CN^-. For the oxygenated complexes the following

Table 6.3. Cobalt coupling constants (in gauss) obtained from ESR data on cobalt(II) corrinoids and their oxygenated derivatives

Complex: References: Temp: Probable ligand X^b	Cockle et al. (1969) 100°K	$[X.Co^{II}]$ Schrauzer and Lee (1968) 90°K	Bayston et al. (1969) 77°K	$[X.Co^{III}.O_2^-]$ Bayston et al. (1969) 77°K (see note^g)
H_2O	144 137–151^e	(108)^f		
MeOH			144	16, 19
DMF			140	16, 21
PPh$_3$ (in DMF)^c			130	16, 20.5
NCS$^-$			129	15, 18
Uracil		114		
Adenine		108	117	14, 18
Adenine^a	114			
2-Methyladenine^a	112			
2-Thiomethyladenine^a	112			
Isoquinoline			114	13, 16.5
Pyridine	110	108	113	13, 16
5,6-Dimethylbenzimidazole			113	13, 16.5
5,6-Dimethylbenzimidazole (Bzm)^a	107–111	108	110	13–17
5-Hydroxybenzimidazole^a	108			
5-Methoxybenzimidazole^a	108			
PPh$_3$ (in MeOH)^c			92, 95	
RNC (R = cyclohexyl)		87		
CN$^-$			84	9.5, 11.5

^{a} Base incorporated into the nucleotide side-chain.
^{b} See comments in text.
^{c} Probably one PPh$_3$ co-ordinated in DMF, two in MeOH.
^{d} Units of cm^{-1} used in Cockle et al. (1969).
^{e} Cobalamin-cobalt(II) at pH 0; Bzm is protonated.
^{f} Probably in error; see comments in Cockle et al. (1969).
^{g} Cobalt hyperfine structure resolved for both $g_\perp$ and $g_\parallel$.

order is observed: $PPh_3 \geqslant MeOH$, $DMF > NCS^- \geqslant$ adenine > isoquinoline $\sim$ pyridine $\sim$ Bzm $> CN^-$. There is a close parallel between the two orders. Comparison of the two series suggests that the cobalt(II) corrinoid with PPh_3 in DMF contains one co-ordinated phosphine, while that in MeOH may well contain two phosphines. If we neglect NCS^-, which may co-ordinate through either N or S, then the general order observed in both series is: O-ligands (H_2O, MeOH, probably DMF) $\sim PPh_3 >$ N-ligands (adenine, pyridine, Bzm, etc.) > C-ligands (CN^- and, in the unoxygenated complexes at least, RNC). Bayston *et al.* (1969) have pointed out that the order of decreasing coupling constants is approximately the order of increasing strength of binding of the other axial ligand. But, since we are here dealing with a ground-state and not a thermodynamic *trans*-effect, it is much more relevant that the ligand order observed by e.s.r. spectroscopy in cobalt(II) corrinoids is similar to that observed in cobalt(III) corrinoids by, for example, absorption spectroscopy (see previous section), which in turn can be correlated with the σ-donor power of the axial ligand.

In spite of all the uncertainties in experimental and theoretical interpretation, therefore, e.s.r. spectroscopy can provide an interesting insight into the way in which the electron density distribution of the unpaired electron is affected by the push and pull of the axial ligands. It appears that the cobalt coupling constant (which is related to the cobalt s-character of the orbital occupied by the unpaired electron) can be reduced by either (1) increasing the donor power of one axial ligand ($H_2O <$ nitrogeneous bases $< CN^-$) or (2) the presence of an axial ligand (O_2) with low-lying unfilled orbitals. A decrease in the cobalt s-character could be due to several causes. If, for example, we assume the unoxygenated complexes to be five-co-ordinate, then one might expect that increasing the donor strength of the lone pair of the axial ligand would repel the unpaired electron more and more to the other side of the cobalt, i.e. increase its p-character at the expense of its s- and d-character. But other causes cannot be excluded.

F. SUMMARY

All the above-mentioned techniques provide evidence of strong electronic interaction between the conjugated corrin ring, the cobalt ion and the axial ligands. Each technique, even e.s.r. studies of the cobalt(II) corrinoids and their oxygen adducts, reveals essentially the same order of ligands. For the most commonly studied ligands we find the order: $H_2O <$ Bzm, $HO^- < CN^- <$ vinyl $<$ methyl $<$ ethyl. For the much wider range of ligands studied by absorption spectroscopy, we find that the ligand order depends to a first approximation on the nature of the donor atom: N, O, Cl, Br and C in CN^- and RNC $<$ S, Se, I and C in organo-ligands. The following conclusions can be drawn about the nature of this interaction. The most important property of the axial ligand is its σ-donor power (shown by absorption spectroscopy). As the σ-donor power increases, it places more electron density on the cobalt ion and on the other ligands (theoretical interpretation of absorption spectra), the other cobalt-ligand bond-lengths increase in both *cis*- and *trans*-positions (X-ray analysis), and the other ligands become more like the free bases in structure (infrared, CN^-).

These results provide an interesting picture of the ground-state *cis*- and *trans*-effects of the axial ligands within the corrinoids. There are, unfortunately, no comparable data for the effect of substituents at C_{10} on the properties of the axial ligands, i.e. for the *cis*-effect of the equatorial ligand.

Other physical techniques which have been applied to the study of the cobalt ion in corrinoids include X-ray absorption edge (Boehm *et al.*, 1954) and Mössbauer spectroscopy (Nath *et al.*, 1968) as well as measurements of magnetic susceptibility (see Chapter 7).

Section 3

Equilibria

7

THE COBALT ION: VALENCY, SPIN-STATE AND STEREOCHEMISTRY

Various types of corrinoids may be produced from the simple cobalt(III) complexes such as aquo- and cyano-cobalamin by reduction (e.g. B_{12r} and B_{12s}) or by further reaction of these reduced corrinoids (e.g. DBC and methyl-cobalamin). For each compound one needs to establish the structure of:

1. the cobalt ion: valency and magnetic properties (number of unpaired electrons). The cobalt ion has 8, 7 and 6 d-electrons in its uni-, di- and tri-valent states respectively.
2. the axial ligands: the complex may possess 2, 1 or 0 axial ligands i.e. be six-, five- or four-coordinate.
3. the corrin ring; whether the ring has been modified by the addition of H^+, H_2O, etc.

Problems frequently arise when trying to apply to the corrinoids the standard techniques of co-ordination chemistry such as titration, chemical analysis, measurement of absorption spectra (d–d spectra) and magnetic susceptibility. Examples of such complications and difficulties are:

(1) the very small amounts of material (e.g. B_{12}, DBC) available when the first experiments were carried out,
(2) the occurrence of side-reactions such as the liberation of H_2 by B_{12s},
(3) the high molecular weight and the presence of a large amount of water of crystallization, which makes analysis of, for example, co-ordinated CH_3^- difficult or impossible,
(4) the intense absorption bands due to transitions within the corrin ring, which prevent the observation of d–d transitions and

(5) the presence of paramagnetic impurities, even in crystalline samples of corrinoids, which complicates the measurement of magnetic susceptibilities (see for example Diehl *et al.* (1950a) and Wallman *et al.* (1951) in the case of cyanocobalamin and Hill *et al.* (1962) for references to early work on DBC).

Spurious results have been obtained and false conclusions drawn on, for example, the valency of cobalt in vitamin B_{12r} and DBC, the presence of a hydride ligand in vitamin B_{12s} and of additional hydrogen atoms in the corrin ring of DBC. These false trails will not be pursued in this book.

Very few of the corrinoids, apart from those like cyanocobalamin dealt with in Section I, have been fully characterized. In particular, the presence or absence of a co-ordinated solvent molecule can only be finally proved by X-ray analysis. Of the complexes which may have a vacant axial co-ordination site, only the dimeric iodo-cobalt(II) complex has so far been subjected to X-ray analysis (see Section IV). X-ray analysis does not always locate the hydrogen atoms and therefore cannot establish whether, for example, the corrin ring has been altered by the addition of hydrogen atoms in the conversion of cyanocobalamin to DBC or to the dimeric iodo-cobalt(II) complex. One can, however, exclude the possibility of addition of hydrogen atoms by determining the number of protons liberated or consumed during reduction or reaction.

Problems of a more theoretical kind arise when one of the axial ligands is a very polarizable group such as CH_3^- (written here as the anion). It may be possible to determine the overall charge for the (cobalt + axial ligand) unit, but the division of charge between the cobalt and the ligand involves a certain measure of arbitrariness. This is discussed in Section II.

The evidence for the valency, spin-state and stereochemistry of the cobalt ion is presented as follows: Section I, cobalt(III) corrinoids with simple ligands such as cyanide and water; Section II, cobalt(III) corrinoids with very polarizable such as organo-ligands; Section III, B_{12r} and analogous monomeric cobalt(II) complexes; Section IV, the recently discovered dimeric and diamagnetic cobalt(II) corrinoid with a bridging iodide ligand and Section V, B_{12s} and other cobalt(I) corrinoids. The corrin ring appears not to be reduced or otherwise modified in any of these groups of compounds.

The redox potentials of corrinoids, almost all of which have been obtained polarographically, are summarized in Section VI. Redox reactions such as disproportionation, chemical oxidation and reduction and the catalytic evolution of hydrogen, are dealt with in Chapter 11.

The corrinoids provide a good example of the general rule that an increase in the number of electrons on the metal (or a decrease in the valency) is accompanied by a decrease in the co-ordination number, from six in the typical Co(III) corrinoids, through five and six in the Co(II) complexes to four in the Co(I) corrinoids.

I. COBALT(III) CORRINOIDS WITH SIMPLE LIGANDS, E.G. CYANOCOBALAMIN

The structure of B$_{12}$ or cyanocobalamin (see Fig. 1.1) has been established by the X-ray analysis of two crystalline modifications ("wet" and "dry"), which differ in the amount of water of crystallization. The cobalt ion is six-co-ordinate with an approximately octahedral configuration. For references and details of the structure of the cobalt co-ordination sphere see Chapter 6, Section I.

B$_{12}$ is diamagnetic, though some paramagnetism is often observed due to the presence of para- and ferro-magnetic impurities (Grün and Menassé, 1950; Diehl et al., 1950a; Wallman et al., 1951). Cyanocobalamin is therefore a cobalt(III) complex. In agreement with this the complex is uncharged in neutral solution (Smith et al., 1952a); the triple charge of the cobalt(III) cation is balanced by the negative charges of the cyanide, the corrin ring and the phosphate of the nucleotide side-chain. Polarography also fully substantiates the assignment as a cobalt(III) complex (see Section VI). The close similarity between the reflection spectrum of the solid and the absorption spectrum of the solution shows that the chromophore has the same structure in both solid and solution (Hill, J. A. et al., 1964).

Other corrinoids which have been shown to be diamagnetic are aquo- or hydroxo-cobalamin (Wallman et al., 1951; Hill, J. A. et al., 1964), nitrito-cobalamin (Smith et al., 1952b) and dicyanocobalamin (Hill, J. A. et al., 1964).

The identity of the axial ligands of cobalt(III) corrinoids can be established by several means such as: similarities in absorption spectra; the existence of an equilibrium involving anion, base or proton which relates them to aquo-, cyano- or dicyano-cobalamin; X-ray analysis; and infra-red spectra. For details see Chapter 4 and Chapter 8, Section IV.

II. ORGANOCORRINOIDS

X-ray analysis showed that the structure of DBC differed from that of cyano-cobalamin in that cyanide had been replaced by 5-deoxyadenosine (Lenhert, 1968; Lenhert and Hodgkin, 1961) which can be considered as a carbanion. Since the hydrogen atoms were not located, this did not establish either the valency of the cobalt ion or whether the corrin ring contained the same number of double bonds as it did in cyanocobalamin. The red crystals of DBC dissolve in water to give a red solution which turns yellow on acidification ($pK_a = 3.3$); the Bzm is co-ordinated and protonated in the yellow form (Ladd et al., 1961; Hill et al., 1962). Comparison of the absorption spectrum of the red solution with the reflection spectrum of the solid indicated the presence of the same chromophore in each case (Hill, J. A. *et al.*, 1964; Firth *et al.*, 1968a), so that experimental results relating to solutions and to the solid state can be compared directly. Solutions of DBC are diamagnetic in both red and yellow forms (Hill, J. A. *et al.*, 1962, 1964). DBC gives no e.s.r. signal either as the crystalline solid or in frozen aqueous solution, in agreement with its diamagnetism (Hogenkamp *et al.*, 1963). Electrophoresis showed that DBC is uncharged in aqueous solution over the range of pH 5–10 (Ladd *et al.*, 1961), as is cyanocobalamin (Smith *et al.*, 1952a). The cobalt ion is, therefore, diamagnetic and the cobalt ion and organo-ligand together carry a net charge of +2. DBC can therefore be regarded as a complex of cobalt(III) with a carbanion.

Alkylcobalamins are, like DBC, uncharged in neutral aqueous solution (Müller and Müller, 1962b), have similar absorption spectra (see Chapter 5, Section I) and can be synthesized by analogous methods (see Chapter 13, Section I); they clearly have the same electronic structure as DBC. The possible presence of additional hydrogen atoms in the corrin ring of methylcobalamin has been excluded by examining the following set of reactions:

$$[Co^{III}OH_2] + 2\ominus \rightarrow Co^I + H_2O$$

$$Co^I + CH_3I \rightarrow [Co^{III}CH_3^-] + I^-$$

Cobalamin-cobalt(I) is produced in the absence of excess reducing agent by controlled potential reduction; it then reacts with methyl iodide to give methylcobalamin without any change in pH (Hill, H. A. O. *et al.*, 1964; Das *et al.*, 1967, 1968). The corrin ring must, therefore, have the same structure in aquo- as in methylcobalamin, and hence in cyanocobalamin and DBC. It has also been shown that vinyl- and ethinyl-cobalamin give no e.s.r. signal in frozen aqueous solution and carry no set charge in neutral solution. They can, therefore, both be regarded as cobalt(III) complexes with the carbanions $CH_2{=}CH^-$ and $HC{\equiv}C^-$ and not, for example, as π-complexes with the uncharged $CH_2{=}CH_2$ or $HC{\equiv}CH$ (Hayward *et al.*, 1965). All other organo-corrinoids so far reported can be related to the above complexes by equilibria in solution and/or by similarities in their absorption spectra.

Some organo-corrinoids appear to be five-co-ordinate. The evidence for five co-ordination and the effect of the nature of the organo-ligand on the position of the equilibrium between the five- and six-co-ordinate complexes are discussed in Chapter 8, Section III.

All organocorrinoids, whether five- or six-co-ordinate, show a proton magnetic resonance (see Chapter 6, Section III), which is additional strong evidence that they are all diamagnetic cobalt(III) complexes.

One could consider these organo-corrinoids to be complexes of either (1) cobalt(III) and a carbanion, (2) cobalt(II) and a free radical with antiferromagnetic coupling of the spins or (3) cobalt(I) and a carbonium ion. Their reactions do in fact proceed through transition states corresponding to each of these formulations (see Chapter 13, Sections I and II) and if we vary the axial ligand in the series CN^-, $HC{\equiv}C^-$, $CH_2{=}CH^-$, $CH_3CH_2^-$, we find that the stereochemistry and formation constants (see Chapter 8, Sections III and IV) change from those typical of a cobalt(III) complex (six-co-ordinate, high formation constant for the binding of CN^- etc.) to those typical of a cobalt(II) complex (five-co-ordinate, low formation constants). The usual correlation between stereochemistry and valency and the division into valencies has broken down; this is discussed further in Chapter 8, Section III. Since, however, these complexes form a continuous series with gradually changing properties, it is inconvenient to draw any arbitrary dividing line between cobalt(III) and cobalt(II) complexes and it is simplest to treat them all as cobalt(III) complexes with cyanide or a carbanion.

Various other ligands such as SO_3^{2-}, $S_2O_3^{2-}$, thiolates, I^- and $NCSe^-$ have effects similar to those of organo-ligands on the absorption spectra (see Chapter 5, Section I) and on equilibria in the *trans*-position (see Chapter 8, Sections III and IV) and similar arguments could be made about valency. But since these complexes are formed reversibly from the aquo-complex and the free ligand in solution, it is only natural to treat them as normal cobalt(III) complexes.

III. MONOMERIC COBALT(II) CORRINOIDS

Cobalt(II) corrinoids can be prepared by various means including:

(1) Reduction of cobalt(III) complexes chemically (see Chapter 11, Section IV), at an electrode as in polarography (see Section VI), by controlled potential reduction (see below) or at the expense of the organic part of the molecule in the process of "self-reduction" (see Chapter 11, Section II); reduction may proceed to the cobalt(I) stage, depending on the reducing agent and the conditions.

(2) Oxidation of cobalt(I) complexes by reaction with oxygen, cobalt(III) complexes etc. or by the liberation of hydrogen on acidification (see Chapter 11).

(3) Photolysis of organocorrinoids and certain other complexes (see Chapter 14, Section II).

Kaczka, Wolf and Folkers (1949) were the first to report that the reduction of solutions of cyanocobalamin with hydrogen and a platinum oxide catalyst caused a change in colour from red to dark brown; the brown solution was readily oxidized on contact with air to give aquocobalamin. They concluded that the cobalt had been reduced in the brown complex, but did not attempt to isolate the product or determine the valency of the cobalt. Diehl and Murie (1952) were the first to study this brown compound, which they called vitamin B_{12r}. Potentiometric titration with ferricyanide in neutral solution showed that the oxidation of B_{12r} required one equivalent and that it therefore contains cobalt(II). The presence of cobalt(II) has been fully confirmed by the stoichiometry of

(1) the oxidation of vitamin B_{12r} with I_2 in $N/5$ H_2SO_4 (Brierly et al., 1953),
(2) the reduction of aquo- and cyano-cobalamin by polarography (Jaselskis and Diehl, 1954) and by controlled potential reduction (Tackett et al., 1963; Hill, H. A. O. et al., 1964; Das et al., 1967, 1968) and
(3) the reduction of hydroxo- and methyl-cobalamin with H_2 and a platinum catalyst (Dolphin et al., 1964b).

Very little work has been reported on solid cobalamin-cobalt(II) (B_{12r}). Diehl and Murie (1952) prepared a brown-black solid, contaminated with potassium sulphate, by the evaporation of a solution of cyanocobalamin containing potassium sulphate which had been catalytically reduced. Yamada, Shimizu and Fukui (1966b) photolysed a solution of methylcobalamin in isopropanol under nitrogen; concentration of the solution and addition of acetone slowly precipitated a dark brown amorphous powder. The solid proved to be fairly stable to oxygen when dry, but readily oxidized when moist. Solutions in ethanol gave the spectrum of cobalamin-cobalt(II). No analysis or magnetic susceptibility measurements were reported, but the solid does give an e.s.r. signal (intensity not estimated). The brown colour and the e.s.r. signal suggest that the cobalt(II) complex has the same structure in the solid and in solution.

Evidence on the spin-state of the cobalt(II) ion comes from e.s.r. measurements, which were first carried out by Hogenkamp, Barker and Mason (1963). They found that frozen solutions of cobalamin-cobalt(II) at $-165°$ gave a signal centred at $g = 1.96$ with a superhyperfine splitting of six lines (instead of the eight expected for interaction with the nuclear spin of Co^{59} $I = 7/2$). The concentration of unpaired electrons was found by comparison with aqueous solutions of $CuSO_4$ and EDTA to be 0.89 unpaired electrons per cobalt. Bayston and Winfield (1967) also obtained a value of 0.8 unpaired spins per cobalt in B_{12r} prepared by the reduction of B_{12a} with CO at $35°$. The d^7 cobalt(II) ion, therefore, has a low-spin configuration (one unpaired spin). It has been pointed out (Hogenkamp et al., 1963; Schrauzer and Lee, 1968; Cockle et al., 1969) that the g-values of cobalt(II) corrinoids are also consistent with those of other low-spin cobalt(II) complexes such as cobalt(II) phthalocyanine.

Evidence about the nature and number of the axial ligands is incomplete.

Ligands which can co-ordinate to the cobalt(II) ion in corrinoids include various nitrogenous bases (Bzm, adenine, pyridine etc.) NCS^-, CN^-, cyclohexylisocyanide and triphenylphosphine (for references see Chapter 6, Section III and Table 6.5) and iodide. Five-co-ordination has been established by X-ray analysis for the dimeric iodide-bridged complex described in the next section, while e.s.r. measurements have established that two pyridines may be co-ordinated to cobinamide-cobalt(II) at high pyridine concentrations to give a six-co-ordinate complex; the presence of five lines in the superhyperfine structure indicates that the unpaired electron interacts with two nitrogen atoms in the axial positions (Schrauzer and Lee, 1968; Cockle et al., 1969). The presence of only three lines in the superhyperfine structure shows that only one molecule of the other nitrogenous bases is co-ordinated. In the case of cyanide and isocyanides, where the donor atom does not give rise to a superhyperfine splitting, it is impossible to state whether one or two molecules are co-ordinated, except by studying the variation of the e.s.r. signal with ligand concentration; this has not yet been done. For the same reason it is very difficult to establish the presence or otherwise of a co-ordinated solvent molecule (H_2O, MeOH) and hence the co-ordination number of cobalt in cobinamide- and cobalamin-cobalt(II).

The absorption spectra of cobalamin- and cobinamide-cobalt(II) have been studied in aqueous solution at room temperature over the range of pH 0–14. Cobinamide-cobalt(II) shows no change from pH 0 to 14 (Hill et al., unpublished results), while cobalamin-cobalt(II) (B_{12r}) shows a change with a pK of ~2.5; the position of the absorption bands of Bzm and comparison with cobinamide-cobalt(II) shows that Bzm is co-ordinated in the neutral form, but displaced and protonated in the acid form (Hill et al., 1965a). In agreement with this, both the cobalamin and the cobinamide give virtually identical e.s.r. signals in acid solution, but differ in neutral solution (Cockle et al., 1969). The absorption spectrum of B_{12r} is shown in Fig. 7.1 and the reported values of wavelengths and extinction co-efficients of monomeric cobalt(II) corrinoids are given in Table 7.1. In view of the small difference observed in the absorption spectra of cobalt(III) corrinoids when Bzm is replaced by H_2O compared to the very large change seen when H_2O is removed to form the (presumed) five-co-ordinate complex (see Chapter 5, Section I), the close similarity between the absorption spectra of cobinamide- and cobalamin-cobalt(II) suggests that they both have the same structure, i.e. are both five-co-ordinate (with H_2O and Bzm respectively as the single axial ligand) or both six-co-ordinate (with an additional co-ordinated solvent molecule). It is also suggestive that the spectra of the cobalt(II) corrinoids resemble those of the five-co-ordinate organo-cobalt(III) corrinoids far more than the normal six-co-ordinate cobalt(III) corrinoids (see Chapter 5, Section I); but one obviously cannot draw any definite conclusions from these comparisons. It is a pity that the absorption spectra of the undoubtedly six-co-ordinate bispyri-dine-cobalt(II) complexes are not available for comparison. It is quite likely that the change in free energy for the binding of a sixth ligand by the five-co-ordinate complex is small and that a displacement of the equilibrium might be brought about by a slight change in conditions (solvent, temperature).

As can be seen in Fig. 7.1, B_{12r} absorbs out to about 800 nm; it is likely that some of the bands of low energy and low intensity are d–d transitions.

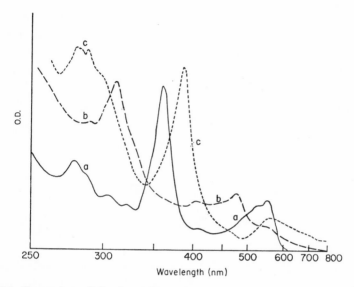

Fig. 7.1. Comparison of the absorption spectra of B_{12} (——), B_{12r} (— — —) and B_{12s} (----). From Beaven and Johnson (1955)

It has been shown that when unbuffered solutions of B_{12a} at a pH of approximately 5.5 or 7 (i.e. in the form of aquocobalamin) are reduced to B_{12r} practically no change in pH is observed, i.e. no H^+ or HO^- is involved in this reaction (Das *et al.*, 1968). This means not only that the second axial ligand must be H_2O or absent, but that the corrin ring in B_{12r} has not been protonated.

Bayston, King, Looney and Winfield (1969) have shown that cobalt(II) corrinoids will react with oxygen at low temperature to form monomeric adducts which are probably better represented as cobalt(III) complexes with the superoxide anion (O_2^-) than cobalt(II) with oxygen; for further details see Chapter 6, Section III.

Table 7.1. *Spectra of cobalt(II) Corrinoids*

Cobalamin-cobalt(II)					References
λ		312.5	405	473	Diehl and Murie, 1952
O.D.		2.83	0.80	1.00	
$E_{1\%}^{1cm}$		153	43	54	
λ		312	405	473	Tackett *et al.*, 1963
O.D.		2.83	0.78	1.00	
$E_{1\%}^{1cm}$		190	52	67	
λ		311	405	473	Brady and Barker, 1961
O.D.		2.96	0.82	1.00	
$\epsilon \times 10^{-4}$		2.28	0.63	0.77	
λ	288	311	402	473	Pratt, 1964; Hill *et al.*,
O.D.		2.98	0.81	1.00	unpublished results
$\epsilon \times 10^{-4}$		2.75	0.75	0.92	

[Cobalamin (BzmH$^+$)]-cobalt(II)				
λ	315	~405	470	Hill *et al.*, unpublished results
O.D.	2.21	0.64	1.00	
$\epsilon \times 10^{-4}$	2.43	0.70	1.10	

Cobinamide-cobalt(II)				
λ	315	~405	470	Hill *et al.*, unpublished results
O.D.	2.21	0.60	1.00	

[Cobyrinic acid heptamethylester]-cobalt(II) in EtOH				
λ	315	~417	469	Werthemann, 1968
O.D.	2.30	0.62	1.00	
$\epsilon \times 10^{-4}$	2.30	0.62	1.00	

λ = wavelength of absorption band in nm.
o.d. = optical density of given band relative to that of the band near 470 nm.
ϵ = molar extinction coefficient in litre. mol^{-1} cm^{-1}.
$E_{1\%}^{1cm}$ = optical density of a 1 % solution in a cell of 1 cm pathlength.

IV. DIMERIC COBALT(II) CORRINOIDS

A completely different type of cobalt(II) corrinoid has been discovered by Werthemann (1968) in his study of complexes of cobyrinic acid heptamethyl ester. Reduction of a benzene solution of the di-iodocobalt(III) complex with aqueous sodium thiosulphate or treating a benzene solution of the cobalt(II) complex with aqueous KI yields a green compound, which can be purified by chromatography to give small green-black needles. Oxidation with iodine,

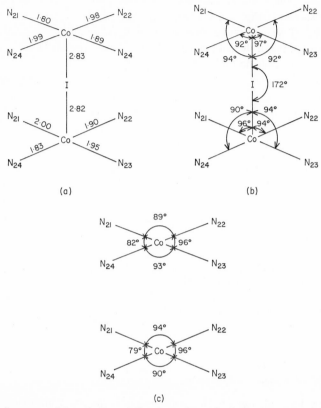

Fig. 7.2. Structure of the cobalt co-ordination sphere of μ-iodo-bis{[cobyrinic acid heptamethyl ester]-cobalt(II)} iodide. (a), bond-lengths. (b) and (c), bond-angles. From Edmond (personal communication).

together with its formation from and dissociation into the cobalt(II) complex (see below), suggested the presence of cobalt(II) in the green compound. Analysis agreed with its formulation as an iodo-cobalt(II) complex. Rather surprisingly, however, magnetic susceptibility measurements showed it to be diamagnetic. Werthemann therefore suggested that the complex was dimerized or polymerized through the formation of iodide bridges between the cobalt ions. X-ray analysis has recently shown that the green compound is indeed dimeric (Edmond, personal communication). It contains one bridging iodide per dimer and both cobalt ions are five-co-ordinate. The second iodide is not co-ordinated. The bond-lengths and angles involving the cobalt and ligand atoms are shown in Fig. 7.2. It can be seen that the configuration around the cobalt is very close to that of a square pyramid; the cobalt is displaced from the least-squares plane of the four nitrogen atoms by 0.13 and 0.11 Å from the top and bottom parts of the molecule respectively.

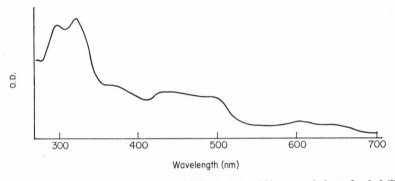

Fig. 7.3. Absorption spectrum of μ-iodo-bis{[cobyrinic acid heptamethyl ester]-cobalt(II)} iodide in benzene. From Werthemann (1968).

The green dimer dissolves in benzene to give a green solution with the spectrum shown in Fig. 7.3. and the following values of λ and ε (Werthemann, 1968):

λ(nm)	299	323	435	492	603
ε × 10⁻⁴	2.05	2.16	0.85	0.76	0.29

Since the solid is also green, this presumably is the spectrum of the chromophore present in the solid state. It dissolves in methanol or ethanol, however, to give a yellow solution of the monomeric cobalt(II) complex, whose λ and ε are quoted in Table 7.1. Since the green dimer can also be formed by treating a solution of the yellow monomer in benzene with aqueous KI there apparently exists an equilibrium of the type:

$$[Co^{II}.I^-.Co^{II}] + 2S \rightleftharpoons [Co^{II}.S] + I^-$$

where S is a molecule of alcohol or some other ligand.

The solid and its green solution in benzene are stable towards oxygen. The yellow solution in dry methanol or ethanol is apparently also stable towards oxygen, while the (? green) solutions in methyl acetate, chloroform and carbon disulphide are oxidized within one day. Other reactions of the dimer include oxidation by I₂ to the di-iodocobalt(III) complex (as already mentioned) and rapid reaction with carbon tetrachloride to give the chloroiodo-cobalt(III) complex; since styrene can be polymerized simultaneously with the latter reaction, the mechanism probably involves the abstraction of a chlorine atom by the cobalt(II) ion to give the CCl_3 radical (Werthemann, 1968).

It will be interesting to see whether other dimeric cobalt(II) corrinoids complexes of this type can be prepared.

V. COBALT(I) CORRINOIDS

Cobalt(I) corrinoids can be formed by the reduction of cobalt(II) and cobalt-(III) complexes at an electrode (see Section VI) or with powerful reducing agents such as Zn, Cr(II), $S_2O_4^{2-}$ and BH_4^- (see Chapter 11, Section IV) and as a by-product in certain photochemical reactions (see Chapter 14, Section III). Cobalt(I) corrinoids can also be produced by the "self-reduction" of cyanocobalamin at high pH (see Chapter 11, Section II).

Schindler (1951) was the first to observe the formation of the complex, subsequently named vitamin B_{12s} (Hill *et al.*, 1962) and shown to be cobalamin-cobalt(I). He found that an aqueous solution of cyanocobalamin was reduced by zinc and ammonium chloride to give a very air-sensitive blue solution and recorded the spectrum (of B_{12s} mixed with B_{12}). Boos, Carr and Conn (1953) also recorded the spectrum of B_{12s} but, as pointed out by Beaven and Johnson (1955), they claimed that this was the spectrum of the brown solution of B_{12r}, produced by the reduction of cyanocobalamin with one equivalent of chromous chloride. It was Beaven and Johnson (1955) who first showed that B_{12s} represented a greater degree of reduction than B_{12r}. The cobalt ion has been shown to be univalent by the number of electrons involved in the reduction of aquo- and cyanocobalamin and cobalamin-cobalt(II) to B_{12s} by controlled potential reduction (Tackett *et al.*, 1963; Hill, H. A. O. *et al.*, 1964; Das *et al.*, 1968). One proton is consumed in the reduction of hydroxocobalamin to B_{12s}, while none is liberated in the reaction of B_{12s} with methyl iodide or ethyl bromide (RX), in agreement with the following equations:

$$[Co(III)OH^-] + H^+ + 2\ominus \rightarrow Co(I) + H_2O$$
$$[Co(I)] + RX \rightarrow [Co(III)R^-] + X^-$$

i.e. the corrin ring has the same structure in B_{12s} (no additional protons) as in B_{12a}; and B_{12s} is a simple cobalt(I) complex and not a cobalt(III) hydride (Hill, H. A. O. *et al.*, 1964; Das *et al.*, 1967, 1968).

The spectrum of B_{12s} has been shown in Fig. 7.1, and the wavelengths and optical density of cobalt(I) corrinoids are given in Table 7.2. The spectra are unusual in showing absorption throughout the visible region, which gives rise to the grey-green colour. It has been suggested that the four bands of lowest

Table 7.2. *Spectra of cobalt(I) corrinoids*

Cobalamin-cobalt(I)

Boos et al., 1953

λ	385	460	554
O.D.	1.00	0.07	0.13
$E_{1\%}^{1\,cm}$	179	12.5	23.6

Tackett et al., 1963

λ	280	286	383	455	553
O.D.	1.07	1.07	1.00	0.09	0.11
$E_{1\%}^{1\,cm}$	250	250	234	22	25

Schrauzer et al., 1965

λ	460	560	697	820
$\log_{10} \epsilon$	3.4	3.5	3.2	3.1

Hill et al., unpublished results

λ	280.5	288	386.5	455	545	680	800
O.D.	1.04	1.05	1.00	0.09	0.10	0.06	0.05
$\epsilon \times 10^{-4}$	2.91	2.94	2.80	0.25	0.28	0.17	0.14

Cobinamide-cobalt(I)

Hill et al., unpublished results

λ	281	294	386.5	455	545	680	800
O.D.	0.92	0.96	1.00	0.11	0.13	0.08	0.066

[Cobyrinic acid heptamethylester]-cobalt(I)

Werthemann, 1968

λ	282	394	465	576
$\epsilon \times 10^{-4}$	3.9	3.8	0.35	0.43

λ = wavelength of absorption band in nm.
o.d. = optical density of given band relative to that of the band near 385 nm.
ε = molar extinction coefficient in litre mol⁻¹ cm⁻¹.
$E_{1\%}^{1\,cm}$ = optical density of a 1% solution in a cell of 1 cm pathlength.

energy are d–d transitions (Schrauzer *et al.*, 1965). It is likely that the spectra will include $\pi-\pi$ transitions of the corrin ring, d–d transitions of the cobalt and one or more bands corresponding to charge transfer from the cobalt(I) ion to the corrin ring.

The spectrum of B_{12s} remains unchanged from pH 5–14 (Das *et al.*, 1967) and is identical (above 300 nm) with that of cobinamide-cobalt(I) (see Table 7.2); and, as pointed out by Beaven and Johnson (1955), the resolution of the absorption bands of Bzm is greater in B_{12s} than in B_{12}. Bzm is therefore not co-ordinated to the cobalt. No other potential ligands have yet been shown to co-ordinate to the cobalt(I) ion in the corrinoids. It appears, therefore, that the cobalt(I) in B_{12s} and its analogues may be four-co-ordinate with a square planar configuration. Because of the effects of the field of the ligands on the splitting of the d-orbitals, we would expect the d^8 Co(I) ion, like the isoelectronic Ni(II), to be spin-paired (i.e. diamagnetic) in a square planar configuration. Magnetic susceptibility measurements have, in fact, been carried out on solutions of B_{12s}, prepared by treating B_{12} in aqueous ammonium chloride with zinc dust, and it was concluded that the cobalt ion was paramagnetic (Grün and Haas, 1956); but the results are too inaccurate to be accepted.

It is conceivable that a hydride is formed in acid solution according to the equilibrium:

$$[Co(I)] + H^+ \rightleftharpoons [Co(III)H^-]$$

and that it is an intermediate in the evolution of hydrogen (see Chapter 11, Section III). An analogous equilibrium is known in the case of the $[Co^{III}(CN)_5H]^{3-}$ ion, which loses a proton in very strongly alkaline solution (Banks and Pratt, 1968; Hanzlík and Vlček, 1969):

$$[Co^{III}(CN)_5H]^{3-} \rightleftharpoons [Co^I(CN)_5]^{4-} + H^+$$

Typical reactions of cobalamin-cobalt(I) include very rapid oxidation by O_2 (see Chapter 11, Section V), reaction with acid to liberate H_2 (Chapter 11, Section III) and with methyl iodide to give methyl-cobalamin (Chapter 13, Section I).

VI. POLAROGRAPHIC AND REDOX POTENTIALS

The published values of the polarographic half-wave potentials for the oxidation and reduction of various corrinoids are listed in Table 7.3. Values are given in volts versus the saturated calomel electrode; they can be converted into potentials versus the standard hydrogen electrode by adding +0.246. It must, however, be noted that these reactions at the dropping mercury

Table 7.3. *Polarographic half-wave potentials* ($E_{1/2}$)

Compound	Solution	Range studied	$E_{1/2}$	n	Notes
(1) Cyanocobalamin	I	+0.2 to −2.0	−1.11	2	
(2) Cyanocobalamin	II	−0.7 to −1.3	−1.021		ir
(3) Aquocobalamin	I	+0.2 to −1.8	−0.06	1	a
			−1.02	1	a
(4) Sulphitocobalamin	I		−1.48		
(5) 5-Deoxyadenosylcobalamin (DBC)	I		−1.52		
(6) 5-Deoxyadenosylcobalamin (DBC)	III	+0.25 to −1.9	−1.2 to	1.5–2	b
			−1.6		
(7) Deaminated DBC	I		−1.51		
(7) Methylcobalamin	I		−1.55		
(7) Ethyl-, propyl-, butyl- and amyl-cobalamin	I		−1.53		
(7) Carboxymethylcobalamin	IV		−1.48		
(8) Dicyanocobalamin	I		−1.33	2	ir
(9) Cyanoaquocobinamide	I		−0.84		
(9) Cyano-*adenine*- [adenylcobamide]	I		−1.03		
(9) 5-deoxyadenosylcobinamide	I		−1.30		
(7) 5-Deoxyadenosyl-[adenylcobamide]	I		−1.49		
(3) Cobalamin-cobalt(II) (B_{12r})	I	+0.2 to −1.8	−0.04	1	an c
			−0.95	1	c
			−1.55	variable	
(10) Cobalamin-cobalt(I) (B_{12s})	II		−0.87		an ir

Potentials are given in volts versus S.C.E.

Solutions: In all cases where the authors have stated the concentrations, the solutions contain $3-5 \times 10^{-4}$ M cobalt and

   I. 0.1 N K_2SO_4
   II. 0.1 M sodium EDTA, pH 9.5 or 9.6.
   III. Solutions various, pH 4.75–11.4
   IV. 0.1 N KCN

Characteristics of the polarographic wave:

   n. number of electrons.
   ir. Reaction *stated* to be irreversible; but it would appear that in fact all the reactions are polarographically irreversible.
   an. Anodic wave, i.e. due to oxidation at the dropping mercury electrode. All other waves are cathodic, i.e. due to reduction.
   a. $E_{1/2}$ stated to be independent of pH, but no details given. Since aquocobalamin forms hydroxocobalamin above pH 8, it is most likely that $E_{1/2}$ of the first wave changes above this pH.
   b. The number (1 or 2), height ($n = 1.5-2$) and $E_{1/2}$ (-1.2 to -1.6) of the waves depend on the pH and composition of the solution.
   c. $E_{1/2}$ invariant over the range of pH 5–10.

References

(1) Diehl *et al.* (1950b, 1951); Jaselskis and Diehl (1954).
(2) Boos *et al.* (1953).
(3) Jaselskis and Diehl (1954).
(4) Bernhauer and Wagner (1963); Bernhauer *et al.* (1964).
(5) Bernhauer *et al.* (1964).
(6) Kratochvil and Diehl (1966).
(7) Müller and Müller (1962b).
(8) Diehl *et al.* (1951).
(9) Bernhauer *et al.* (1964).
(10) Tackett *et al.* (1963).

electrode are probably all irreversible and cannot therefore be used to obtain true standard electrode potentials. Kratochvil and Diehl's study (1966) of the polarography of DBC showed that $E_{1/2}$ can vary considerably with the nature of the other electrolytes present in the solution. Such effects have not been studied for any other corrinoids and it is therefore difficult to know how to compare results obtained under different conditions; compare, for example, the two values obtained for the reduction of cyanocobalamin or the anodic wave of cobalamin-cobalt(I) with the cathodic wave of cobalamin-cobalt(II) (see Table 7.3). Boos, Carr and Conn (1953) reported that cobalamin-cobalt(II) showed an anodic wave at an $E_{1/2}$ of -0.311 volts versus S.C.E.; it was subsequently shown that this wave was due to the oxidation of mercury in the presence of cyanide liberated on the reduction of cyanocobalamin (Collat and Tackett, 1962).

Various comments can be made on the potentials listed in Table 7.3 and certain conclusions can be drawn. The polarographic data are in complete accord with the data of Sections I–V, namely that the cobalt ion can exist in the oxidation states I, II and III. Further reduction, as revealed by the third wave of cobalamin-cobalt(II), seems to involve reduction of the corrin ring (Jaselskis and Diehl, 1954). Since the potential for the reduction of cobalamin-cobalt(II) is less negative than for the reduction of, for example, cyanocobalamin, it is not surprising that cyanocobalamin is reduced in a two-electron step in contrast to aquocobalamin, which has a much less negative potential. The potentials of B_{12a}, B_{12r} and B_{12s} are such that B_{12s} is expected to reduce B_{12a} to B_{12r}, as is observed (see Chapter 11, Section I).

The effect of the axial ligands on $E_{1/2}$ can be seen most readily when the values are tabulated as in Table 7.4, according to the nature of the two axial ligands. We could hardly expect to find any simple pattern or correlation of $E_{1/2}$ values with other effects of the axial ligands, since these potentials are irreversible and are bound to depend on the difference in the binding of the axial ligands by the cobalt(II) and cobalt(III) ions, while we have virtually no information on formation constants involving cobalt(II) corrinoids. Nevertheless, the limited data do show that $E_{1/2}$ becomes more negative as the ligands are changed in the order $H_2O < \underline{Aden} < \underline{Bzm} < CN^- < SO_3^{2-} < R^-$, which is the same order of ligands as is found for cis- and trans- effects (see Chapter 6, Section III and Chapter 8, Section V) and reflects the amount of negative charge donated by the ligand to the cobalt.

Finally, the occurrence of only one polarographic wave over the whole range from approx. $+0.2$ to -2.0 versus S.C.E. for both cyano- and 5-deoxyadenosyl-cobalamin emphasizes the remarkable stability of these corrinoids towards both oxidation and reduction.

Only one attempt has been reported to determine the (reversible) standard redox potential by a method not involving polarography. Schrauzer, Deutsch and Windgassen (1968a) studied the equilibrium between cobalamin-cobalt(I) and cobalt(II) under one atmosphere of hydrogen in the presence of a

Table 7.4. *Effect of the axial ligands on $E_{1/2}$ of cobalt(III) corrinoids*[a]

	H_2O	CN^-	SO_3^{2-}	5-deoxyadenosyl	CH_3
H_2O		−0.84		−1.30	
Aden		−1.03		−1.49	
Bzm	−0.06	−1.11	−1.48	−1.52	−1.55
CN^-	−0.84	−1.33			

[a] Values of $E_{1/2}$ are given in volts versus S.C.E.

platinum catalyst. No experimental details were given, but they stated that equilibrium was observed at pH 9.9 from which they calculated the standard redox potential of the Co(II)/Co(I) couple to be approximately −0.59 volts. This would correspond to a potential of −0.84 volts versus the S.C.E., which agrees reasonably well with the polarographic values of −0.95 v for the reduction of cobalamin-cobalt(II) and −0.87 for the oxidation of cobalamin-cobalt-(I) (see Table 7.3).

8

THE AXIAL LIGANDS AND THEIR EQUILIBRIA IN COBALT(III) CORRINOIDS

I. INTRODUCTION

It is useful to divide the unidentate axial ligands into two groups depending on the mode of formation of the cobalt-ligand bond and on the use which can be made of the ligand in experimental studies. In the first group the ligand can exist free in aqueous solution and the complex may be formed by the displacement of, for example, co-ordinated H$_2$O, i.e.:

$$[Co^{III}OH_2] + X = [Co^{III}X] + H_2O$$

114

The complex can be identified from the stoichiometry of the equilibrium. Examples of such ligands are the usual anions and bases, amino-acids etc. In the second group the ligand cannot exist free in aqueous solution and the complex is prepared by an indirect method, e.g.

$$Co^I + CH_3I = [Co^{III}CH_3{}^-] + I^-$$

This group includes the organo-ligands and similar groups such as Ph_3Si^-, Ph_3Pb^-, R_2As^- etc. In most cases the identity of a complex containing ligands of this second group cannot be accurately established by chemical analysis because the ligand represents too small a fraction of the total molecular weight, and it is therefore deduced from analogies in the absorption spectrum and/or mode of preparation with those of known complexes, such as cyano- and de-oxyadenosyl-cobalamin. Ligands of the second group cannot, of course, undergo reversible ligand substitution reactions. They have, however, proved extremely useful in the study of equilibria for two reasons. Firstly, they are not readily displaced and therefore enable one to study equilibria involving only one co-ordination site. Secondly, they provide a series of ligands (exemplified by NC^-, $HC{\equiv}C^-$, $CH_2{=}CH^-$, $CH_3CH_2{}^-$) which produce markedly different effects on the cobalt ion and the rest of the complex, but in which the ligand atom and the charge remain unchanged; the use of this series of ligands has provided the experimental basis for the study of the *trans*-effect in the cobalt(III) corrinoids. This chapter is concerned almost entirely with reversible ligand substitution reactions involving ligands of the first group.

Quantitative and qualitative studies on equilibria involving the axial ligands provide information of two kinds: the stoichiometry of the formation constant establishes the identity of the complex, while the magnitude of the formation constant and the way in which this depends on, for example, the nature of the ligand in the *trans*-position provides information on the *trans*-effect and other factors. Such studies with cobalt(III) corrinoids have provided a wealth of information of relevance to our understanding of co-ordination chemistry in general. The cobalt corrinoids have, for example, provided the first examples of the co-ordination of ligands such as heterocyclic anions or protonated adenine, and of the further co-ordination of an organo-ligand to another metal (as in $Co{-}CH{=}CH_2$ co-ordinated to Ag(I) ions) and the first (single) step-wise formation constants for ligands such as CH_3NC, SO_3^{2-} or $NCSe^-$. But the most important contribution to co-ordination chemistry has probably come from the measurement of a wide range of stepwise formation constants, from which one has been able to build up a good picture of the thermodynamic *trans*-effect and gain some insight into the factors which are involved in determining the magnitude of formation constants.

In this chapter we are concerned only with equilibria involving the axial ligands in cobalt(III) corrinoids. Equilibrium constants and qualitative observations for the substitution of one axial ligand by another in aqueous solution are summarized in Section IV and the underlying pattern revealed by these formation constants and the factors which determine them are discussed in Section V. Some evidence relating to the equilibria of co-ordinated ligands with protons and Ag(I) ions is also included in Section IV. There are, however, two complicating features of the corrinoids which must be explained before the main body of data are discussed. Firstly, since the corrin ring does not possess a plane of symmetry, stereoisomerism is possible when the two axial ligands are different (Section II). Secondly, when one axial ligand is a very strong donor, such as $CH_3CH_2^-$, the other axial ligand may apparently become displaced with the formation of a five-co-ordinate complex (Section III). The formation and composition of ionic salts of cobalt(III) corrinoids in the solid state and of ion-pairs in non-aqueous solvents are discussed in Section VI. Equilibria observed in strong acids such as concentrated sulphuric acid, however, are entirely different from those observed in aqueous solution and are treated separately (Chapter 9, Section III).

No equilibria appear to have been studied in non-aqueous solvents except those between five- and six-co-ordinate organo-corrinoids (see Section III). But the use of non-aqueous solvents might offer certain advantages over water and reveal interesting differences in behaviour. The use of dimethylsulph-oxide instead of water, for example, stabilizes certain organo-ligands towards displacement by cyanide and increases the formation constants for the binding of cyanide in the *trans*-position (Firth *et al.*, 1968d). A second good example is provided by the cobalt(II) corrinoids (see Chapter 7, Section IV); the green iodide-bridged dimeric form of [cobyrinic acid heptamethyl ester]-cobalt(II) can be formed and studied in benzene but is decomposed by methanol or ethanol to the monomer, i.e.:

$$[Co^{II}.I^-.Co^{II}] + 2S \underset{\text{alcohol}}{\overset{\text{benzene}}{\rightleftharpoons}} 2[Co^{II}S] + I^-$$

where S is a molecule of alcohol or some other ligand. The solubility of corrinoids in different solvents and the effects of hydrogen-bonding between corrinoids and other molecules, including proteins, are mentioned in Chapter 6, Section II.

The study of certain equilibria may be complicated by the occurrence of further reactions. Some organo-ligands are displaced or altered by acid (e.g. loss of $-CH=CH_2$ to give ethylene and conversion of $-C\equiv CH$ to $-COCH_3$), alkali (e.g. loss of $-COCH_3$ to give Co(I) and CH_3COOH) or cyanide (e.g. displacement of 5-deoxyadenosyl); these reactions are discussed in Chapter 13, Section II. Diaquocobinamide and aquocobalamin are parti-cularly prone to undergo side-reactions, e.g. the reduction of cobalt(III) by thiols and other ligands or in very alkaline solution by the side-chains of the corrin ring, the autoxidation of iodide to iodine catalyzed by aquocobalamin (all discussed in Chapter 11) and the uptake of SO_2 from the atmosphere to give the sulphite complex (Bernhauer and Wagner, 1963; Hayward et al., 1965; Firth et al., 1968b).

The small amount of evidence relating to equilibria in cobalt(II) corrinoids is given in Chapter 6, Section III, Chapter 7, Sections III and IV. Cobalt(I) corrinoids are apparently always four-co-ordinate (Chapter 7, Section V).

Finally, it is worth considering the advantages offered by the cobalt(III) corrinoids over other groups of transition metal complexes for the study of ligand substitution equilibria. The main advantages are that

1. ligand substitution in the axial positions is usually very rapid and that
2. the number of co-ordination sites undergoing substitution is limited to two by the presence of the corrin ring and can be further limited to one by the presence of a carbanion or Bzm in the trans-position; contrast other labile metal cations such as Cu(II) (and, outside the transition metals, Ag(I)) where one often has to determine the overall stability constant for the substitution of all ligands.

The very high rate of ligand substitution in the cobalt(III) corrinoids facilitates equilibrium studies, but makes it very hard to obtain kinetic data—in complete contrast to the situation with most other groups of cobalt(III) complexes. In addition,

3. the corrinoids are soluble in aqueous solution and stable over a very wide range of pH and
4. they have absorption spectra which are very sensitive to changes in the axial ligands and therefore provide a quick and easy means of studying equilibria.

One might expect that the cobalt(III) phthalocyaninetetrasulphonate complexes, for example, might offer similar advantages for the study of ligand substitution equilibria; but very little attention has as yet been paid to this group of complexes. One could, therefore, add one further advantage:

5. their biochemical interest has provided the incentive for the study of the cobalt(III) corrinoid complexes.

II. STEREOISOMERISM INVOLVING THE AXIAL LIGANDS

A. INTRODUCTION

The corrin ring does not possess a plane of symmetry, i.e. it has an "upper" and a "lower" side. Stereoisomers are, therefore, theoretically possible whenever the two axial ligands are different. The absence of a plane of symmetry is due to two factors.

1. The presence of the single bond between rings A and D and the relative orientation of the tetrahedral carbon atoms, C_1 and C_{23}, forces this part of the corrin ring out of the plane. In fact the whole corrin ring is buckled and distorted and a different conformation has been found for each structure determined by X-ray analysis. For further details of the structure of the corrin ring see Chapter 6, Section I.

2. All the acetamide side-chains project towards one side of the corrin ring, which we shall call the "upper" side, and all the propionamide side-chains towards the "lower" side. Asymmetry of this type is present in all naturally occurring corrinoids. One could, however, envisage corrinoids in which all the substitutents on the exocyclic ring were identical (or absent); in this case the only cause of asymmetry would be (1).

Stereoisomerism has been established for corrinoids where $X = CN^-$, CH_3^- and $CH_2CH_3^-$ and Y is H_2O (or absent). The relative orientation of some of these isomers has been established, rough values of equilibrium constants obtained and the absorption and circular dichroism spectra of some of the isomeric pairs reported. There are, however, several limitations on the range of corrinoids in which stereoisomerism might be detected. The cobalamins, for example, possess a nucleotide side-chain which projects downwards and terminates in the heterocyclic base 5,6-dimethylbenziminazole (Bzm), which is usually co-ordinated to the cobalt. In all the cobalamins so far studied by X-ray analysis ($X = CN^-$, NCS^-, $NCSe^-$, NO_2 (Hodgkin, 1958) and 5-deoxyadenosyl (Lenhert, 1968)) Bzm is co-ordinated to the lower side of the cobalt, and it appears unlikely that the side-chain is long enough to swing around and allow the base to co-ordinate to the upper side of the cobalt ion. No isomers are, therefore, expected for cobalamins in which Bzm can and does co-ordinate to the cobalt. Secondly, isomers will only be separable when the rate of isomerization is very low, as is the case with organo-ligands which do not normally dissociate, and with cyanide co-ordinated in the position *trans-* to ligands such as H_2O and Bzm, where the formation constants for the binding of cyanide are very high and the rates of dissociation immeasurably slow.

The stereoisomerism of cyanoaquocorrinoids is discussed in Section II,A, that of organocorrinoids in Section II,B. The possibility of stereoisomerism involving certain other ligands such as NH_3 and SO_3^{2-} is also mentioned briefly in Section II,A.

As explained in the chapter on nomenclature (Chapter 2, Section II) the prefixes u- and l- denote the isomers in which the first named axial ligand (cyanide, methyl and ethyl in the corrinoids of interest to this section) is co-ordinated in the "upper" or "lower" position respectively. Much of our knowledge of these stereoisomers is due to Friedrich and his co-workers, who use a different nomenclature, viz.

Our u-isomer = Friedrich's b-isomer

Our l-isomer = Friedrich's a-isomer

Friedrich has used a wide range of corrinoids which differ in the number and position of the amide and carboxylic acid side-chains on positions a–e and g of the corrin ring and in the presence or absence of an aminopropanol and phosphate on position f (see p. 18). The IUPAC–IUB nomenclature for many of these derivatives is lengthy and inconvenient (see Chapter 2, Section I) and Friedrich has therefore used many "trivial" names. Since much of this section relates to work done by Friedrich and his co-workers it would probably be even more confusing to replace Friedrich's nomenclature by any other. We have therefore used Friedrich's nomenclature (anglicized where necessary) as far as possible in this section (Section II) and the following is a guide to his nomenclature. The nature of the side-chains at positions a–g on the corrin ring together with the IUPAC–IUB and Friedrich's names are given in Table 8.1. As pointed out in Chapter 2 these IUPAC–IUB names do strictly speaking include the axial ligands, while in the nomenclature proposed in this book the IUPAC–IUB names given in Table 8.1 cover the nature of the equatorial ligand only. For example, Friedrich's "cobyramide" is "cobyrinic acid hepta-amide" in the IUPAC–IUB nomenclature, but cyanoaquo-[cobyrinic acid hepta-amide] in our nomenclature. But, since all the complexes to be discussed in Section II,B are cyanoaquocorrinoids, it is not necessary to specify the nature of the axial ligands. Isomers are possible wherever the corrin ring possesses both acid and amide side-chains on positions a–e and g. In most cases the nature and positions of the different side-chains are not known and Friedrich identifies the different isomers by the use of the suffixes L, M, S, β, γ and δ (Friedrich, 1965; Friedrich and Moskophidis, 1968).

B. STEREOISOMERS OF CYANOAQUO COMPLEXES

Friedrich (1965) observed that certain corrinoids, which contain carboxylic acid side-chains together with cyanide and water as the axial ligands, gave two orange-red bands in approximately equal amounts when passed through a chromatography column. He concluded that a propionic acid side-chain was necessary to produce the two components but, although he noted that they were interconverted by the action of HCN, he did not make any suggestion as to the structural difference between the two. He later found that cyanoaquo-cobinamide and cyanoaquocobyramide, which do not contain a propionic acid side-chain, could also be separated into two components; and he suggested that these two components were the two stereoisomers involving the axial ligands H_2O and CN^- (Friedrich, 1966a). There can now be no reasonable

5

Table 8.1. *Comparison of IUPAC–IUB and Friedrich's nomenclature*

IUPAC–IUB	Friedrich	Nature of side-chains at positions:	
		f	a–e and g
Cobyrinic acid		Acid	Acids
Cobyrinic acid n-amide	(7-n)carbonsäure	Acid	Acids + Amides
Cobyric acid	Cobyrsäure (or Faktor V$_{1a}$)	Acid	Amides
Cobyrinic acid f-monoamide		Amide	Acids
Cobyrinic acid n-amide	Cobyramid(7-n)carbonsäure	Amide	Acids + Amides
Cobyrinic acid hepta-amide	Cobyramid	Amide	Amides
Cobinic acid		Aminopropanol	Acids
Cobinic acid n-amide	Cobinamid(6-n)carbonsäure	Aminopropanol	Acids + Amides
Cobinamide	Cobinamid (or Faktor B)	Aminopropanol	Amides
O-phospho-cobinic acid n-amide	Cobinamidphosphorsäure Analog	Phosphate	Acids + Amides
O-phospho-cobinic acid	Cobinamidphosphorsäure	Phosphate	Amides

n etc. = mono-, di- etc.

Side-chains at f: acid —CH$_2$.CH$_2$.COOH, amide —CH$_2$.CH$_2$.CO.NH$_2$, aminopropanol —CH$_2$.CH$_2$.CO.NH.CH$_2$.CHOH.CH$_3$,
phosphate—CH$_2$.CH$_2$.CO.NH.CH$_2$.CHMe.OPO$_3$H$_2$.

For further explanations see the text.

doubt of this interpretation. It would, however, be interesting to carry out an X-ray analysis of a pair of isomers, if only to obtain evidence on the effect of a change in the relative orientation of the axial ligands on the details of the structure of the equatorial ligand.

The present position is that virtually all the corrinoids so far studied in which the two axial ligands are CN^- and H_2O have been separated into two components by techniques such as paper, column and thin layer chromatography and by electrophoresis (Friedrich, 1966a; Friedrich et al., 1967; Friedrich and Moskophidis, 1968; Firth et al., 1968b,c). Cyanoaquocobinamide has also been shown to be present as a mixture of two components by proton magnetic resonance spectroscopy (Hill et al., 1968a; Firth et al., 1968a). The cyano-aquocorrinoids studied include those where the equatorial ligand is cobin-amide, cobinamide-phosphoric acid, cobyramide and a wide range of other derivatives with one, two, three or four carboxylic acid side-chains; a few compounds such as Friedrich's cobinamide monocarboxylic acid $\beta(S)$ and cobyramidemonocarboxylic acid S have not yet been resolved (Friedrich, 1966a; Friedrich et al., 1967; Friedrich and Moskophidis, 1968). Certain monocyanide complexes of nucleotide-containing corrinoids can also be separated into two isomers, at least in solutions of acetic acid; under these conditions the base is obviously displaced and protonated, so that here also the two axial ligands are CN^- and H_2O (Friedrich, 1966a).

The presence of isomers was originally detected because of their different R_f values in chromatography. Friedrich (1965) designated the slower moving component as the a isomer, the faster moving as the b isomer. Further work showed that for all the isomeric pairs studied the a isomers shared certain features in common, such as R_f value, basicity and acidity, absorption and circular dichroism spectra (see below), which distinguished them as a group from the b isomers.

Two pieces of evidence have been obtained for the relative orientation of the axial ligands in the two isomers. The first, provided by Friedrich (1966a; Friedrich et al., 1967), is based on arguments relating the effect of the position of a carboxylic acid side-chain on the properties of the two isomers to the steric requirements for the formation of a hydrogen-bond between the carboxylate anion of the side-chain and H_2O co-ordinated in the lower position, see below. The second and more direct approach involves cyanoaquocobyric acid (Factor V_{1a}), which has been shown by X-ray analysis to be the l-isomer (i.e. cyanide co-ordinated in the lower position). It was shown by thin layer chromato-graphy that the isomer present in a crystalline sample of Factor V_{1a} was the slower-moving (or a-) isomer; unless different crystalline samples happen by chance to contain different isomers, then Friedrich's a-isomers can be identified as those with cyanide co-ordinated in the lower position, i.e. the l-isomer (Firth et al., 1968c). Since both approaches give the same result, one can be reasonably certain that the relative orientation of the two ligands has been established.

The rate of interconversion of the isomers is increased by heat, light, bases, CO (compared to H$_2$, N$_2$ or CO$_2$ as the gas phase), HCN and increased concentration, but is inhibited by O$_2$ (Friedrich, 1965, 1966a; Friedrich and Bieganowski, 1967; Friedrich and Moskophidis, 1968; Friedrich et al., 1967). Isomerization, at least in some cases, requires the presence of free cyanide and proceeds through the intermediate formation of the dicyanide complex (Firth et al., 1968c).

Friedrich and co-workers (Friedrich et al., 1967; Friedrich and Moskophidis 1968) have studied the equilibrium shown by certain pairs of isomers in aqueous solution over the range of pH 2.5–8. For compounds which lack the aminopropanol side-chain at position f in the corrin ring, but possess a carboxylic acid side-chain at some other position, the proportion of the l- (or a-) isomer is 50–70% at pH $\leqslant$3 (where the carboxylic acids are undissociated, i.e. —COOH) but falls to a lower value at pH $\geqslant$5 (i.e. —COO$^-$), the proportion depending on the number of carboxylate groups, viz. ~35% for one, ~30% for two, ~25% for three and ~20% for four (studied out to pH 12 in this case). They explained this behaviour by suggesting that the u- (or b-) isomer is stabilized by the formation of a hydrogen-bond between the H$_2$O co-ordinated in the lower position and the anionic form of a downward-projecting propionic acid side-chain. By contrast, those compounds which possess both the aminopropanol and phosphate residue at position f in the corrin ring (cobinamide-phosphoric acid and derivatives containing a carboxylic acid side-chain) all contain 50–60% of the l-isomer at equilibrium and the proportion does not vary with pH. They explained this observation by suggesting that the phosphate can interact equally with both sides of the corrin ring. They must, of course, also assume that the phosphate interacts with co-ordinated H$_2$O far more strongly than does the carboxylate. Another possibility is, however, that the phosphate does not interact with the co-ordinated H$_2$O at all, but that the aminopropanol forms a hydrogen-bond to the carboxylate and thereby suppresses the latter's effect on the equilibrium between the isomers. There can be little doubt that such effects of the nature and stereochemistry of the side-chains on equilibria involving the axial ligands can be ascribed to changes in hydrogen-bonding; but with such complex molecules it is difficult to identify the site of these hydrogen-bonds with complete certainty. Nor can one exclude the possible effects of hydrogen-bonds to the axial ligands at pH $\leqslant$2. Other examples of such effects of hydrogen-bonding in corrinoids are mentioned in Section V,G. The above results show that in every case the concentrations of isomers a and b are fairly similar. The equilibrium constant $K = $ [a]/[b] ranges from 1.5 (60% a) to 0.25 (20% a), i.e. K varies by a factor of only 6 and log$_{10}K$ by a factor of only 0.8. This is small compared to the variations discussed in

Section IV and suggests that the formation constants for the substitution of co-ordinated H_2O by CN^- in the two different axial positions of the diaquo complex do not differ by more than a factor of 10 at most.

Both isomers of a tetracarboxylic acid, probably cyanoaquo-[cobyrinic acid a, c, g-triamide], have been isolated in crystalline form (Friedrich, 1966a; Friedrich et al., 1967). The two isomers have very different crystal habits; the l- (or a-) isomer forms short, rhombic rods, the u- (or b-) isomer long, fine hairs. The l-isomer appears to be the more soluble in water. As expected, no isomerization is observed in the solid state.

There is some information available on the difference in physical properties between pairs of isomers. Friedrich has published data on the absorption spectra of the isomeric pairs of the cyanoaquo complexes of cobinamide, cobinamide-phosphoric acid, cobyric acid and a tetracarboxylic acid (Friedrich, 1966b). The spectra of all four a-isomers appear to be the same within experimental error; similarly, the spectra of all the b-isomers are the same. The following data show the relative positions of the α, β and γ bands (in nm) together with molar extinction coefficients ($\times 10^{-3}$) in brackets for the two sets of isomers. The data represent the average of those given by Friedrich (1966b) for the four pairs of isomers.

	γ	β	α
a-isomers	353.5 (28)	495 (9.1)	527 (8.5)
b-isomers	355 (27)	496 (8.7)	528 (8.2)

The absorption spectra from 250 to 600 nm of the two isomers of the tetra-carboxylic acid have also been published together with slightly modified tabulated data (Friedrich et al., 1967). The circular dichroism spectra appear to be more sensitive to changes in structure than the absorption spectra; relatively greater differences are observed between the a- and b-isomers and differences are also noted with changes in the equatorial ligand. The circular dichroism spectra of the two isomers of cobinamide-phosphoric acid from 400 to 600 nm have been published (Friedrich et al., 1967) together with tabulated data for four pairs of isomers (see Table 8.2). The two isomers of cyanoaquo-cobinamide show a slightly different proton magnetic resonance due to the proton on C_{10} of the corrin ring (τ-values of 3.47 and 3.53 in D_2O at 0–20°), but it is not known which isomer gives which signal (Hill et al., 1968a; Firth et al., 1968a). The infrared spectra of the two isomers of the tetracarboxylic acid, on the other hand, show no significant differences and in both cases the cyanide stretching frequency occurs at 2136 cm^{-1} (Friedrich et al., 1967). The absorption and proton magnetic resonance spectra both suggest that the electron density in the corrin ring is slightly different in the two isomers; it may be that the cyanide is more electronegative in the l- (or a-) isomer (Friedrich *et al.*, 1967).

One might expect all corrinoids where the two axial ligands are different to be capable of showing stereoisomerism, unless precluded by steric factors such as the structure of the nucleotide side-chain, which allows Bzm to co-ordinate only in the lower position. But since most other ligands have much lower formation constants than cyanide, the free ligand may be formed more easily and isomerization proceed more rapidly, which would make it difficult to establish the existence of two isomers. SO_3^{2-} and NH_3 are two other ligands where isomers might be observed, since the formation constants can be high and the rates of substitution low. It has, in fact, been suggested that slight

Table 8.2. *Circular dichroism spectra of isomeric pairs of cyanoaquocorrinoids*

| | | Maxima ($\Delta\epsilon$) at | | |
Equatorial ligand	Isomer	430 nm	490 nm	550 nm
Cobinamide	a	+16.0	−6.8	+3.3
	b	+12.5	−6.1	
Cobyric acid	a	+14.6	−7.4	+3.2
	b	+11.7	−6.3	
Tetracarboxylic acid	a	+14.3	−7.4	+3.8
	b	+11.8	−6.4	
Cobinamidephosphoric acid	a	+16.6	−5.6	+4.6
	b	+11.5	−4.4	

Data from Friedrich *et al.* (1967) and Friedrich (1966b). Friedrich's nomenclature has been used. For the structures of the equatorial ligands see Table 8.1 and the discussion in Section II,A. Friedrich's a- and b-isomers are the l- and u-isomers respectively.

variations in the spectra of sulphitocobinamide and sulphitocobalamin in acid solution may be due to the existence of stereoisomers (Firth *et al.*, 1969).

C. STEREOISOMERS OF ALKYLCORRINOIDS

From the historical point of view, interest in the possibility of stereoisomerism involving the axial ligands was focused on the alkylcorrinoids before attention turned to the cyanoaquocorrinoids, but isolation of both stereoisomers was achieved later in the case of the alkylcorrinoids. Both Müller and Müller (1963) and Zagalak (1963) looked unsuccessfully for the existence of isomers amongst alkylcorrinoids and determined the position of the alkyl ligand in the single known isomer. It was Friedrich and Nordmeyer (1968) who demonstrated the existence of two isomers in the case of methylcobalamin; since then Friedrich and co-workers have established the existence of several other pairs of isomers.

The simplest type of isomerism one can envisage for organocorrinoids is that involving the exchange of the two axial ligands, as shown schematically in A and B (see Fig. 8.1). In this section the organocorrinoids are all treated as being six-co-ordinate, although in fact they are probably present in aqueous solution as a mixture of the five-co-ordinate complex and the six-co-ordinate

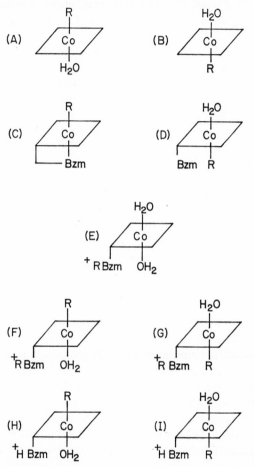

Fig. 8.1. Possible isomers of organocorrinoids. R is an alkyl ligand.

complex with co-ordinated H_2O (see Section III). In the case of the cobalamins, true isomerism involving simply the exchange of the two axial ligands is impossible since Bzm is apparently unable, for steric reasons, to co-ordinate to the cobalt in the upper position. The two "isomers" of organocobalamins are represented in C and D. Since organocorrinoids are prepared by alkylating cobalt(I) corrinoids, additional products may be formed by the alkylation of sites other than the cobalt atom. In the cobalamins, for example, the N_3 of Bzm may also be alkylated. We, therefore, have the possibility of a cobalamin alkylated only on N_3 (E) and of another pair of "isomers" involving alkylation of N_3 as well as the cobalt atom (F and G). Finally the acidification of solutions C and D will give the compounds H and I, in which Bzm has been protonated. Examples of all these types are now known (see below). A carboxylic acid side-chain may also be alkylated to give the ester (Friedrich and Messerschmidt, 1969).

Müller and Müller (1963) prepared butylcobinamide (in 74% yield) by reducing cyanoaquocobinamide with zinc dust and ammonium chloride solution and alkylating the cobalt(I) complex with n-butyl iodide, and claimed that no mixture of isomers was formed; but it is probably safer to conclude that one isomer was formed preferentially ($\geqslant 74\%$). They also showed that cultures of *Propionibacterium shermanii* convert butylcobinamide into butylcobalamin (and more slowly into DBC): if one excludes the unlikely possibility of the isomerization of butylcobinamide *in vivo*, then this means that the butyl ligand occupies the same position in the cobinamide as in the cobalamin, i.e. the u-position. They also showed that three different ways of preparing 5-deoxy-adenosylcobinamide (cobinamidecoenzyme), viz. (1) alkylation of cobin-amide-cobalt(I) (61% yield), (2) biosynthesis using *Propionibacterium shermanii* and (3) removal of the side-chain from DBC by treating with cerous hydroxide, all gave products which were shown to be identical by chromatography, electrophoresis and absorption spectroscopy; again this shows that both synthetic and biosynthetic methods produce mainly or entirely the u-isomer.

Zagalak (1963) prepared several alkylcobinamides (from methyl to decyl) by a standard method involving the reduction of cyanoaquocobinamide with zinc and magnesium in ammonium chloride solution, followed by alkylation with an alkyl halide; in addition he prepared methylcobinamide under different conditions of pH, reducing agent and alkylating agent (MeI, Me_2SO_4). Yields of 80–90% were obtained in all cases. No isomers were, he claimed, observed; but here again it is probably safer to say that one isomer is formed preferentially ($\geqslant 90\%$). The position of the methyl ligand was established by removing the nucleotide side-chain from methylcobalamin in two different ways, viz.

1. treatment with 65% $HClO_4$ at room temperature for three hours (almost complete conversion) and
2. reaction with cerous hydroxide at 95° for 30 minutes (30% conversion).

Both products were identical with the methylcobinamide prepared by alkylation of cobinamide-cobalt(I) and the methyl ligand in the cobinamide must therefore occupy the u-position as in the cobalamin.

Very recently Friedrich and his co-workers have demonstrated the existence of several pairs of isomers. As examples of the simple u- and l-isomers represented by A and B (see Fig. 8.1), they obtained the two isomers of both methyl- and ethyl-[cobyric acid] (Friedrich and Messerschmidt, 1969). They failed, however, to resolve a methyl-[tetracarboxylic acid] and methyl-[cobinamide-phosphoric acid] into two isomers (Friedrich and Nordmeyer, 1969) and have apparently made no attempt to separate the two possible isomers of any alkyl-cobinamides. The cobalamins present a more complicated picture. The two isomers (C and D) of both methyl- and ethyl-cobalamin and the pairs of isomers methylated on the N_3 of Bzm as well as cobalt (F and G) have all been isolated (Friedrich and Nordmeyer, 1968, 1969); the monocyanide derivatives of E, in which the N_3 but not the cobalt is methylated, is produced together with

Table 8.3. *Absorption spectra of isomers of organocorrinoids*

Compound	Structure	Main absorption bands (nm)		
u-Methyl-[cobalamin(BzmH$^+$)]	H	305	376	462
u-Methyl-[cobinamide]	A	305		462
u-Methyl-[cobyric acid]	A	305		464
l-Methyl-[cobalamin(BzmH$^+$)]	I	308		492
l-Methyl-[cobyric acid]	B	307		491
u-Ethyl-[cobalamin(BzmH$^+$)]	H	303	385	444
u-Ethyl-[cobinamide]	A	303	385	444
u-Ethyl-[cobyric acid]	A	304	383	444
l-Ethyl-[cobalamin(BzmH$^+$)][a]	I	307		478
l-Ethyl[cobyric acid][a]	B	305		474

Data taken from Friedrich and Messerschmidt (1969) except that those marked[a] have been corrected in accordance with a personal communication. For diagrams of structures see Fig. 8.1. The u- and l-isomers correspond to Friedrich's b and a isomers respectively. Further details, e.g. of extinction coefficients, are given in the original paper.

the last pair of isomers (F and G), but this may of course be produced from F and G by, for example, photolysis.

The relative orientations of the two isomers of methyl- and ethyl-[cobyric acid] have been established by comparison of their spectra with those of the cobalamins. Some of the relevant spectroscopic data are given in Table 8.3. The data demonstrate that changes in the side-chains (i.e. outside the chromophore) have very little effect on the spectrum, but that exchange of the position of the axial ligands has a very noticeable effect. Comparison of the spectra provides therefore an excellent means of identifying the stereoisomers of organocorrinoids.

Friedrich and co-workers have shown that the stereoisomers can be inter-converted. The most complete and interesting information relates to the isomers of methyl-[cobyric acid] (Friedrich and Messerschmidt, 1969). The two isomers can be interconverted in solution either by (1) heating at 95° in an atmosphere of CO for one to several hours or by (2) photolysis at 20° in an atmosphere of CO. Use of either isomer as the starting material gave the same equilibrium mixture containing 7–8% of the l-isomer (the a isomer in Friedrich's nomenclature). They also made the interesting observation that roughly the same ratio of isomers is obtained from the methylation of the cobalt(I) complex, i.e. under apparently non-equilibrium conditions. The two isomers of methylcobalamin may also be interconverted by heating at 85–95° for several hours in an atmosphere of N_2 or CO; some by-products such as aquocobalamin are also formed (Friedrich and Nordmeyer, 1968, 1969). The effect of light has apparently not been studied in this case. The equilibrium mixture contains 2.5% of the l-isomer (Friedrich's "a" isomer); again this is similar to the ratio of isomers obtained from the methylation of cobalamin-cobalt(I). They were able to show by the use of methylcobalamin labelled with ^{14}C in the methyl ligand that an exchange of methyl ligands occurred when a solution of methylcobalamin and methylcobinamide was heated at 95° under nitrogen, but that no reaction was observed at 50° (Friedrich and Nordmeyer, 1968, 1969). On the other hand, heating a solution of either isomer of methylcobalamin at 85° for 6 hours (gas not stated, but presumably CO or N_2) gave no cyanoaquo-[cobalamin($N_3CH_3^+$)] (after separation involving the use of cyanide), which indicates that the methyl group cannot be transferred from the cobalt to the N_3 atom of Bzm; they also found that heating a solution of the u-isomer of methyl-Bzm-[cobalamin($N_3CH_3^+$)] under the same conditions gave no cyanocobalamin or methylcobalamin (Friedrich and Nordmeyer, 1969).

Two questions arising from the above results are

1. what is the mechanism of isomerization and
2. what determines the position of the equilibrium between the two isomers?

Since both light and heat (~90°) promote isomerization, while light is known to cause homolytic cleavage of the Co–C bond (see Chapter 14) and heating probably has the same effect (see Chapter 14, Section II,A), one may conclude that isomerization occurs via the reversible formation of methyl radicals and cobalt(II) complexes, i.e.

$$CH_3{-}Co \xrightleftharpoons{\text{heat or light}} CH_3. + Co(II)$$

Friedrich and Messerschmidt (1969) noted the interesting fact that the percentage of the l-isomer of, for example, the cobyric acid complexes, varied with the nature of the axial ligand as follows:

—CN 50% (at equilibrium)
—CH₃ 8% (at equilibrium and from methylation of cobalt(I))
—CH₂CH₃ 1% (from ethylation of cobalt(I) only).

From these figures we can obtain rough values of the equilibrium constants $K = $ [u-isomer]/[l-isomer], as follows:

—CN $K = 1$ $\log_{10} K = 0$
—CH₃   11.5   ~1
—CH₂CH₃   ~100   ~2

This is both the order of increasing donor power of the ligand X (see Section V) and of increasing size. Müller and Müller (1963) suggested that the apparently exclusive alkylation at the upper position was due to the fact that the lone pair of electrons on the cobalt(I) ion (or the hydride ion, if it picked up a proton) was located on the upper side—a distortion due presumably to some subtle, but unspecified, effect of the non-planarity of the corrin ring. Hodgkin (1964), on the other hand, has pointed out that access to the lower site is hindered by the presence of the methyl group CH₃ 24 on C1. This steric repulsion between CH₃ 24 and ligands in the lower co-ordination site is clearly shown by X-ray analysis and is discussed in Chapter 6, Section I. It provides a natural explanation why the lower position becomes less favoured as the size of the ligand increases.

Friedrich has pointed out that the difference in the absorption spectrum between the two isomers is smaller when X is cyanide (i.e. when the difference in stability is smallest) than when X is methyl or ethyl (Friedrich and Messerschmidt, 1969). He has also noted that the spectra of the l-isomers of methylcorrinoids are less "abnormal" (i.e. the first absorption band occurs at longer wavelength, nearer the usual position of the $\alpha\beta$ bands; see Table 8.3) than those of the u-isomers, and concluded that the methyl ligand acts as a poorer donor in the l-isomer in agreement with the lower stability of this isomer (Friedrich and Nordmeyer, 1969); the difference in spectra could, however, also be due to different proportions of the five- and six-co-ordinate complexes (see Chapter 5, Section I).

There are very few references to other possible isomers of organocorrinoids. Smith and co-workers reported (Smith et al., 1964) that acetylcobalamin apparently exists in two forms. The form which they obtained (from the reaction of cobalamin-cobalt(I) with acetyl chloride or acetic anhydride, but conditions not stated) is yellow at all pHs, but turns red on photolysis, while its solution in aqueous acetone slowly deposits orange-red crystals of the second form. This second form, which has been obtained directly in other laboratories, gives a red solution which turns yellow below pH 4.5. It is possible that the red and yellow forms may be the u- and l-isomers respectively.

III. FIVE-CO-ORDINATE COBALT(III) CORRINOIDS

Although the vast majority of cobalt(III) complexes whether corrinoids or others are octahedral, it has been found that organocobalt(III) complexes as a class may also adopt a square pyramidal configuration or, in one case at least, achieve an octahedral configuration by the dimerization of two square pyramidal units. For examples of other structures adopted by cobalt(III) complexes (tetrahedral, square planar, trigonal bipyramidal, trigonal prismatic) see the review by Pratt and Thorp (1969). Evidence for five-co-ordination is more complete for certain non-corrinoid complexes and these will be discussed first.

Costa and co-workers (Costa et al., 1966) reported that the solid complexes [R.Co.BAE.H$_2$O] where R is Me, Et or Ph could lose H$_2$O on heating or on standing over P$_2$O$_5$ to give complexes which dissolved in benzene as diamagnetic monomers. Further examples where R is propyl, vinyl, etc., were reported later (Costa and Mestroni, 1968). They suggested that these complexes had a five-co-ordinate, i.e. square pyramidal, structure. Proof of this structure was provided by an X-ray analysis of the structure of [CH$_3$.Co.BAE] by Brückner et al. (1969). The configuration around the cobalt atom is a square pyramid; the cobalt atom is situated 0.12 Å above the basal plane comprising the two oxygen and two nitrogen ligand atoms. The structure of [Vinyl.Co. BAE.H$_2$O] has also been determined by X-ray analysis (Brückner et al., 1968); in this case the cobalt atom is six-co-ordinate and lies very nearly in the plane of the two oxygen and two nitrogen atoms of the BAE ligand.

Schrauzer and Windgassen (1966a) reported that when they distilled solutions in benzene of the complexes [R.Co(DMG)$_2$.H$_2$O], where R is Me or Et but not Pr, solids of composition [R.Co(DMG)$_2$] were deposited. They suggested that these complexes were associated in the solid state by interaction between the cobalt atom of one complex with an oxime oxygen of a neighbouring complex. Ludwick and Brown (1969) subsequently determined the molecular weight of [CH$_3$.Co(DMG)$_2$] in methylene chloride and found that it corresponded to that of a dimer. The postulated structure is similar to that found in bis-dimethylglyoximato-copper(II), in which the two M(DMG)$_2$ units lie parallel and one oxygen atom of each M(DMG)$_2$ unit is co-ordinated (by interaction of the p-orbital of the planar O atom) to the M of the other unit to give a centrosymmetric dimeric unit (see C below). The n.m.r. spectrum at low temperature is apparently in agreement with this structure (Ludwick and Brown, 1969).

The organo-cobalt(III) complexes can therefore adopt three different structures, represented schematically below: monomeric octahedral (A), monomeric square pyramidal (B) and dimeric (C).

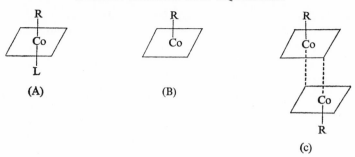

(A)   (B)

(c)

Although B has been shown to occur in the BAE complexes and C in DMG complexes, there is probably little difference in energy between B and C and both structures might well be shown by the same complex under slightly different conditions.

Costa and co-workers also found evidence for unusual structures, presumed to be five-co-ordinate, amongst the organo-cobalt(III)-salen complexes (Costa *et al.*, 1967). In addition, a few equilibrium constants have been reported for the binding of pyridine by five-co-ordinate organo-cobalt(III)-BAE complexes (Hill *et al.*, 1968b), and it has been shown that ligand substitution reactions of certain other organo-cobalt(III) complexes proceed via the formation of five-co-ordinate intermediates (Costa *et al.*, 1970) (see also Chapter 12, Section I).

Finally, certain equilibria were observed in organocobinamides (and some organocobalamins), both in solution and in the solid state, which were ascribed to equilibria between six- and five-co-ordinate monomeric complexes (Firth *et al.*, 1967b, 1968a). Since the dimeric structure C can be excluded because this equilibrium is independent of concentration and the square pyramidal structure has been proved to exist in the BAE complexes, it seems reasonable to accept the occurrence of a square pyramidal structure amongst the organo-corrinoids. But conclusive proof by X-ray analysis would be welcome.

The discovery of this equilibrium between six- and five-co-ordinate corrinoids arose from attempts to establish that B_{12} and DBC retained the same structure in solution as already established by X-ray analysis for the solid state by comparison of the absorption spectra of their solutions in different solvents with the reflection spectra of the solids. The absorption and reflection spectra of B_{12} were very similar and scarcely affected by the nature of the solvent, while those of DBC showed much greater variation (Hill, J. A. *et al.*, 1964). Further study, involving the effect of temperature on the absorption spectrum in solution and the effect of varying the water content of the solid on the reflection spectrum of the solid, suggested the existence of some chemical equilibrium. Since the effect of any variable (such as temperature or solvent) on displacing the position of an equilibrium would be superimposed upon the background of its usual effects on spectra (as observed, for example, in aromatic hydrocarbons), a wide range of compounds and conditions were studied (Firth *et al.*, 1968a). The compounds studied were: cyano-, vinyl-, methyl-, ethyl-, isopropyl- and sulphito-cobinamide; dicyanocobinamide in the presence of excess cyanide (where no change in the nature of the axial ligands could occur); and aquo-, cyano-, ethinyl-, vinyl-, methyl-, ethyl- and 5-deoxyadenosyl-(DBC)-cobalamin. Experiments were carried out to determine the effect of

1. temperature on the absorption spectra (from $-180°C$ in a glass to $+95°$ in water),
2. different solvents on the absorption spectra at room temperature (H_2O, EtOH, dimethylsulphoxide, pyridine),
3. varying the water content of the solid on the reflection spectra of the solids and
4. temperature on the proton magnetic resonance of the methine hydrogen of the corrin ring C_{10}-H and the hydrogens of co-ordinated methyl Co-CH$_3$ (from $-50°C$ in CD$_3$OD to $+95°$ in D$_2$O).

No significant changes in the absorption, reflection or p.m.r. spectra were observed for either dicyanocobinamide or cyanocobalamin, where the identity of the two axial ligands is known and no change is likely. Significant changes were, however, observed in many other cases, and these can most readily be interpreted by reference to the known *trans*-effect order of ligands (see Section V), i.e.

$$H_2O < CN^- < \text{ethinyl} < \text{vinyl} < \text{methyl} < \text{ethyl} < \text{isopropyl}$$

In the case of the cobinamides it was found that:

1. Significant changes in the absorption, reflection and p.m.r. spectra were observed when X is vinyl or methyl (see Fig. 5.3), none when X is cyanide (except for partial conversion to cyanohydroxocobinamide on drying the solid), ethyl (except for a change in absorption spectrum at very low temperature) and isopropyl. Furthermore, the high temperature forms of vinyl- and methyl-cobinamide have similar absorption spectra and τ-values to those of isopropylcobinamide, the low-temperature forms to those of cyanoaquocobinamide (see Table 8.4.) This suggests that the cobinamides as a group can exist in two forms; the end-members (cyano- and isopropyl-cobinamide) exist in one form only, while the intermediate members (vinyl-cobinamide etc.) are present as an equilibrium mixture.
2. The effect of varying the water content of the solid on the reflection spectrum shows that H_2O (whether co-ordinated or not) is involved in the equilibrium in the solid state. The role of water cannot be studied directly in solution, but the similar positions of the absorption bands and isosbestic

points show that the equilibria observed in solution and in the solid state are analogous.

3. It was furthermore found that the equilibrium shown by vinylcobinamide did not involve the co-ordination of O_2 or dimerization and that the equilibrium shown by methylcobinamide did not involve the co-ordination of any amide side-chain.

Hence we can conclude that the equilibrium involves the removal of co-ordinated H_2O (or some other solvent molecule) to give the five-co-ordinate square pyramidal cobinamide, i.e.

$$[X.Co.corrin.H_2O] \rightleftharpoons [X.Co.corrin] + H_2O$$

and that cyanoaquocobinamide exists entirely as the six-co-ordinate complex under all conditions so far investigated, while isopropylcobinamide exists entirely as the five-co-ordinate complex. Vinyl- and methyl-cobinamide exist as equilibrium mixtures of the two forms in aqueous solution at room temperature. Sulphitocobinamide can also give the two forms. Data from Firth *et al.* (1968a) relating to the equilibria and the τ-values and absorption bands of the five- and six-co-ordinate cobinamides are given in Table 8.4.

Changes were also observed in the case of certain cobalamins on varying the temperature, the solvent or the water content of the solid. The degree of change varied with the ligand X in the order: CN^-, ethinyl, vinyl (no significant change) $\leqslant$ methyl $\ll$ 5-deoxyadenosyl $\sim$ ethyl. It was shown that the high-temperature form in solution and the "dry" form in the solid had the same absorption spectrum as the cobinamide, i.e. the observed equilibrium involved the displacement of Bzm from co-ordination to the cobalt. Aqueous solutions of ethyl- and 5-deoxyadenosyl-cobalamin at 20° contain ~15 and 10% of the high-temperature form respectively (Firth *et al.*, 1968a). The organo-cobalamins can therefore exist in solution as an equilibrium mixture of three species represented schematically below in A (the expected six-co-ordinate complex in which Bzm is co-ordinated), B (six-co-ordinate; Bzm replaced by H_2O, but not protonated) and C (five-co-ordinate):

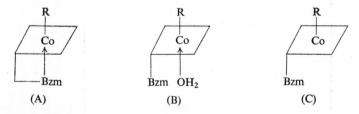

The possibility that some of the equilibria of organocorrinoids discussed above might involve changes in the spin state of the cobalt(III) ion was considered but rejected, both because p.m.r. spectra were observed in every case

Table 8.4. *Data relating to the equilibria between five- and six-co-ordinate cobinamides*

Ligand X	%5-c.n. present in[a]		Thermodynamic data[a]		Main absorption bands[b] of		τ-values of C$_{10}$-H	
	EtOH at −180°	H$_2$O at +20°	ΔH (Kcal/mole)	ΔS (e.u.)	6-c.n. form (EtOH, −180°)	5-c.n. form (H$_2$O, +95°)	6-c.n. (CD$_3$OD, 50°)	5-c.n. (D$_2$O, 95°)
CN⁻	0	0	0	—	320, 353, (385), 404, (470), 498, 531	—	3.47, 3.53[c]	—
CH$_2$=CH—	5	70	4.5 ± 2.0	15.5 ± 7	299, (313), 333 (350), 363, (467), 495 (518)	266, 284, 325, 451	3.60–3.70[d]	3.10–3.20[d]
CH$_3$—	20	90	4.4 ± 2.0	16 ± 7	313, 337, (352), 369, (467), 503, (529)	306, 373, 458, (at 65°)	3.45–3.65[d]	3.03–3.15[d]
CH$_3$CH$_2$—	30	100			301, 339, (356), (373), 503	305, 383, 445–455	—	3.04
Me$_2$CH—	100	100			—	266, 306, 444, (488) (at 20°)	—	3.03
SO$_3^{2-}$	5	95			(308), 326, 351, 418, 485, 514	(313), 322, 360, 445		

Data taken from Firth *et al.* (1968a).

5-c.n. and 6-c.n. are the five- and six-co-ordinate forms.

[a] For formation of 5-c.n. from 6-c.n. in CD$_3$OD.

[b] Wavelengths in nm. Shoulders given in brackets.

[c] Two signals due to the presence of two isomers involving the axial ligands (CN⁻, H$_2$O).

[d] Extrapolated values.

and because of the absence of any large shift in τ-values, which one would expect as a consequence of a contact shift due to delocalization of unpaired spin from the cobalt onto the corrin ring (Firth *et al.*, 1968a).

Other organo-corrinoids are expected to behave similarly to the organo-cobinamides and cobalamins discussed above; acidified solutions of organo-cobalamins, in which the Bzm has been displaced and protonated, will of course behave like the analogous cobinamides. The spectrum of cyclohexyl-cobinamide (Brodie, 1969) is almost identical to that of isopropylcobinamide (Firth *et al.*, 1968a) and therefore presumably exists entirely as the five-co-ordinate complex. The spectrum of 5-deoxyadenosyl-[adenylcobamide] (AC) is the same in both acid and alkaline solution as that of DBC in acid, i.e. the adenine is not co-ordinated (Bernhauer *et al.*, 1960a; Ladd *et al.*, 1961) and AC is probably present almost entirely as the five co-ordinate complex (Hill *et al.*, 1970b). Five-co-ordinate complexes may also be formed by corrinoids with certain ligands other than organo-ligands. The effect of temperature on the spectrum of sulphitocobinamide, for example, is similar to that observed with the organocobinamides (Firth *et al.*, 1968a); the relevant data are given in Table 8.4. It was also suggested that solutions of cobinamides containing very polarizable ligands such as $S_2O_3^{2-}$, thiolates, I^- or $NCSe^-$, which are similar to SO_3^{2-} and organo-ligands in their effect on other properties of the corrinoids, might in fact contain five-co-ordinate complexes (Firth *et al.*, 1968a). Solutions of organocorrinoids in strong acid (e.g. concentrated sulphuric acid) are also likely to contain five-co-ordinate complexes (see Chapter 9, Section III).

We can use the data of Tables 8.4 and 8.8 to derive equilibrium constants for the binding of several ligands Z by the five-co-ordinate corrinoid, i.e..

$$K_{5/6} = \frac{[X-Co-Z]}{[X-Co][Z]} \quad \text{(in units of M}^{-1}\text{)} \tag{8.1}$$

The results are given in Table 8.5. The ligands X are arranged in the order of their *trans*-effect, as discussed in Section V. Columns 2 and 3 give the ratios of the six-co-ordinate to the five-co-ordinate complexes under the experimental conditions indicated, i.e. in water at 20°

$$K_{H_2O} = \frac{[X-Co-H_2O]}{[X-Co]} \tag{8.2}$$

and in ethanol at −180°, assuming that the sixth ligand is EtOH,

$$K_{EtOH} = \frac{[X-Co-EtOH]}{[X-Co]} \tag{8.3}$$

The values of 0 and 100% taken from Table 8.4 have been treated as ≤2 and ≥98% in these calculations. Columns 4–8 give the equilibrium constants $K_{5/6}$ defined as above for the binding of the stated ligand Z. The constant for

$Z = H_2O$ is obtained by dividing K_{H_2O} by the molarity of H_2O in the pure solvent (viz. 56). The other constants have been derived as follows. The formation constants listed in Table 8.8 are the "observed" formation constants

$$K_{obs} = \frac{[X—Co—Z]}{([X—Co] + [X—Co—OH_2])[Z]} \qquad (8.4)$$

i.e. the aquocorrinoid is treated as though it exists in solution as only one species and no account is taken of the formation of five-co-ordinate complexes. If we substitute (8.2) into (8.4) we obtain

$$K_{obs} = \frac{[X—Co—Z]}{[Z]([X—Co] + K_{H_2O}[X—Co])} \qquad (8.5)$$

Hence $K_{5/6} = K_{obs}(1 + K_{H_2O})$ (8.6)

Table 8.5. *Equilibria between five- and six-co-ordinate corrinoids*

Trans-ligand X	K_{EtOH} (in EtOH at $-180°$)	K_{H_2O} (in water at $+20°$)	$\log_{10} K_{5/6}$ for Z =				
			H_2O	Bzm	NH_3	HO^-	CN^-
CN^-	$\geqslant 50$	$\geqslant 50$	$\geqslant 0$	$\geqslant 6.3$	$\geqslant 5.1$	$\geqslant 4.7$	$\geqslant 9.7$
SO_3^{2-}	19	0.053	-3.0	2.7	~ 0.6	-0.7	4.4
$CH_2{=}CH—$	19	0.43	-2.1	2.4		<-0.9	2.9
$CH_3—$	4	0.11	-2.7	2.0	-1.0	<-1	2.1
$CH_3CH_2—$	2.33	$\leqslant 0.02$	$\leqslant -3.4$	0.8		<-1	
$Me_2CH—$	$\leqslant 0.02$	$\leqslant 0.02$	$\leqslant -3.4$	<-1			

For definitions of equilibrium constants see text.

Several points can be made about the effect of X on the magnitude of the equilibrium constants in Table 8.5. If we consider only the carbanions, it appears that the same order of ligands ($CN^- >$ vinyl > methyl > ethyl > isopropyl) is observed for each equilibrium. The same order is observed not only when studying the effect of the trans-ligand X on the binding of an additional ligand by a five-co-ordinate complex (Table 8.5), but also on the substitution of one ligand by another in purely six-co-ordinate complexes or in the mixed equilibria represented by K_{obs} (Tables 8.7 and 8.8). The position of SO_3^{2-} is, by contrast, variable; it may lie between cyanide and vinyl (for $Z = CN^-$, HO^- and Bzm), at the same place as vinyl (K_{EtOH}) or between methyl and ethyl (for $Z = H_2O$). The varying position of sulphite relative to the carbanions shows that one or more additional factors are involved, which would probably include a steric factor. Comparison of the known structures of $[CH_3.Co.BAE]$ and $[vinyl.Co.BAE.H_2O]$ (see above) shows that the cobalt lies in the plane of the equatorial ligand atoms in the six-co-ordinate vinylaquo complex, but is situated about 0.12 Å above the plane in the five-co-ordinate organo-complex. Since carbon and sulphur have very different atomic radii (0.77 and 1.04 Å respectively), one might expect to find differences between C-ligands as a group and S-ligands as a group when dealing with equilibria between five- and six-co-ordinate complexes. It would be interesting to see whether other S-ligands such as thiosulphate and thiolates behave similarly to sulphite in this respect.

No five-co-ordinate sulphito-cobalt(III) complexes have yet been reported other than sulphitocobinamide. In fact the only other unidentate ligand (apart from sulphite and the organo-ligands) giving rise to a group of complexes, which show both five- and six-co-ordination and which could formally be written as cobalt(III) complexes, is nitric oxide (NO), complexes containing which are called nitrosyls; for examples and references see Pratt and Thorp (1969). These cobalt nitrosyls are prepared by the reaction of cobalt(II) complexes with nitric oxide (NO). The resulting complexes might be considered as $Co(III) + NO^-$, $Co(II) + NO$ (spins paired) or $Co(I) + NO^+$. They are usually diamagnetic, and are five- or six-co-ordinate. There is clearly an interesting parallel between the nitrosyls and the organo complexes. But because the Co-alkyl bond can only be a σ-bond, while the Co-NO bond probably consists of σ- and π-bonds, the organo-cobalt(III) complexes provide the simplest and most convincing demonstration of the change in stereochemistry from six- to five-co-ordination without any obvious change in valency.

The most interesting aspect of these organo-cobalt(III) complexes, and of the organocorrinoids in particular, is probably that they provide a good illustration of the way in which the concept of formal oxidation states breaks down (Pratt and Thorp, 1969). By varying only one ligand in the series $CN^-\ldots CH_3CH_2^-$ we can pass from a typical cobalt(III) complex to one which is more characteristic of a low-spin cobalt(II) complex. Cobalt(III) complexes are characterized by an octahedral configuration and high formation constants for the substitution of H_2O by NH_3, CN^- etc. Low-spin cobalt(II) complexes, on the other hand, show a balance between six- and five- (and four-) co-ordination and the formation constant for the substitution of, for example, H_2O by CN^- in $[Co^{II}(CN)_5H_2O]$ is very low. Like the nitrosyls, these organo-cobalt complexes could be considered as, for example, $Co(III) + CH_3^-$, $Co(II) + CH_3$ (with antiferromagnetic interaction between the spins of the metal ion and the organic radical) or $Co(I) + CH_3^+$. The usual correlation between stereochemistry and valency and the division into valencies clearly breaks down when we are dealing with very polarizable ligands such as the alkyls, whose oxidation state is not well defined: the term "balanced valency" has been used to describe this situation (Firth $et\ al.$, 1967b). Conversely if we vary the ligands in the order $CH_3CH_2^-\ldots CN^-$, we see how the five-co-ordinate complexes bind different ligands with different formation constants and how these formation constants increase in magnitude at different rates (see Table 8.5); until we observe only six-co-ordinate complexes and can obtain only equilibrium constants for the substitution of one ligand by another (the subject of Sections IV and V).

IV. SUMMARY OF EQUILIBRIUM CONSTANTS IN AQUEOUS SOLUTION

A very large number of equilibrium constants have been determined for the substitution of one axial ligand (Y) by another (Z) in cobalt(III) corrinoids. The corrinoids are probably unique in providing such a large number of step-wise equilibrium constants (K) as distinct from overall equilibrium constants (β), which are often the only experimentally obtainable equilibrium constants. For example, many values of the overall equilibrium constants β ($=K_1K_2$) have been determined for the Ag(I) ion,

$$\beta = \frac{[AgL_2]}{[Ag][L]^2}$$

but values of β are not so readily amenable to theoretical interpretation as values of K. The large amount of experimental information available for the corrinoids reveals a fairly simple underlying pattern, from which deductions can be made about the nature of the factors which determine the magnitude of the equilibrium constants and the stereochemistry (five- or six-co-ordination). All the available equilibrium constants and most of the qualitative observations relating to the binding of different ligands in the axial position of cobalt(III) corrinoids are given in this section. The general pattern shown by the constants and the factors which determine them are discussed in Section V.

The possible permutations of the axial ligands (X, Y and Z) together with the side-chains and substitutents in the corrin ring are immense. Happily, from the point of view of presenting the data, virtually all the equilibrium constants so far determined refer to cobalamins or cobinamides; the only exceptions are cyanoaquo-[cobyric acid] (Factor V_{1a}) and cyano-adenine-[adenylcobamide] (ψ-B_{12}). The entropy and enthalpy changes have only been determined in a very few cases; these are listed in Table 8.6. The remainder of the equilibrium constants are given in Table 8.7. Further qualitative observations are mentioned at the end of this section.

Almost all these equilibrium constants have been determined by spectrophotometry; only a very few have been determined by other methods such as pH-titrations or the effect of pH on ionophoretic mobility (see, for example, Ladd et al., (1961)). All constants have been determined in aqueous solution and most in unthermostated solutions at room temperature, though the exact

Table 8.6. *Thermodynamic data for ligand substitution equilibria in cobalt(III) corrinoids*

Compound	$pK°$	$\Delta G°$ (Kcal/mole)	K (litre/mole)	ΔG (Kcal/mole)	ΔH (Kcal/mole)	ΔS (e.u.)
(1) Ionization of co-ordinated H_2O						
Factor B	⌈10.95 ± 0.02	15.01 ± 0.02			11.0 ± 0.6	−13 ± 2[a]
	⌊10.96	14.95			9.25 ± 0.5	−19 ± 2[b]
Factor V$_{1a}$	11.04	15.06			6.18 ± 0.5	−30 ± 2[b]
Aquocobalamin	7.65	10.43			4.60 ± 0.5	−19 ± 2[b]
(2) Substitution of co-ordinated H_2O by imidazole						
Factor B			1.22×10^4	5.58	−6.30 ± 0.5	−2.4 ± 1.7[b]
Aquocobalamin			3.90×10^4	6.26	−7.30 ± 0.5	−3.5 ± 1.7[b]
			3.90×10^4	6.26	−7.20 ± 0.6	−3.2 ± 2.0[c]
(3) Ionization of co-ordinated imidazole ($C_3H_4N_2°$) to imidazolate ($C_3H_3N_2^-$)						
Cyanoimidazole-cobinamide	11.38	15.50			12.0 ± 1.0	−12 ± 3[b]
Imidazolecobalamin	⌈10.25	14.00			10.4 ± 1.0	−12 ± 3[b]
	⌊10.25 ± 0.02				10.5 ± 1.0	−12 ± 3[c]

References.
[a] Offenhartz and George (1963).
[b] Hanania and Irvine (1964a).
[c] Hanania and Irvine (1964b).

Table 8.7. *Equilibrium constants for ligand substitution in cobalt(III) corrinoids in aqueous solution**

Y	Z	X	pK	K	$\log_{10} K$	References
H$_2$O	F$^-$	Bzm		+	+	Pratt and Thorp (1966)
		CN$^-$		−	−	George et al. (1960)
H$_2$O	Cl$^-$	H$_2$O		3.3	0.5	Hayward et al. (1965)
		Bzm		1.3	0.1	Pratt and Thorp (1966)
		CN$^-$		+	+	Firth et al. (1969)
		—CH=CH$_2$		+	+	Firth et al. (1969)
		—CH$_3$		+	+	Firth et al. (1969)
		—CH$_2$CH$_3$		+	+	Firth et al. (1969)
H$_2$O	Br$^-$	Bzm		1.9	0.3	Pratt and Thorp (1966)
H$_2$O	I$^-$	Bzm		32	1.5	Pratt and Thorp (1966)
		CN$^-$		+	+	Firth et al. (1969)
		—CH=CH$_2$		1	0	Firth et al. (1969)
		—CH$_3$		+	+	Firth et al. (1969)
		—CH$_2$CH$_3$		+	+	Firth et al. (1969)
H$_2$O	HO$^-$	H$_2$O	6.0		8.0	Hayward et al. (1965)
		Bzm	6.9		7.1	Buhs et al. (1951)
			7.5		6.5	Smith et al. (1952b)
			7.65		6.35	Hanania and Irvine (1964a)
			7.72		6.3	Hanania and Irvine (1964b)
			7.8		6.2	Hayward et al. (1965)
		CN$^-$	11		3	George et al. (1960)
			10.95		3.05	Offenhartz and George (1963)
			11.0		3.0	Hayward et al. (1965)
		SO$_3^{2-}$	(14.7)	0.2	−0.7	Firth et al. (1969)
		—CH=CH$_2$	>15		<−1	Firth et al, (1968d)
		—CH$_3$	>15		<−1	Hayward et al. (1965)
		—CH$_2$CH$_3$	>15		<−1	Firth et al. (1968d)
H$_2$O	ClO$_4^-$	Bzm			<−1	Pratt and Thorp (1966)

H_2O	NO_3^-	Bzm		<-1	Pratt and Thorp (1966)
H_2O	PO_4^{3-}	Bzm		—	Hayward et al. (1965)
		CN^-		—	George et al. (1960)
H_2O	$CH_3CO_2^-$	Bzm	4.5	0.7	Firth et al. (1969)
H_2O	$C_6H_5O^-$ (phenolate)	Bzm		2.9	Hill et al. (1970b)
		CN^-		—	George et al. (1950)
H_2O	NH_3	H_2O		$\geqslant 9$	Hayward et al. (1971)
		Bzm		7	Hayward et al. (1971)
		NH_3		$+$	Hayward et al. (1971)
		HO^-		$+$	Hayward et al. (1971)
		CN^-		3.35	Hayward et al. (1971)
		SO_3^{2-}	~ 4	~ 0.6	Hayward et al. (1971)
		$-CH_3$	0.1	~ -1	Pailes and Hogenkamp (1968)
				$\leqslant -0.7$	Brodie (1969)
H_2O	$NH_2.CH_2.CO_2^-$ (glycine)	Bzm	~ 0.1	~ -1	Hayward et al. (1971)
				5.8	Hill et al. (1970b)
H_2O	Piperidine	$-CH_3$	<0.01	<-2	Pailes and Hogenkamp (1968)
H_2O	$NH_2.CH_2.CH_2OH$	$-CH_3$	0.03	-1.5	Pailes and Hogenkamp (1968)
H_2O	Pyridine	Bzm		$+$	Bauriedel et al. (1956)
		CN^-		2.6	Hill et al. (1962)
		SO_3^{2-}		$+$	Hayward et al. (1971)
		$-CH_3$	6	0.8	Bernhauer and Wagner (1963)
				$\leqslant 1$	Pailes and Hogenkamp (1968)
H_2O	Imidazole	H_2O	3.9×10^4	7.5	Brodie (1969)
		Bzm	$+$	4.6	Hayward et al. (1971)
		Imidazole		$+$	Hanania and Irvine (1964a)
		CN^-	1.2×10^4	4.1	Hayward et al. (1971)
				4.7	Hanania and Irvine (1964a)
		SO_3^{2-}		$+$	Hayward et al. (1971)
		$-CH_3$	11	1.0	Hill et al. (1962)
					Pailes and Hogenkamp (1968)

Table 8.7. (*continued*)

Y	Z	X	pK	K	$\log_{10} K$	References
H_2O	1-methylimidazole	—$CH_2CH_2CH_3$		0.1	−1	Pailes and Hogenkamp (1968)
H_2O	Histidine	—CH_3		5	0.7	Pailes and Hogenkamp (1968)
H_2O	Benzimidazole	Bzm			5.8[a]	Bauriedel (1956)
		CN^-			+	George et al. (1960)
		Bzm			2.3	Hill et al. (1962)
H_2O	Adenine	CN^-			+	Hayward et al. (1971)
		SO_3^{2-}			−	Hill et al. (1962)
		CN^-			−	Hayward et al. (1971)
		SO_3^{2-}			−	Hill et al. (1962)
H_2O	$CO(NH_2)_2$ (urea)	CN^-			−	George et al. (1960)
H_2O	Bzm	H_2O	−2.4		7.1	Hayward et al. (1965)
		NH_3	<0		>4.7	Pratt and Thorp (1966)
		Cl^-	<0		>4.7	Pratt and Thorp (1966)
		CH_3NC	−(i.e. <0)		>4.7	Firth et al. (1969)
		CN^-	~0		~4.7	Beaven et al. (1950)
		—$C{\equiv}CH$	0.1		4.6	Hayward et al. (1965)
		—CH_2COOH	0.7		4.0	Hayward et al. (1965)
			1.05		3.65	Dolphin et al. (1963a)
			1.50		3.2	Dolphin et al. (1964a)
		SO_3^{2-}	2.20		2.5	Hogenkamp et al. (1965)
			2.0		2.7	Hill et al. (1962); Firth et al. (1969)
		—CH_2COOCH_3	2.25		2.45	Hogenkamp et al. (1965)
		—$CH{=}CH_2$	2.4		2.3	Hayward et al. (1965)
		—$CH_2CH_2NH_3^+$	2.45		2.25	Hogenkamp (1966b)
		—$CH_2CH_2NMe_3^+$	2.61		2.1	Hogenkamp (1966b)
		—CH_3	2.7		2.0	Dolphin et al. (1963a)
			2.72		2.0	Hogenkamp et al. (1965)

Ligand			Reference
2'3'-Isopropylidene-5'-deoxyadenosyl	2.5	2.2	Hayward et al. (1965)
	2.94	1.8	Dolphin et al. (1963a)
—CH₂CH₂CN	2.95	1.75	Hogenkamp et al. (1965)
—CH₂CH₂OCH₃	3.10	1.6	Hogenkamp et al. (1965)
—CH₂CH₂OH	3.15	1.55	Hogenkamp et al. (1965)
—CH₂CH₂COOH	3.25	1.45	Hogenkamp et al. (1965)
—CH₂CH₂COOCH₃	3.27	1.4	Hogenkamp et al. (1965)
2'5'-Dideoxyadenosyl	3.3	1.4	Hogenkamp and Oikawa (1964)
5'-Deoxyadenosyl (DBC)	3.3–3.5	~1.3	Ladd et al. (1961)
	3.35	1.35	Hill et al. (1962); Hayward et al. (1965)
	3.52	1.2	Johnson et al. (1963a); Dolphin et al. (1963a)
5'-Deoxythymidyl	3.5	1.2	Hogenkamp and Oikawa (1964)
—CH₂CH₃ (ethyl)	3.87	0.8	Hogenkamp et al. (1965)
n-Propyl	3.84	0.8	Hogenkamp et al. (1965)
n-Butyl	3.93	0.8	Dolphin et al. (1963a)
n-Heptyl	4.01	0.6	Dolphin et al. (1963a)
—CO.CH₃ (acetyl)	~4.5	approx. −0.2	Johnson et al. (1963a)
—CHMe₂ (isopropyl)	Probably >5	Probably ≤−1	Firth et al. (1968a)
Br⁻	0–1	~4	Pratt and Thorp (1966)
I⁻	0–1	~4	Pratt and Thorp (1966)
SC(NH₂)₂	0–1	~4	Pratt and Thorp (1966)
NCS⁻	~2	~2.5	Pratt and Thorp (1966)
Thioglycollate (RS⁻)	>0	<4.7	Hayward et al. (1965)
Cysteinate (RS⁻)	>0	<4.7	Hayward et al. (1965)
?HS⁻	>0	<4.7	Hayward et al. (1965)

Table 8.7. (*continued*)

Y	Z	X	pK	K	log$_{10}$ K	References
H_2O		$S_2O_3^{2-}$	>0		<4.7	Hayward et al. (1965)
		p-Toluene-sulphinate	≥0		<5	Dolphin and Johnson (1965b)
H_2O	Adenine	CN^-			~3[b]	Hill et al. (1970b)
		5'-Deoxyadenosyl			<-1	Hill et al. (1970b)
H_2O	N_3^-	Bzm		7.2×10^4	4.9	Firth et al. (1969)
		CN^-		4.8×10^2	2.7	Firth et al. (1969)
		$-CH=CH_2$		3.8	0.6	Firth et al. (1969)
		$-CH_3$			<-1	Firth et al. (1969)
		$-CH_2CH_3$			<-1	Firth et al. (1969)
H_2O	NO_2^-	Bzm		2.3×10^5	5.4	George et al. (1960)
		CN^-		+	+	George et al. (1960)
H_2O	NCO^-	Bzm		530	2.7	Pratt and Thorp (1966)
H_2O	NCS^-, $NCSe^-$	See below				
H_2O	$[Fe(CN)_6]^{4-}$	CN^-		+	+	George et al. (1960)
H_2O	$[Fe(CN)_6]^{3-}$	CN^-		+	+	George et al. (1960)
H_2O	$[Co(CN)_6]^{3-}$	CN^-		+	+	George et al. (1960)
H_2O	CH_3CN	CN^-		–	–	George et al. (1960)
H_2O	$C_3H_3N_2^-$ (imidazolate)	Bzm		–	7.8[c]	Hanania and Irvine (1964a,b)
		CN^-			6.2[c]	Hanania and Irvine (1964a)
H_2O	Benzimidazolate	CN^-			~8	Hayward et al. (1971)
H_2O	Adeninate	CN^-			5	Hayward et al. (1971)
H_2O	CN^-	H_2O			4	Hayward et al. (1971)
		Bzm			≥14[d]	Hayward et al. (1965)
		CN^-			≥12[d]	Hayward et al. (1965)
		$-C\equiv CH$			8	George et al. (1960)
		SO_3^{2-}			6.7[e]	Firth et al. (1969)
					4.3	Firth et al. (1969)

H_2O		$-CH=CH_2$		2.7	Firth et al. (1968d)
		$-CH_3$		2.1	Firth et al. (1968d)
H_2O	CH_3NC	Bzm	230	2.4	Pailes and Hogenkamp (1968)
		CN^-	7×10^4	4.8	Firth et al. (1969)
		$-CH=CH_2$	4×10^2	2.6	George et al. (1960)
		$-CH_3$	6.2×10^2	2.7	Firth et al. (1969)
		$-CH_2CH_3$	4.2	0.6	Firth et al. (1969)
H_2O	$SC(NH_2)_2$	Bzm		<-1	Firth et al. (1969)
		CN^-, CH_3		<-1	Firth et al. (1969)
		$-CH_2CH_3$	13	1.1	Firth et al. (1969)
H_2O	Me_2S	Bzm, CN^-		<-1	Firth et al. (1969)
		$-CH=CH_2, -CH_3$		<-1	Firth et al. (1968a)
		$-CH_2CH_3$		<-1	Firth et al. (1968a)
H_2O	NCS^-	Bzm	1.2×10^3	3.1	Pratt (1964); Pratt and Thorp (1966)
		CN^-	$+$	$+$	George et al. (1960)
		$-CH_3$	$-$	$-$	Pailes and Hogenkamp (1968)
H_2O	HS^-	Bzm	$+$	$+$	Firth et al. (1969)
		CN^-	$+$	$+$	George et al. (1960)
H_2O	$CH_3CH_2S^-$	Bzm	$+$	$+$	Dolphin and Johnson (1965b); Adler et al. (1966)
H_2O	$^-SCH_2CHNH_2.CO_2^-$ (cysteinate)	Bzm		6.0 or 8.3[f]	Hill et al. (1970b)
H_2O	Glutathionate	CN^-	$+$	$+$	Firth et al. (1969)
		$-CH_3$	$-$	$-$	Pailes and Hogenkamp (1968)
H_2O		Bzm		4.9 or 5.8[f]	Adler et al. (1966)
H_2O	SO_3^{2-}	H_2O		~11	Firth et al. (1969)
		Bzm	2.2×10^7	7.3	Firth et al. (1969)
		CN^-	4×10^4	4.6	Firth et al. (1969)

Table 8.7. (*continued*)

Y	Z	X	pK	K	log K	Reference
H_2O	$S_2O_3^{2-}$	SO_3^{2-}			<-1	Firth et al. (1969)
H_2O	$NCSe^-$	$-CH=CH_2$			<-1	Firth et al. (1969)
H_2O	$SeC(NH_2)_2$	$-CH_3$			<-1	Firth et al. (1969)
H_2O	PPh_3	$-CH_2CH_3$			<-1	Firth et al. (1969)
		Bzm		7.3×10^3	3.9	Pratt and Thorp (1966)
		Bzm		8.3×10^3	3.9	Pratt and Thorp (1966)
		Bzm, CN^-		?+	?+	Firth et al. (1969)
		$-CH=CH_2$			<-1	Firth et al. (1969)
		$-CH_3$			<-1	Firth et al. (1969)
		$-CH_2CH_3$			<-1	Firth et al. (1969)
Bzm	CN^-	CN^-		$\sim 3 \times 10^3$	3.5	Diehl and Sealock (1952)
					4	George et al. (1960)
		$-C\equiv CH$			3.8	Firth et al. (1968d)
		$-CH=CH_2$			2.7	Hayward et al. (1965)
		$-CH_3$			0.7	Hayward et al. (1965)
		$-CH_2CH_3$			0.1	Hayward et al. (1965)
		CN^-			<0	Firth et al. (1968d)
Bzm	HO^-	CN^-			<-0.5	Hill et al. (1970b)
Bzm	NCS^-	NCS^-			≈ 1	Pratt, 1964; Pratt and Thorp (1966)
Aden	CN^-	CN^-			5.1	Hill et al. (1970b)
	HO^-	CN^-	13.8		0.2	Hill et al. (1970b)
	Aden H^+[g]	CN^-	2.3			Hill et al. (1970b)
Imidazole ($C_3H_4N_2$)	Imidazolate ($C_3H_3N_2^-$)	Bzm	10.25			Hanania and Irvine (1946a,b)
		CN^-	11.38			Hanania and Irvine (1964a)
Benzimidazole	Benzimidazolate	CN^-	~ 11			Hayward et al. (1971)
		CN^-	9.5			Hayward et al. (1971)

* Equilibria are of the general type (axial ligands only given)

$$[X-Co-Y] + Z \rightleftharpoons [X-Co-Z] + Y$$

where Y is substituted by Z, while X is the non-substituted ligand in the trans-position. For definitions and units of K, pK (and K') see pp. 150–2. For details of experimental conditions consult the original papers.

[a] Calculated from the published value of K' using the value of 9.2 (Sillén and Martell, 1964), for the pK_b of histidine.

[b] If one assumes that equilibrium constants determined for the cobinamides will not be significantly altered by the presence of the unco-ordinated adenosine side-chain, then one can calculate a value for the given equilibrium constant as the product of the equilibrium constants for either (1) the substitution of H_2O in cyanoaquocobinamide by HO^- ($\log_{10} K = 3.0$) and the substitution of HO^- by aden in ψ-B_{12} (-0.2), giving $\log_{10} K = 2.8$ or (2) the substitution of H_2O in cyanoaquocobinamide by CN^- (8) and the substitution of CN^- by aden in ψ-B_{12} (-5.1), giving $\log_{10} K = 2.9$.

[c] Calculated from the published value of the pK_a of co-ordinated imidazole using the method of (Hayward et al., 1971) and the value of 14.5 (Albert, 1959) for the pK_a of free imidazole.

[d] Previously reported values (George et al., 1960) were later shown to be based on a false interpretation of the equilibria observed.

[e] This value has not been determined experimentally, but calculated as the product of the constants for the substitution of H_2O by Bzm and of Bzm by CN^- ($X = -C \equiv CH$) (Firth et al., 1969).

[f] It is not certain which of the pKs of cysteine (8.2 and 10.5) or of glutathione (8.6 and 9.5) correspond to the ionization of the thiol group (Elson and Edsall, 1962; Wallenfels and Streffer, 1966) hence the two values of K.

[g] The adenine remains co-ordinated and the site of protonation is probably the $-NH_2$ group.

conditions are often not stated; for details of the experimental conditions, where available, see the original papers.

In certain cases the nature of the observed equilibrium cannot be specified unambiguously. The evidence concerning the nature of the ligand atom and the possible existence of linkage isomers is discussed below. Two major sources of ambiguity are the possible existence of stereoisomers and of five-co-ordinate complexes. Stereoisomers are theoretically possible whenever X and Y are different (except in the case of the cobalamins, where it is probably impossible for Bzm to be co-ordinated in the u-position for steric reasons). Cyanoaquo complexes, for example, are usually present as a mixture of the two isomers unless obtained as crystalline, while one isomer is the major product for organocobinamides; for a fuller discussion see Section II. Virtually all equilibria involving cobinamides are therefore subject to uncertainty as to whether we are dealing with one or two equilibria involving the formation of the two possible stereoisomers or, if only one, which. However, it has been shown that cyanoaquocorrinoids are present at equilibrium as a mixture of the two isomers in very nearly equal concentrations so that the formation constants for the binding of cyanide by the diaquo complex in the upper and lower positions must be almost identical (see Section II). The possible existence of stereoisomers has therefore been neglected in this section. It is also now known that certain corrinoids where one ligand is a strong donor such as CH_3^- or SO_3^{2-} are present as a mixture of five- and six-co-ordinate complexes (see Section III). In the binding of a ligand Z by, for example, methylcobinamide, the experimentally observed formation constant K_{obs} will therefore differ from the true formation constant, which refers only to six-coordinate complexes, since

$$K_{obs} = \frac{[\text{X—Co—Z}]}{([\text{X—Co—OH}_2] + [\text{X—Co}])[\text{Z}]}$$

where X—Co is the five-coordinate complex. Values of K reported in the Table have not been corrected for the presence of five-co-ordinate complexes, since in most cases the ratio of the six-co-ordinate aquo complex to the five-coordinate complex is not known or known only with low accuracy.

Many equilibria have been studied experimentally as the variation of some property (usually the spectrum) with pH. In most cases the interpretation of the nature of such equilibria is straightforward. Equilibria which involve a change in the spectrum must, of course, involve a change in the chromophore (the corrin ring, the cobalt ion, the co-ordinated atoms of the axial ligands and any other atoms which interact strongly with the latter). Such changes may involve the displacement of one ligand by another (e.g. the displacement of Bzm by H_2O in the cobalamins or of simple bases by H_2O due to protonation of the base, or of adenine in ψ-B_{12} by HO^-) or the ionization of a co-ordinated ligand (e.g. H_2O or imidazole). On the other hand, the ionization of Co—CH_2COOH has only a slight effect on the spectrum (Firth *et al.*, 1968d) and is a border-line case, while the protonation of adenine in 5'-deoxyadenosyl (the organo-ligand present in DBC and other coenzymes) has no effect on the spectrum (Ladd *et al.*, 1961); equilibria of this type are mentioned again in Section IV. It had at one time been suggested (Hill *et al.*, 1962) that the corrin ring could also be reversibly protonated under certain conditions, e.g. in very strong acid and in corrinoids such as methylcobinamide, whose spectra were very different from those of the typical red corrinoids. It still remains to be proved whether the corrin ring can or cannot be protonated in strong acid, but there is now no doubt that the ring is not protonated with the commoner ligands and over the usual range of pH covered by the data of Table 8.7. Equilibria and reactions involving the corrin ring are dealt with in Chapters 9 and 15.

A. THERMODYNAMIC DATA

Table 8.6 lists the thermodynamic data which have been determined for ligand substitution reactions of corrinoids. Values of $pK°$ and $\Delta G°$ were obtained by extrapolation to zero ionic strength. Offenhartz and George (1963) report ΔH for solutions of ionic strength (I) = 0.1. Hanania and Irvine, on the other hand, state that both for the formation and for the ionization of imidazolecobalamin they assume that $\Delta H° = \Delta H$ (determined for I = 0.042) (1964a); for the other equilibria they merely report values of $\Delta H°$ and $T\Delta S°$ without experimental details (1964b), but it seems very likely that here again they assumed $\Delta H°$ to be the same as the experimentally determined value of ΔH. All these values of ΔH have apparently been determined by the variation of K or pK with temperature. Offenhartz and George (1963) compared their results with published thermodynamic data for the ionization of co-ordinated H_2O in other Fe(III) and Co(III) complexes, and concluded that the conjugated porphyrin ring, and to a lesser extent the corrin ring, had important effects on the enthalpy of binding to the metal. Hanania and Irvine (1964a,b) also determined analogous thermodynamic data for ferrimyoglobin complexes and discussed the electrostatic effects of, for example, the negatively charged carboxylate in Factor V_{1a} (compared to Factor B), the stronger ligand field stabilization in Co(III) compared to Fe(III) complexes and the possibility of hydrogen-bonding between the co-ordinated imidazole in the cobalamin and a carbonyl group in a side-chain.

Certain general remarks can be made about thermodynamic data. The value of K is related to the change in free energy, which is in turn made up of changes in enthalpy and entropy

$$-RT \ln K = \Delta G = \Delta H - T\Delta S$$

and it is natural to expect that electronic factors (such as ligand field stabilization, cis- and trans-effects etc.) which affect bond-strengths should be reflected mainly in changes in enthalpy. This is undoubtedly true at absolute zero, where there is no difference between $\Delta G°$ and $\Delta H°$. But at finite temperatures ΔH includes an unknown contribution from the relative change in heat capacities of reagents and products. As Bell (1959) pointed out, $G°$ and $H°$ are "overlaid by a large amount of thermal energy, distributed between many degrees of freedom, and when a solvent is present there will be a considerable contribution from the effect of the system being studied upon the kinetic and potential energy of the solvent molecules. The quantities H and G represent, in effect, different ways of averaging the molecular energies, and it is not at all obvious which is more directly comparable with the model (of electronic changes)". There are, in fact, certain theoretical reasons for believing that electronic changes may be reflected better in ΔG than in ΔH, and this is undoubtedly so in the most thoroughly studied cases of the dissociation constants of substituted acetic and benzoic acids. For a fuller discussion see Bell (1959) and Hambly (1965). It is, therefore, probably not useful to try and analyse the data in Table 8.6 too deeply.

B. EQUILIBRIUM CONSTANTS

Table 8.7 lists the equilibrium constants relating to cobalamins, cobinamides and ψ-B_{12}, grouped according to the nature of the ligands Y and Z involved in the equilibrium. All the equilibria where one of X, Y or Z is Bzm are cobalamins; Y is aden in the three equilibria involving ψ-B_{12}. All other equilibrium constants involve cobinamides. The ligands Y are arranged in the order: H_2O, nucleotide bases (Bzm, aden), other ligands which can ionize while remaining co-ordinated (e.g. imidazole). The ligands Z are arranged in groups depending on the nature of the ligand atom: halides, O, N (including NO_2, even though the identity of the ligand atom is not known), C, S, Se and P. For any given set of Y and Z, the ligands X are usually given in the order of decreasing value of the equilibrium constant; as will be discussed in Section V, this is essentially the order of the trans-effect or increasing donor power of X.

The equilibrium constants reported in Table 8.7 are stoichiometric equilibrium constants, i.e. they refer to the concentrations, not the thermodynamic activities, of the species under the experimental conditions. The commonest equilibrium involves the substitution of H_2O (=Y) by a second ligand Z according to (8.7)

$$K = \frac{[\text{X—Co—Z}]}{[\text{X—Co—OH}_2][\text{Z}]} \tag{8.7}$$

The constant is expressed in units of M^{-1}, and the concentration of free H_2O is neglected.

Equilibrium constants are quoted as the pK_a when the co-ordinated ligand can lose (or gain) a proton. There are several types of such equilibria:

1. Where both forms of the ligand can exist free in solution. In this case the pK can be used to derive a value of the equilibrium constant, e.g. the pK_a for the ionization of Co—OH_2 to Co—OH can be converted into the equilibrium constant K, where

$$K = \frac{[X—Co—OH]}{[X—Co—OH_2][HO^-]} \tag{8.8}$$

using the relationship $\log_{10} K = 14 - pK_a$. Similar considerations apply to the ionization of co-ordinated imidazole and benzimidazole; the pKs can be used to derive the equilibrium constants for the substitution of co-ordinated H_2O by the heterocyclic anion, provided the formation constant for the substitution of H_2O by the uncharged base is known (see Hayward *et al.* 1971)).

2. No equilibrium constant can, however, be derived from the pK in cases such as the protonation of aden in ψ-B_{12}, which still remains co-ordinated, or the ionization of Co—$\overline{CH_2COOH}$ to Co—CH_2COO^-.

3. In the displacement of co-ordinated Bzm by H_2O with simultaneous protonation according to (8.9):

$$\tag{8.9}$$

the concentration of free H_2O is again neglected and the equilibrium constant is usually reported as the pK_a ($=-\log_{10} K$ in units of M^{-1}). These pKs can be converted into equilibrium constants for the equilibrium (8.10),

$$\tag{8.10}$$

in which co-ordinated H_2O is displaced by the unprotonated Bzm of the nucleotide side-chain, by making two reasonable assumptions. The pK of 1-β-D-ribo-5,6-dimethylbenzimidazole has been determined as 4.7 (Davies *et al.*, 1951); however, the base which is present in the nucleotide side-chain of the cobalamins has the α-link. If one assumes that the change of the β

6

to the α link and the proximity of the corrinoid molecule do not significantly alter the value of the pK, then when the observed $pK_a \leqslant 3.7$ we can write

$$K = \frac{[\overline{X-Co-Bzm}]}{\underset{\displaystyle Bzm}{[X-Co-OH_2]}} = \frac{[\overline{X-Co-Bzm}]}{\underset{\displaystyle {}^+HBzm}{[X-Co-OH_2]}} \cdot \frac{[BzmH^+]}{[Bzm]} \tag{8.11}$$

or $\log_{10} K = 4.7 - pK_a$. In these equilibria K is expressed as a ratio. If the observed pK_a is closer to 4.7, a more complex expression must be used, which leads to $\log_{10}(K+1) = 4.7 - pK_a$.

Some equilibrium constants have been studied at pHs below the pK_b of the free ligand (or, more specifically, of the functional group of the ligand which is to be co-ordinated) and equilibrium constants (K') have been reported which do not allow for the protonation of the free ligand, i.e.

$$K' = \frac{[X-Co-Z]}{[X-Co-OH_2]([Z]+[ZH])} \tag{8.12}$$

When $pH \ll pK_b$, K and K' are related by equation (8.13),

$$\log_{10} K = \log_{10} K' + pK_b - pH \tag{8.13}$$

which has been used to convert the reported values of K' into the values of K listed in the Table. The value of the pK of the ligand used is given in a footnote to the Table. In the case of cysteine and glutathione it is not known with certainty which pK corresponds to the ionization of the thiol group and two values have therefore been given.

Where qualitative observations have been made that a given complex can be formed but no formation constant reported or data given from which a calculation can be made, this is indicated in the Table by $+$. These observations are only listed either where

(1) there is at least one formation constant available for the same combination of Y and Z or where

(2) the ligand contains a single donor function of a type which is not otherwise represented except in multifunctional groups (e.g. PR_3, EtS^-).

Earlier qualitative observations of this sort are not mentioned where a formation constant has been reported subsequently. The possible co-ordination of gaseous molecules (CO, NO, O_2) is dealt with separately in Section IV,D.

There are many reports that a given ligand does not complex. Since virtually all known ligand substitution reactions of corrinoids are extremely fast (see Chapter 12, Section II), failure to detect co-ordination is probably due to a low formation constant rather than to kinetic inertness. It can also be assumed that $\geqslant 10\%$ complexing would be detected by spectrophotometry, except in those few cases where very little change in spectrum is expected, e.g. the substitution of H_2O by carboxylates or of Bzm by NH_3. If the concentration of the ligand (and the pH, if the ligand is the conjugate base of a weak acid) is mentioned, then a maximum value for the formation constant can be calculated; e.g. if no complexing is observed in the presence of 1 M ligand, then $K < 0.1$ or $\log_{10} K < -1$. Where such calculations cannot be made the failure to observe complexing of the ligand is indicated in the Table by a dash (—).

C. IDENTITY OF THE LIGAND ATOM AND THE POSSIBILITY OF LINKAGE ISOMERS

Whether or not Bzm (or any other nucleotide base) is co-ordinated to the cobalt can be established by either

1. comparing the absorption spectrum above 300 nm with that of, for example, the corresponding cobinamide or
2. examining the absorption spectrum below 300 nm, which contains bands due to Bzm.

The first absorption band of Bzm occurs at 288 nm when the base is neither protonated or co-ordinated, at 285 nm when protonated and at 288.5 nm when co-ordinated to the cobalt; the bands are less well resolved when Bzm is co-ordinated (Beaven et al., 1949, 1950); the pK of Bzm is 4.7 (see the discussion in Section IV,B).

Many of the ligands given in Table 8.7 can potentially co-ordinate through more than one atom; these include simple ligands, such as NCS^- or NO_2^-, as well as more complex ligands with several separate functional groups as in the amino-acids and peptides. There are two factors which make the identification of the ligand atom more difficult for cobalt(III) corrinoids than for most other cobalt(III) complexes. Firstly, virtually all ligand substitution reactions of the corrinoids are instantaneous; one can therefore never be certain that the evidence obtained for the solid (X-ray, infrared spectra), applies to the complex in solution as well. Secondly, the intense $\pi-\pi$ transitions of the corrin ring completely obscure the d–d transitions of the cobalt ion, which could provide evidence as to whether NO_2^-, for example, is co-ordinated through N or O. Certain conclusions can, however, be drawn from the effect of the ligand on the $\pi-\pi$ transitions (see below). The evidence as to the identity of the ligand atom can be summarized as follows.

X-ray analysis has shown that NCS^- and $NCSe^-$ are bonded through S and Se respectively in the cobalamins in the solid state (Hodgkin, 1958, personal communication). Infrared spectra have been used to show that SO_3^{2-} is also bonded through S in the cobalamin in the solid state (Dolphin et al., 1963b).

Similarities in the u.v.-visible absorption spectra in solution provide evidence that most sulphur-containing ligands such as SO_3^{2-}, $S_2O_3^{2-}$ and thiols are co-ordinated through S (Hill *et al.*, 1962; Pratt and Thorp, 1966; Adler *et al.*, 1966; Cavallini *et al.*, 1968a; Hill *et al.*, 1970b) and $NCSe^-$ through Se (Pratt and Thorp, 1966). No firm conclusions can be drawn from the spectra about the binding of NCS^- in solution, though it has been assumed (Pratt and Thorp, 1966) that the co-ordination through S observed in the solid state is also pre-served in solution; there is, in fact, evidence for the existence of isomers in solu-tion (see below). Similar spectroscopic evidence leads to the conclusion that gly-cine is bound through N rather than O (Hill *et al.*, 1970b), but spectroscopic data cannot be used to decide whether histidine binds through the amine N or the imidazole N (Hill *et al.*, 1970b). Since, however, histidine has a higher formation constant at pH 7 ($\log_{10} K' = 3.6$) than glycine ($\log_{10} K' = 3.1$) (Hill *et al.*, 1970b) and histidine alone out of the twenty amino-acids tested reacted with aquocobalamin under the experimental conditions (Bauriedel, 1956), it seems reasonable to conclude that histidine is co-ordinated through the imida-zole nitrogen. No conclusion can be drawn about the identity of the ligand atom in NO_2^-, since NO_2^- is known to be able to co-ordinate to other cobalt(III) complexes through either N or O and we cannot predict the dif-ference in spectrum between the two cobalamin isomers. NCO^- is apparently always co-ordinated through N and the same was assumed for the cobalamin (Pratt and Thorp, 1966). There is little or no evidence concerning the site of co-ordination of free adenine or adenosine as a unidentate ligand by metal ions in general (Phillips, 1966). X-ray analysis has, however, shown that the adenine present in the nucleotide side-chain of ψ-B_{12} is co-ordinated to the cobalt through N_9 (Hodgkin, 1958). It also seems reasonable to assume that the free adeninate anion is co-ordinated through N_9, since co-ordination through the other nitrogen atom N_7 in the negatively-charged imidazole ring would lead to considerable steric hindrance from the exocyclic —NH_2 group (Hill *et al.*, 1970b).

There is evidence for the existence of linkage isomers in cobalamins contain-ing NCS^- and SO_3^{2-}. Thusius (1968) found evidence from kinetic studies for the existence of a rapidly-established equilibrium in solutions of thiocyanato-cobalamin, which was not shown by the azide and iodide complexes and which he ascribed to linkage isomerization. The kinetic data implied that the equili-brium mixture at 25°C contained 5–10% of one isomer and 90–95% of the other, and it was assumed that the major component was the Co—SCN isomer and the minor component the Co—NCS isomer; but there is no direct evidence as to the nature of the bonding of the major component in solution. The rate constants of liganding and isomerization are given in Chapter 12, Section II. Sulphite ion reacts rapidly with hydroxocobalamin at pH 14 to give some intermediate which slowly yields the known S-bonded sulphitocobalamin, and it has been suggested that the intermediate may be the O-bonded isomer (Firth *et al.*, 1969).

Finally, the data of Table 8.7 show that the formation constants in neutral solution for functional groups such as RNH_2, imidazole and RS^- are the same, within an order of magnitude or so, and it has been pointed out (Hill *et al.*, 1970b) that cobalamins containing amino-acids such as histidine or cysteine probably exist as a mixture of isomers, although one isomer will predominate.

D. GASES: CO, NO, NO⁻, O_2, O_2^-

No complexes are formed by the reaction in aqueous solution at room temperature of CO or O_2 with aquocobalamin (X = Bzm) or cobinamides with $X = CN^-$, $—CH{=}CH_2$, $—CH_3$ or $—CH_2CH_3$ (George *et al.*, 1960; Firth *et al.*, 1969) or of NO with aquocobalamin (Firth *et al.*, 1969). CO will, however, reduce aquocobalamin when the solution is heated (Bayston and Winfield, 1967); there is conflicting evidence as to whether this reaction proceeds via the initial formation of a cobalt(III) carbonyl complex, and this is discussed in Chapter 11, Section IV. Many cobalt(II) complexes react with NO to give cobalt nitrosyls which can be considered as cobalt(III) complexes with NO^- as a ligand (for references see (Pratt and Thorp, 1969)), but no such complex was formed by the reaction of NO with cobalamin-cobalt(II) even after three hours (Firth *et al.*, 1969).

O_2 reacts reversibly with cobalt(II) corrinoids in the crystalline state or in solution (e.g. methanol) at low temperature. This reaction was discovered by Bayston, King, Looney and Winfield (1969), using electron spin resonance spectroscopy. They found that when cobalamin-cobalt(II) was oxygenated the coupling constant for interaction of the unpaired electron with the cobalt nucleus was decreased by a factor of nine, while the superhyperfine structure due to interaction with the nitrogen atom of Bzm disappeared completely. They concluded that in the oxygenated complex the unpaired spin density was no longer located principally on the cobalt but on the O_2 ligand and that the new complex was better represented as a cobalt(II) complex of the superoxide anion (O_2^-) i.e.

$$[Co^{II}] + O_2 \rightleftharpoons [O_2^-{\rightarrow}Co^{III}].$$

They therefore proposed that it should be called "superoxocobalamin". They did not, unfortunately, report the absorption spectrum, which could have provided some means of comparing the electron density on the cobalt as seen by the corrin ring in the superoxide complex with that in corrinoids containing other, more common ligands. Superoxide complexes with other ligands in the *trans*-position were prepared by the reaction of O_2 with cobinamide-cobalt(II) alone or in the presence of potential ligands (see also Chapter 6, Section III and Chapter 7, Section III).

It has been suggested that aquocobalamin reacts with O_2 to form a dimeric complex (Jaselskis and Diehl, 1958); but the evidence is circumstantial and cannot be accepted.

E. AMINES, HETEROCYCLES AND AMINO-ACIDS

Cooley *et al.* (1951) were the first to report that a simple nitrogeneous base (NH_3) and an amino-acid (histidine) could be co-ordinated by aquocobalamin. Most of the other amines, heterocycles, amino-acids and peptides subsequently reported as ligands for corrinoids have been listed in Table 8.7. In addition, $MeNH_2$ and $EtNH_2$ are co-ordinated by methylcobinamide (Brodie, 1969); the α-, β- and γ-picolines are co-ordinated by aquocobalamin and the difference in the spectra of the cobalamins shows the effect of steric hindrance in the case of α-picoline (Hill *et al.*, 1962); and histamine, carnosine and histidyl-histidine are also co-ordinated by aquocobalamin (Bauriedel, *et al.* 1956). Amino-acids and related compounds which have been reported not to complex under the experimental conditions include: aquocobalamin with twenty (unspecified) common amino-acids, except histidine which did complex (Bauriedel, 1956); aquocobalamin with methionine, cysteine and oxidized glutathione (Adler *et al.*, 1966); and methylcobinamide with cysteine, methionine, tyrosine, lysine and caprolactam (Pailes and Hogenkamp, 1968). In none of these cases were the concentrations and pH reported and it would seem likely from the data in Table 8.7 that most of these amino-acids should co-ordinate through the amine nitrogen atom at some suitable concentration and pH. Yurkevich *et al.* (1965) reported that they found slight changes in the spectrum of cyanocobalamin in water in the presence of imidazole and the amino-acids histidine, lysine and tyrosine (as well as p-nitrophenol). They ascribed these changes to the displacement of Bzm by tyrosine (and p-nitrophenol) and of CN^- by the others. But this explanation has been criticized on the basis of known equilibria and reactions and it was suggested that the observed changes in spectra were probably caused by the formation of hydrogen-bonds between the reagents and various parts of the corrinoid molecule (Hill *et al.*, 1970b).

F. HETEROCYCLIC BASES IN THE NUCLEOTIDE SIDE-CHAIN

A wide range of analogues of vitamin B_{12} have been prepared or isolated in which the 5,6-dimethylbenziminazole of the nucleotide side-chain (Bzm) has been replaced by some other heterocyclic base. For references see the review by Mervyn and Smith (1964) and Chapter 9 of the monograph by Smith (1965). It is generally assumed that the base is co-ordinated to the cobalt, at least in those cases where the second axial ligand is cyanide. These analogues therefore provide examples, in many cases the first known examples, of the co-ordination of a variety of heterocyclic bases (see Fig. 8.2). The best known analogues are cyano-adenine-[adenylcobamide] (adenylcobamidecyanide or ψ-B$_{12}$) and 5-deoxyadenosyl-[adenylcobamide] (adenylcobamidecoenzyme or AC), which both contain adenine in the side-chain and for which some equilibrium

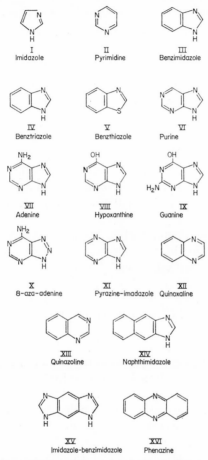

Fig. 8.2. Examples of parent heterocycles and derivatives which (except for pyrimidine(II)) can be incorporated into the nucleotide side-chain of corrinoids.

constants have been reported (see Table 8.7). Little is known, however, about the equilibria and reactions of the other heterocyclic bases.

Vitamin B$_{12}$ is only one member of a large group of corrinoids which occur naturally. The naturally occurring corrinoids are termed "complete" if they possess a complete nucleotide side-chain (i.e. phosphate + ribose + heterocyclic base) and "incomplete" if part or all of the nucleotide is missing. Since the heterocyclic base is present at the end of the side-chain, we are interested only in the "complete" analogues. Several different bases may be synthesized and incorporated by a given organism. In addition, the organism may incorporate artificial bases which have been added to the culture; this method is termed "guided biosynthesis". One can also prepare analogues by chemical synthesis starting from an incomplete corrinoid or by chemical modification of some complete corrinoid. But by far the largest number of analogues have been obtained by guided biosynthesis. These analogues have been prepared and studied in the hope (so far in vain) of finding analogues of vitamin B_{12} which are either

1. much more active than B_{12} itself in the treatment of pernicious anaemia etc. or
2. potent antagonists of B_{12}, which might offer the possibility of interfering with the metabolism of cancerous cells.

The analogues are produced *in vivo* as the coenzymes, i.e. with the axial ligand 5-deoxyadenosyl; but since the organo-ligand is readily removed by the action of light, acid and cyanide, the corrinoid is usually isolated as the monocyanide complex.

Naturally occurring coenzymes (i.e. $X = 5'$-deoxyadenosyl) have been isolated with the following bases in the nucleotide: 5,6-dimethylbenzimidazole (as in Vitamin B_{12} itself), benzimidazole(III), adenine(VII) and 2-methyladenine. The following additional bases have been incorporated by adding the appropriate base, i.e. by "guided biosynthesis": benzimidazole derivatives with CH_3, CF_3, NH_2 and NO_2 in the 5 or 6 position, adenine and 2,6-diaminopurine.

The number of bases present in the nucleotide side-chain of corrinoids isolated as the monocyanide complex is much greater. The naturally occurring analogues invariably contain a benzimidazole(III) or purine(VI) base, e.g. benzimidazole, 5-methylbenzimidazole, 5,6-dimethylbenzimidazole (B_{12} itself), 5-hydroxybenzimidazole, naphthimidazole(XIV), adenine (VII), 2-methyladenine, 2-methylthioadenine, guanine(IX), hypoxanthine(VIII) or 2-methylhypoxanthine. Bases which can be incorporated through guided biosynthesis include the following parent heterocycles and/or their derivatives (for full details see the references given above): 4,5-dimethylimidazole (parent imidazole shown as I); benzimidazole(III) and derivatives containing substituents such as Me, Et, Pr, CF_3, CH_2OH, $CONH_2$, OH, OMe, OEt, NH_2, NO_2, Cl and Br; benztriazole(IV); benzthiazole(V); purine(VI); 8, azaadenine(X); pyrazine-imidazole(XI); quinoxaline(XII); quinazoline(XIII); 5,6-imidazole-benzimidazole(XV); phenazine(XVI). Strangely enough, pyrimidines(II) are not incorporated and it appears that no other monocyclic bases have been tested except for 5,6-dimethylimidazole, which is incorporated.

Chemical modifications which can be made to existing analogues include:

1. Deamination, e.g. of 5-methyladenine by reaction with nitrous acid to give 5-methylhypoxanthine.
2. Alkylation, e.g. of 5-hydroxybenzimidazole to give 5-ethoxybenzimidazole.

There are interesting differences in structure between the free nucleotides and the nucleotides present in the side-chains of corrinoids. In the former the purine base is linked to the sugar by a β-glycosidic linkage involving N_9; in the latter, however, the purine is attached by the unique α-linkage through N_7. There is one corrinoid which contains yet another type of nucleotide structure. Two different corrinoids have been reported which contain the base guanine; one (isolated from sewage sludge) is a normal corrinoid in that guanine is linked through N_7, while the other (from *Nocardia*) contains guanine linked through N_9 *and* contains pyrophosphate instead of phosphate.

G. OTHER S-ANIONS

Thiolates (RS^-). A very wide range of thiols have been used as ligands in addition to ethanethiol, cysteine and glutathione listed in Table 8.7, e.g. 2-mercaptoethanol, thioglycollate, ω-mercaptotoluene, homocysteine and cysteamine (see, for example, Hill *et al.*, (1962), Dolphin and Johnson (1965b) and Cavallini *et al.* (1968a)). In most cases these lignads have been added to aquocobalamin to give the S-bonded thiolatocobalamin. Pailes and Hogenkamp (1968) have, however, studies the reaction of thiols with methylcobinamide. They failed to observe any change in the spectrum of methylcobinamide in the presence of 1–2 M cysteine; they did, however, observe a change in the presence of 2 M mercaptoethanol and 2 M NaOH, which might be due to the formation of the [CH_3—Co—SR] complex, but irreversible changes prevented any quantitative study.

Sulphinates ($ArSO_2^-$). Bernhauer and Wagner (1963) reported that cyano-aquocobinamide reacts with benzene- and p-toluene-sulphinic acid to give complexes, which can probably be regarded as S-bonded sulphinatocobinamides. The second product was also formed by the reaction of cobinamide-cobalt(I) with p-toluene-sulphonyl chloride (see Chapter 13, Section III). New complexes were also formed by treating cyanocobalamin with benzene- or p-toluene-sulphinate. All these complexes were reported to be unstable; it appears that the formation constants are rather low. Cobalamins can be obtained by analogous methods, e.g. by the reaction of cobalamin-cobalt(I) with p-toluene-sulphonyl chloride (Dolphin and Johnson, 1965b) or simply by treating aquocobalamin with benzenesulphinate ion in aqueous solution (Pratt, unpublished observations).

Sulphoxylates (SO_2^{2-}). George *et al.* (1960) treated cyanoaquocobinamide with dithionite ($S_2O_4^{2-}$) and considered the product to be cobinamide-cobalt(II). The spectrum they reported is not, however, that of cobinamide-cobalt(II) (see Chapter 7, Section III). In unpublished work by Pratt, it has been shown that the same absorption spectrum (above 300 nm, i.e. excluding the region where Bzm absorbs) can be obtained by several different routes such as treating aquocobalamin with either sodium dithionite ($S_2O_4^{2-}$) or form-aldehyde-sulphoxylate ($HOCH_2SO_2^-$) and cyanoaquocobinamide with dithionite; reaction proceeds further under certain conditions to give the cobalt(I) complex. One possible formulation for the complex, which would represent the common denominator of all the methods of formation, is a cobalt(III) corrinoid in which one axial ligand is the sulphoxylate ion (SO_2^{2-}) and the other is H_2O or is absent as in the five-co-ordinate ethyl- or sulphito-cobinamide (see Section III).

H. PHOSPHINES

Firth *et al.* (1969) studied the possible co-ordination of triphenylphosphine by corrinoids with X = Bzm, CN^-, —CH=CH_2, —CH_3 and —CH_2CH_3 in ethanol; as recorded in Table 8.7, they found that no significant changes in spectrum were caused by the presence of up to 1 M PPh_3 and concluded that co-ordination of the phosphine did not occur. Yurkevich, Rudakova and Pospelova (1969), however, obtained a 1:1 complex from the reaction of cyanocobalamin with PPh_3 in ethanol. The phosphine was not removed by evaporation under vacuum or by extraction with n-hexane; but the complex was decomposed by water. The presence of PPh_3 had no significant effect on the absorption spectrum above 300 nm (γ-band unchanged at 361 nm) and only a small effect on the cyanide stretching frequency. They also observed an inter-action of 5-deoxyadenosylcobalamin with PPh_3. In both cases they concluded that the phosphine had displaced Bzm from co-ordination to the cobalt. It has been pointed out (Hill *et al.*, 1970b), however, that it is also possible for phosphines to interact with parts of the corrinoid molecule other than the cobalt ion, e.g. the amide side-chains; the formation of such compounds of the clathrate type is discussed in Chapter 6, Section II.

I. GAIN OR LOSS OF PROTON BY/FROM A CO-ORDINATED LIGAND

The simplest example is the ionization of co-ordinated H_2O to give HO^-; many pKs and equilibrium constants have been determined and are listed in Table 8.7. Heterocyclic bases such as imidazole and benzimidazole may also lose a proton to give the corresponding anion while remaining co-ordinated.

On the other hand, the adenine present in the nucleotide side-chain of cyano-adenine-[adenylcobamide] may be protonated ($pK = 2.3$), while still remaining co-ordinated, and it was suggested that the site of protonation was the exocyclic —NH_2 group (Hill et al., 1970b). These equilibria have also been included in the Table. Randall and Alberty (1967) studied the forward and reverse reactions between aquocobalamin and azide as a function of pH and obtained evidence that $HN_3°$ as well as N_3^- was involved in the ligand substitution reactions, although no evidence could be obtained for the Co—N_3H complex under equilibrium conditions. No evidence has yet been obtained for the protonation of other anions such as CN^- or SO_3^{2-}.

Many organo-ligands can lose or gain a proton. The ionization of the ligand Co—CH_2COOH has not yet been studied quantitatively, though some of its effects have been noted. Marked differences are observed in the R_f values in thin layer chromatography in acidic and basic solvents (relative to cyano-cobalamin and other cobalamins) (Firth et al., 1968b) and small differences have been noted in the absorption spectra at pH 4 and 9 (Firth et al., 1968d), both of which can probably be ascribed to the ionization of the carboxylic acid with a pK between 4 and 9. Hogenkamp, Rush and Swenson (1965) concluded from indirect evidence that the pKs of the cobalamins with the ligands —CH_2COOH and —CH_2CH_2COOH were greater than 2.25 and 3.25 respectively. The adenine moiety of the organo-ligand 5-deoxyadenosyl, present in the coenzymes (AC, BC and DBC), can be protonated with a pK of 3.3–3.4 (Ladd et al., 1961). (DBC and BC also undergo a second protonation with $pK = 3.5$, in which the heterocyclic base of the nucleotide side-chain is displaced and protonated, but in AC the adenine of the nucleotide side-chain is never co-ordinated. This second protonation is revealed by changes in the absorption spectrum, while the first is only detected by pH-titration and the effect of pH on the mobilities in paper ionophoresis.) Many organo-ligands such as 5-deoxyadenosyl, ethynyl, vinyl and β-hydroxyethyl are removed or irreversibly changed by the action of strong acid, presumably through initial protonation, e.g. of the σ-vinyl complex to give a π-ethylene complex; these reactions are discussed in Chapter 13, Section II.

Finally, ligands such as amino-acids and peptides which contain several basic functional groups can undoubtedly exhibit one or more pKs while remaining co-ordinated. Direct evidence is, however, available only in the case of the cobalamin containing glutathione; the spectrum indicates that the ligand is co-ordinated through the S atom, i.e. as the thiolate (RS^-) (Adler et al., 1966). Wagner and Bernhauer (1964) showed by electrophoresis that the glutathione complex was uncharged at pH 2, had one negative charge over the range of pH 4–7 and two negative charges at pH 11. At pH 4–7 the co-ordinated glutathione has, therefore, lost two protons, presumably from the carboxylic acid and thiol groups. The pK between 7 and 11 is presumably due to the

—NH_2 group, that between 2.5 and 4 could be due to either protonation of the carboxylate or to the displacement and protonation of Bzm.

J. EQUILIBRIA INVOLVING METAL IONS

A few equilibria involving metal ions and related Lewis acids have been reported. An axial ligand may, firstly, be displaced from co-ordination to the cobalt by complexing with the added Lewis acid. $HgCl_2$ will, for example, remove one cyanide from dicyanocobinamide to give cyanoaquocobinamide, though the second cyanide is not attacked (Firth *et al.*, 1968c). Bzm can be displaced from co-ordination to the cobalt in cyano- and organo-cobalamins by the addition of Ag(I) or Hg(II) ions (Hill *et al.*, 1970a), i.e.

The axial ligand may also be co-ordinated to a second metal ion while remaining co-ordinated to the cobalt. Ethynylcobalamin and vinylcobalamin and cobinamide show reversible equilibria with Ag(I) ions which have been ascribed to equilibria such as:

$$Co—C≡CH + Ag^+ \rightleftharpoons Co—C≡C—Ag + H^+$$

But no equilibrium constants have been determined (Hill *et al.*, 1970a). These appear to be the first equilibria of co-ordinated ethynyl and vinyl groups reported for any organometallic complexes. As noted in Table 8.7, other binuclear complexes with a bridging cyanide have been obtained from the reaction of cyanoaquocobinamide with the anions $[M(CN)_6]^{n-}$ where M = Fe(II), Fe(III) and Co(III) (George *et al.*, 1960).

Several reactions are known which involve metal ions; these are discussed in more detail elsewhere. Ag(I) ions will remove CN^- from cyanocobalamin, and Hg(II) ions will remove CH_3 and other organo-ligands from organo-cobalamins and cobinamides (see Chapter 12, Section II and Chapter 13,

Section II). Cu(II) ions will catalyze the conversion of thiolatocobalamins into cobalamin-cobalt(II) (see Chapter 11, Section IV,E).

V. FACTORS WHICH DETERMINE THE MAGNITUDE OF THE EQUILIBRIUM CONSTANTS

The large number of equilibrium constants K available for the corrinoids has enabled certain conclusions to be drawn regarding the factors which determine their magnitude. In this section we present data from Section IV, selected in order to demonstrate the general pattern observed, and discuss the factors involved. Additional information relating to the nature of the metal-ligand bond, such as the effect of the axial ligand on the rest of the corrinoid molecule as shown by the absorption spectrum or the stretching frequency of co-ordinated cyanide, has been discussed in Chapter 5, Section I and Chapter 6, Section III.

Table 8.8 presents the equilibrium constants for the substitution of co-ordinated H_2O in cobalt(III) corrinoids by various ligands Z, with several different ligands X in the *trans*-position, for those combinations of X and Z where there is sufficient quantitative information available to show a definite trend. The ligands X are arranged in the order of their effect on the magnitude of K, i.e. in the order of their *trans*-effect (see below). The ligands Z are grouped broadly into neutral bases, monobasic anions and dibasic anions. It must be stressed that these equilibrium constants (K_{obs}) have not been corrected for the presence of five-co-ordinate complexes, i.e.

$$K_{obs} = \frac{[X—Co—Z]}{([X—Co—OH_2] + [X—Co])[Z]}$$

The amount of five-co-ordinate cobinamide (X—Co) present in equilibrium with the six co-ordinate aquocobinamide (X—Co—OH$_2$) is only significant when X is an organo-ligand, SO_3^{2-} or perhaps some other very polarizable ligand containing S, Se or I as the ligand atom (see Section III). Since the constant for the equilibrium between these two types of complex is known either rather inaccurately (e.g. when X = CH_3) or not at all (e.g. when X is CH_3CH_2), it is simplest to leave all the formation constants uncorrected, The equilibrium between the five- and six-co-ordinate complexes and the influence of X on this equilibrium has been discussed in Section III.

The data of Table 8.8 show that we are dealing with large changes and differences in equilibrium constants and energies. For example, the equilibrium constant for the substitution of H_2O by CN^- can be changed by a factor of over 10^{13} simply by changing the *trans*-ligand X, while the equilibrium constants for the binding of the two monobasic anions CN^- and Cl^- when

Table 8.8. *Selected formation constants for the substitution of co-ordinated H_2O by various ligands Z with different ligands X in the trans-position*

X	NH₃	Py	Imid	Bzm	CH₃NC	HO⁻	N₃⁻	CN⁻	Cl⁻	I⁻	SO₃²⁻
H₂O	≥9		7.5	7.1		8.0		≥14	0.5		~11
Bzm	7	+	4.6	4.6	4.8	6.3	4.9	≥12	0.1	1.5	7.3
CN⁻	3.35	2.6	4.1	4.0	2.7	3.0	2.7	8	+	+	4.6
—C≡CH											
SO₃³⁻	~0.6	+	+	2.7	0.6	−0.7	0.6	6.7			
—CH=CH₂				2.3	<−1	<−1	<−1	4.3	+	0	<−1
—CH₃	−1	0.8	1.0	2.0	<−1	<−1	<−1	2.7	+	+	<−1
—CH₂CH₃				0.8		<−1		2.1	+	+	<−1
—CH₂CH₂CH₃			−1	0.9							<−1

The formation constants are taken from Table 8.7 and expressed as $\log_{10} K$ in units of litre. mol⁻¹ except for Z = Bzm where the constant is a ratio.

$X = H_2O$ differ by more than 10^{13}. The most important features of the pattern of equilibrium constants can be discussed in terms of

1. the *trans*-effect of X and
2. the effect of the nature of Z.

(One could consider the effect of both Y and Z, but in this discussion it is assumed that Y is always H_2O, and that any equilibrium constant where $Y \neq H_2O$ can be considered as the product of the constants for the equilibria H_2O/Y and Z/H_2O). As will be seen below, a simple pattern is observed for (1), which can be explained satisfactorily; but the same is not true for (2).

In neither the changes nor the differences in equilibrium constant does charge appear to play any major role. Compare the very close parallel between CH_3NC and N_3^-, as examples of ligands Z which differ in charge, and note the constancy of the position of the doubly charged SO_3^{2-} between the singly charged $HC{\equiv}C^-$ and $CH_2{=}CH^-$ even when the ligands Z differ in charge (e.g. Bzm and CN^-).

Other factors which may influence the equilibrium constants, such as steric hindrance, chelation, and the formation of hydrogen-bonds, are mentioned briefly at the end of this section.

A. THE *TRANS*-EFFECT OF X

The main conclusions to be drawn (see Firth *et al.* (1968d, 1969)) are:

1. There is a single order of ligands X observed for all the different Z. This order includes ligands co-ordinated through O, N, C and S; it is particularly interesting that SO_3^{2-} occupies the same position *vis-à-vis* the organo-ligands (which have a different charge and ligand atom) in all the equilibria studied. The position of SO_3^{2-} is, however, different if we compare formation constants for the binding of H_2O by the five-co-ordinate cobinamides (see Section III).
2. All the equilibrium constants change in the same direction, i.e. the equilibrium constants for the substitution of H_2O by another ligand Z fall as X becomes a better σ-donor (down the column) and approach those expected for ion-pairs with non-transition metals, i.e. low values with no marked preference for C or N as the ligand atom. The rates of change of equilibrium constant with X do, however, depend markedly on the nature of Z (see below).
3. The order of ligands X observed for this thermodynamic *trans*-effect (Table 8.8) is the same as that observed for the "ground-state" *cis*- and *trans*-effects, i.e. for the effect of X on the absorption spectra due to transitions within the corrin ring (see Chapter 5, Section I), on the proton magnetic

resonance of the C_{10}-H in the corrin ring (Chapter 6, Section III). The correlation between the effect of X on the equilibrium constants and on the cyanide stretching frequency, i.e. between the thermodynamic and ground-state *trans*-effects, is shown graphically in Fig. 8.3. It has been pointed out already (see Chapter 5, Section I and Chapter 6, Section III) that this order of ligands ($H_2O...CN^-...CH_3CH_2^-$) represents the order of the increasing σ-donor power of the ligand X; it shows a positive correlation with the order of ligands in the nephelauxetic series, but not in the spectro-chemical series.

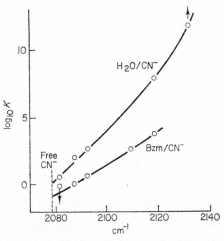

Fig. 8.3. Correlation between the stretching frequency of co-ordinated cyanide (in cyanoco-balamins) and the equilibrium constant for the substitution by CN^- of H_2O in cobinamides and of Bzm in cobalamins. The ligands X (taken from left to right) are: ethyl, methyl, vinyl, CN^-, Bzm and H_2O. From Firth *et al.* (1968d)

B. QUALITATIVE EVIDENCE ON THE *TRANS*-EFFECT OF OTHER LIGANDS X

There are many other ligands X, where an equilibrium constant is available for one Z only or where even this equilibrium has only been studied qualitatively. Such information can, however, provide useful qualitative evidence as to the position of certain other ligands in the order of *trans*-effect.

Values of the pK for the displacement and protonation of Bzm, and hence equilibrium constants for the substitution of H_2O by Bzm, have been determined for a large number of organo-ligands (see Table 8.7). If we include only the simplest types of organo-ligands, the order of pK and hence the position in the *trans*-effect order is as follows:

	pK
CN⁻	0.1
—C≡CH	0.7
—CH₂COOR (R = H, Me)	~2
—CH=CH₂	2.4
—CH₂CH₂NR₃⁺ (R = H, Me)	2.4–2.6
—CH₃	2.7
—CH₂CH₂R (R = CN, OH, OMe, COOH, COOMe)	2.9–3.3
—CH₂CH₂R (R = H, Me)	3.8–4.0
—COCH₃	~4.5

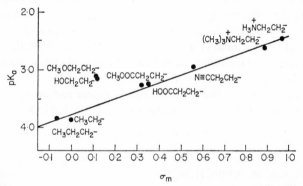

Fig. 8.4. Relation between Hammett *meta* substituent constants (σ_m) and pK_a values for the protonation of Bzm in organocobalamins containing a β-substituted ethyl ligand. From Hogenkamp (1966b).

Hogenkamp and colleagues have pointed out (Hogenkamp, 1966b; Hogen-kamp *et al.*, 1965) that there is a linear relationship between the pK for the displacement of Bzm when X is a substituted ethyl group (Co—CH₂CH₂R) and the Hammett meta-substitutent constant of R, as shown in Fig. 8.4. The ligands —CH₂CH₂OH and —CH₂CH₂OMe do not, however, fall on the line. They also found that the substituted methyl ligands —CH₃, —CH₂COOH and —CH₂COOMe showed a similar linear correlation; the line was different from that for the substituted ethyl ligands, but showed the same slope. As they point out, these results show that

1. the substituents R affect the pK by their ability to donate or withdraw electrons and that
2. the inductive effect of R can be transmitted to the cobalt ion through two carbon atoms.

It is, however, rather strange that the slopes should be identical for both substituted methyl and ethyl ligands, which suggests that the effect of substituents is transmitted equally well to the cobalt through either one or two carbon atoms. There may be additional effects such as hydrogen-bonds with the substituted alkyl ligands (see below) which could upset a true correlation.

Two secondary alkyl ligands have been reported, viz. isopropyl in both co-balamin (Firth *et al.*, 1968d) and cobinamide (Firth *et al.*, 1968d; Hill *et al.*, 1970a) and cyclohexyl in the cobinamide (Brodie, 1969). Isopropylcobalamin proved to be too unstable to isolate and purify, but its spectrum appeared to be the same as that of the cobinamide, i.e. Bzm is not co-ordinated and $\log_{10} K$ for the co-ordination of Bzm is probably $\leqslant -1$. This indicates that the isopropyl ligand has the strongest *trans*-effect of any organo-ligand so far studied. No studies have yet been reported for the binding of ligands by isopropylcobin-amide. It is clear from Brodie's (1969) results that cyclohexylcobinamide binds CN$^-$ weakly if at all and $\log_{10} K \leqslant -1$; the cyclohexyl ligand is therefore also a very powerful donor. Since the spectra of iso-propyl- and cyclohexyl-cobinamide are very similar (Firth *et al.*, 1968a; Brodie, 1969), the two ligands probably exert a very similar *trans*-effect. Both complexes appear to exist entirely as the five-co-ordinate complex (see Section III).

Qualitative data are available for the displacement and protonation of Bzm in cobalamins with the following ligands (data from Table 8.7):

	pK
Cl$^-$, NH$_3$ (and probably CH$_3$NC)	<0
Br$^-$, I$^-$, thiourea	0–1
NCS$^-$	~2
HS$^-$, thiolates (from cysteine and thioglycollate), S$_2$O$_3^{2-}$	>0

These data do not establish the position of all these ligands in the *trans*-effect order with certainty. Firstly, these equilibria were studied in the presence of excess ligand X. Only in the case of Br$^-$ and NH$_3$ (Pratt and Thorp, 1966) has it been shown that the equilibrium involves the simple displacement of Bzm by H$_2$O and not by a second molecule of X. The same is probably true for HS$^-$, thiols and S$_2$O$_3^{2-}$ since their acidified solutions are all yellow, as are the known sulphito-cobinamide and acidified sulphitocobalamin (Firth *et al.*, 1968a, 1969). Secondly, the displacement of Bzm may also be coupled with isomerization of the ligand, e.g. from S-bonded to N-bonded NCS$^-$. However, the above pKs may probably be accepted provisionally as evidence for the position of these ligands in the *trans*-effect order. If we include the ligands of Table 8.8, which have been established quantitatively, then the general order of the *trans*-effect of X becomes:

H$_2$O, NH$_3$, Cl$^-$, CH$_3$NC (probably) < CN$^-$ < all organo-ligands,
thiourea, NCS$^-$, HS$^-$, RS$^-$ (thiols), S$_2$O$_3^{2-}$, I$^-$

All the ligands with the more electronegative and less polarizable ligand atoms appear on the left (O, N, Cl), those with the more polarizable ligand atoms on the right (C, S, I).

C. THE EFFECT OF THE NATURE OF THE LIGAND Z

The data of Table 8.8 show that the rate of change of the value of $\log_{10} K$ with a change in X (i.e. the sensitivity of K) varies tremendously with the nature of Z. This difference in sensitivity can lead to a change in the relative order of binding of two different axial ligands Z as X is varied; for example, NH_3 is bound more strongly than imidazole when X is H_2O, but the converse is true when X is CH_3^-. There is, therefore, no single order of ligands Z which can be determined from the magnitude of the formation constants and which applies whatever the nature of X; this contrasts with the ligands X which can be placed in a single order which applies to all Z. It means that each ligand Z must be defined by two (or more) parameters, the nature of which can perhaps be made clearer in the following way. If one could plot for each Z the values of $\log_{10} K$ along the y-axis against the σ-donor power of X along the x-axis, then these two parameters would correspond to the "slope" of the plot (which is the same as the sensitivity of $\log_{10} K$ to a change in X) and the "intercept" at some arbitrary value of the σ-donor power of X (e.g. when X = Bzm or CH_3^-); such a plot cannot be constructed at present because there is no independent measure of the σ-donor power of the particular ligands of interest.

The "slope" (i.e. the sensitivity of $\log_{10} K$ to the nature of X) varies with the nature of Z in the following rough order: $SO_3^{2-} \sim CN^- \sim HO^- \sim NH_3 > N_3^-$ $= CH_3NC > imid > Bzm \geqslant py > I^- \geqslant Cl^- > H_2O$. The following points can be made about this order of ligands Z.

1. Even such a closely related group of ligands as the nitrogeneous bases can show very different slopes.

2. There is no correlation between the position of ligands in the above order and the position of ligands in either the spectrochemical series ($CN^- \geqslant SO_3^{2-} > NH_3 \sim py > H_2O > HO^- > N_3^- > Cl^- > I^-$) or the nephelauxetic series (which to a first approximation depends on the nature of the ligand atom: $I \sim S > C > Cl > N \sim O$), or the position of the ligand in the *trans*-effect order.

3. There is no change between class (a) and class (b) character as X is varied. Class (a) cations are those in which the formation constants for the binding of halides fall in the order $F^- > Cl^- > Br^- > I^-$, while class (b) cations show the reverse order (Ahrland *et al.*, 1958). The cobalt(III) cation in aquo-cobalamin shows mild class (b) character: cf. the formation constants with

I^- 32, Br^- 1.9, Cl^- 1.3, F^- just detectable (Pratt and Thorp, 1966). Whatever the factors are that determine the balance between class (a) and class (b) character, they appear to remain constant in the cobalt(III) corrinoids, whatever the nature of X.

4. There is no detectable effect which can be attributed to π-bonding between the cobalt ion and the ligand Z by back-donation from the d-orbitals of the cobalt(III) ion into unfilled orbitals on the ligand. This is shown most clearly by the very close parallel in formation constants between CH_3NC, which is expected to favour π-bonding, and N_3^-, which is not. A similar comparison can be made between CN^-, which is often accused of being a π-acceptor, and HO^-, which can only be a π-donor; both ligands show a similar slope. Since any significant contribution to the energy of complexing from π-bonding would destroy the close parallel between the two pairs of ligands, one can only conclude that π-bonding makes no detectable contribution to the energy of interaction. This conclusion is also supported by the inability of either CO or PR_3 (which only co-ordinate when some π-bonding is possible through back-donation from the metal to the ligand) to co-ordinate to cobalt(III) corrinoids, whatever the nature of X (Section IV).

5. There is, however, a positive correlation between those ligands which show a steep "slope" and those bases which form adducts with aldehydes according to the equation:

$$R.CHO + H^+ + X^- = R.CHOH.X$$

This can be considered as the co-ordination of bases to the $R.CHOH^+$ cation. Bases which can form such adducts with aldehydes and which can exist free in aqueous solution are HO^- (and alkoxides RO^-), HS^-, thiolates RS^-, SO_3^{2-}, NR_3 (adducts with NH_3 or RNH_2, N_2H_4, NH_2OH, etc., react further to lose H_2O) and CN^- (March, 1968; Sander and Jencks, 1968). Recent work has shown that N_3^- can also form a weak adduct, but no adduct could be detected with imidazole (Sander and Jencks, 1968). There is apparently no report of the formation of adducts with pyridine, I^- or Cl^- (except by polyfluorinated aldehydes) (March, 1968). There is, therefore, a positive correlation between those ligands which form adducts with aldehydes (i.e. have relatively high formation constants) and those which show a steep "slope" in their formation constants towards cobalt(III) corrinoids. In both series SO_3^{2-}, CN^-, HO^- and NH_3 (assumed to behave like NR_3) appear at one end, N_3^- is a border-line case and the halides and heterocyclic bases appear at the other end. The most interesting and intriguing conclusion is, therefore, that the same factors appear to govern the magnitude of the formation constants towards both the cobalt(III) ion and the carbonium ion ($RCHOH^+$). This should simplify any interpretation, since one can now concentrate on the carbonium ions and neglect complicating factors such as d-orbitals and crystal field stabilization associated with cobalt(III) ions. It has been suggested that the main factor in both series is the strength of the covalent bond between the cation and the base (Firth *et al.*, 1969), but in fact no satisfactory theory has yet been developed to explain which bases form adducts with aldehydes. It has also been suggested that the smaller slope of the heterocyclic bases compared to NH_3 may be connected with the greater polarizability of the heterocyclic ring and hence greater ease of varying the electron density on the nitrogen atom; the smaller slope of Bzm compared to imidazole may also be due in part to a favourable change in entropy connected with the formation of a chelate ring (Bzm is attached to the equatorial corrin ring by a nucleoside side-chain), which is not expected to vary with the nature of X (Hayward *et al.*, 1971).

Relatively little can be said about the factors which determine the "intercept", i.e. the magnitude of the formation constant for a given ligand X (say Bzm). It is obvious that the existence of differing "slopes" will mean that, as the σ-donor power of X gets weaker (i.e. going from CH_3^- to CN^-, Bzm, H_2O), so the ligands Z with the steepest "slope" will tend to show the highest formation constants. This has already happened for X = Bzm; the four ligands known to show very steep "slopes" (SO_3^{2-}, CN^-, HO^- and NH_3) are all amongst the six most firmly bound ligands (see Table 8.9). Contrast this with the situation when X = CH_3^-, where SO_3^{2-}, HO^- and NH_3 are all bound less firmly than pyridine, imidazole, and probably even Cl^- and I^-. Since the "slope" appears to vary even between such closely related ligands as the heterocycles pyridine and imidazole, it is difficult to know where (i.e. with which X) to look for any correlation between the magnitude of the formation constant and any other property such as the pK of the free ligand.

More formation constants have been determined for X = Bzm than for any other X and these formation constants are listed in Table 8.9. Examination of the data shows, as expected, no simple correlation between the magnitude of the formation constant and factors such as

1. the charge on the ligand,
2. the nature of the ligand atom,
3. the pK_a of the conjugate acid of the ligand or
4. the position of the ligand in either the spectrochemical or nephelauxetic series; but the formation constants are undoubtedly greater for the anionic compared to the neutral form of the same molecule (cf. H_2O with HO^-, and imidazole with the imidazolate anion).

More limited tables of formation constants could be made from the data in Table 8.7 for X = CN^- or CH_3^-; but again there are no obvious correlations.

From the biochemist's point of view the most interesting data relating to this section probably concern the strength of binding of the different heterocyclic bases present in the nucleotide side-chain. Constants have only recently

(Hill *et al.*, 1970b) been determined for equilibria between cyanoadenine-[adenylcobamide], commonly called ψ-B_{12}, and CN^-, HO^- and H^+, from which an approximate value can be derived for the equilibrium constant for the sub-

Table 8.9. *Equilibrium constants for the substitution of co-ordinated H_2O in aquoco-balamin (B_{12a}) compared with the pK_a of the conjugate acid of the ligand*

Ligand Z	Ligand Atom	$\log_{10} K$ (M^{-1})	pK_a of ligand
CN^-	C	>12	9.3
Imidazolate ($C_3H_3N_2^-$)	N	7.8	14.5
SO_3^{2-}	S	7.3	7.0
NH_3	N	7	9.4
Cysteinate (RS^-)	S	6.0 or 8.3	8.2 or 10.5
HO^-	O	6.2	14
Histidine	N (imid)	5.8	9.2
Glycine ($H_2NCH_2COO^-$)	N	5.8	9.7
NO_2^-	N or O	5.3	3.3
Glutathionate (RS^-)	S	4.9 or 5.8	8.6 or 9.5
N_3^-	N	4.9	4.7
CH_3NC	C	4.8	?
$S_2O_3^{2-}$	S	3.9	1.6
$NCSe^-$	Se	3.9	<0
Imidazole ($C_3H_4N_2^\circ$)	N	4.6	7.2
NCS^-	S + N (prob. two isomers)	3.1	<0
Phenoxide ($C_6H_5O^-$)	O	2.9	10.0
NCO^-	N	2.7	3.7
I^-	I	1.5	−9.5
Thiourea	S	1.1	2.0
CH_3COO^-	O	0.7	4.6
Br^-	Br	0.3	−9
Cl^-	Cl	0.1	−7
F^-	F	+	3

Values of the equilibrium constants are taken from Table 8.7. Values of the ligand pK_a are taken from Sillén and Martell (1964) with the exception of the following: imidazole and imidazolate (Albert, 1959), cysteine and glutathione (Wallenfels and Streffer, 1966), NCS^- (Laurence, 1956) and $NCSe^-$ (Hamada, 1961). The exact value of any given pK_a depends very much on the temperature and ionic strength, and the values given above are intended to provide only a rough comparison with the formation constants for binding to the cobalt(III) ion.

stitution of H_2O by aden (see data in Table 8.7). This allows a comparison to be made between the formation constants for the substitution of H_2O by Bzm and aden in two pairs of corrinoids. Compare the following constants (in $\log_{10} K$) taken from Table 8.7:

trans-ligand X	aden	Bzm
CN⁻	~3	4.6
5-deoxyadenosyl	<−1	1.3

Aden is clearly bound less firmly than Bzm in both cases. Additional evidence from studies of the ease of displacing the nucleotide base by CN^- in corrinoids where $X = CN^-$ shows that the Co-nucleotide bond decreases in strength in the order: 5,6-dimethylbenzimidazole (B_{12}) > 5-hydroxybenzimidazole (Factor III) > 2-methylbenzimidazole (Factor A) > adenine $(\psi\text{-}B_{12})$ (Friedrich and Bernhauer, 1956). The combination of the low intrinsic strength of the Co-aden bond together with the strong trans-effect of the 5-deoxyadenosyl ligand leads to the curious situation that 5-deoxyadenosyl-[adenylcobamide] or adenylcobamide coenzyme (AC) exists in solution as a five-co-ordinate complex, in which the base is not co-ordinated (see discussion in Hill et al. (1970b)). Other qualitative evidence on the binding strength of nucleotide bases can be obtained from the adsorption spectra of other coenzymes (i.e. where $X = 5$-deoxyadenosyl) given by Toohey, Perlman and Barker (1961). It appears that 2,6-diaminopurine resembles adenine and is not co-ordinated (i.e. $\log_{10} K < -1$), while benzimidazole and 5-methylbenzimidazole, like 5,6-dimethylbenzimidazole (Bzm), are co-ordinated $(\log_{10} K \geqslant 0)$; the spectra of the coenzymes containing 5-amino-,5-nitro- and 4-trifluoro-benzimidazole are intermediate and may indicate the presence of a mixture of the five- and six-co-ordinate complexes in solution (i.e. $\log_{10} K \sim 0$).

Some interesting information is provided by the electronic spectra of the corrinoids. Chloro- and iodo-cobalamin, for example, have very different absorption spectra, which resemble those of aquo- and vinyl-cobalamin respectively (Pratt and Thorp, 1966) and clearly indicate a great difference in the nature of the Co-halogen bond. It must, therefore, be somewhat fortuitous that the two formation constants are both small and similar (see Table 8.9). Similar large differences in the absorption spectra are observed when $X = CH_3^-$ and Y is H_2O, Bzm and CN^-, even though the formation constants are all small. This serves as a useful reminder that chemical equilibria reflect the resultant small differences between large forces of attraction and repulsion. There are obviously grave difficulties in the way of understanding these small differences until we know more about the magnitude and nature of the large forces.

D. CIS-EFFECTS

A study of the effect of substitution at C_{10} or reaction at C_8 (for examples of these derivatives see Chapter 15, Section I) on equilibria involving the axial ligands would provide interesting information on the thermodynamic cis-effect. Unfortunately, no quantitative data have yet been reported and only a few relevant qualitative observations have been made. A spectroscopic study of the nature of the complexes present in solutions of B_{12} and analogues at pH 7.5 in the presence of 0.005 % HCN showed that the ease of displacing Bzm by CN^- increased in the following order: B_{12} (monocyanide only present) < analogue containing chlorine at C_{10} (50 % each of the mono- and di-cyanide) < analogue containing both chlorine at C_{10} and a lactam ring (dicyanide only) (Wagner and Renz, 1963). The presence of chlorine at C_{10} would be expected to increase the electronegativity of the corrin ring and hence, by analogy with the effect of substituting the *trans*-ligand CN^- by the more electronegative H_2O, to increase the equilibrium constant for the substituion of Bzm by CN^-—as found experimentally.

E. THE EFFECT OF STERIC HINDRANCE

The effects of steric hindrance between an axial ligand and the cobalt ion or the corrin ring have been discussed in Chapter 6, Section I. Although steric hindrance probably will have a detectable effect on certain equilibrium constants, no equilibrium constants have yet been determined for closely related ligands where any observed difference could be ascribed with certainty to steric factors and not, for example, to changes in basicity.

F. THE "CHELATE" EFFECT

It is generally found that chelating (i.e. multidentate) ligands tend to form more stable complexes than unidentate ligands of the same structural type. For example, K_1 for the binding of one mol of ethylenediamine (en) according to equation (8.14) is

$$[ML_4(H_2O)_2] + en = [ML_4en] + 2H_2O \qquad (8.14)$$

usually greater than β_2 ($=K_1K_2$) for the binding of two moles of NH_3 according to equation (8.15).

$$[ML_4(H_2O)_2] + 2NH_3 = [ML_4(NH_3)_2] + 2H_2O \qquad (8.15)$$

This is usually attributed to a more favorable entropy change associated with equation (8.14) than equation (8.15), because the former leads to an increase in the number of free molecules by one (replacing 1 en in solution by 2 H_2O), while the latter does not. This "chelate" effect usually increases $\log_{10} K$ by a factor of 1–2 (at 25°C) (Rossotti, 1960).

Since the nucleotide side-chain of the cobalamins and other corrinoids can be regarded as a chelating ligand, such a "chelate" effect should be operating. It should be possible in principle to compare directly the formation constants for the binding of Bzm in the nucleotide side-chain and of the identical, but un-attached nucleotide and to calculate an effective concentration for Bzm in the cobalamin from the molecular dimensions. Since, however, the nucleotide side-chain carries many functional groups which form hydrogen-bonds to the solvent or to other parts of the corrinoid molecule, it is very likely that the total contribution to the entropy (and enthalpy) of co-ordination from changes in these hydrogen-bonds will completely swamp any possible "chelate" effect.

G. THE EFFECT OF HYDROGEN-BONDS INVOLVING THE AXIAL LIGANDS

The possible effect of hydrogen-bonding between the axial ligands and the side-chains of the corrinoid molecule on equilibria was first discussed by Hanania and Irvine (1964b) and subsequently by Hayward et al. (1971). X-ray analysis has shown the existence in the solid state of intra-molecular hydrogen-bonding between an amide side-chain and an axial ligand, e.g. with CN^- in dry cyanocobalamin (Hodgkin et al., 1962) and with H_2O in Factor V_{1a} (cobyric acid) (Hodgkin, 1965) (see also Chapter 6, Sections I and II). The probability of such intramolecular hydrogen-bonding is greatly reduced in aqueous solution, but may be increased with larger ligands such as imidazole which can place a hydrogen-bonding centre ($\diagup^{N}$—H) closer to the amide side-chain. Such interaction might have a detectable effect on the formation constants and might upset to a small extent any order or correlation based on the trans-effect. The variation in the equilibrium between the l- and u-isomers of cyanoaquocorrinoids with the nature and position of the side-chains is prob-ably due to the preferential formation of hydrogen-bonds between co-ordinated H_2O and particular side-chains (see Section II,B). This might also be the cause of the unexpectedly small difference in formation constant ob-served for Z = imidazole and imidazolate between X = Bzm and CN^-. It would be surprising if co-ordinated amino-acids, and in particular peptides such as glutathione, did not form hydrogen-bonds to the side-chains.

It has been shown that the R_f values of organocorrinoids in thin layer chromatography show little correlation with the pK for the displacement of Bzm (i.e. with the trans-effect of the organo-ligand), but are very sensitive to the presence of electronegative substituents in the organo-ligand which can form hydrogen-bonds (Firth et al., 1968b). Since strong hydrogen-bonding capacity leads to low R_f values the hydrogen-bonds are presumably formed between the organo-ligand and the stationary phase. Changes in the pattern of hydrogen-bonding around the organo-ligand may be one of the factors which upsets the linear correlation between the Hammett meta-substituent constant for substituted ethyl ligands and the pK for displacement and pro-tonation of Bzm (see Fig. 8.4).

The formation of hydrogen-bonds by the amide side-chains probably plays an important role in the binding of corrinoids to proteins and polypeptides (see Chapter 6, Section II).

VI. SALTS AND ION-PAIRS

Surprisingly little work has been done either on the preparation and study of solid salts containing a corrinoid complex (as either cation or anion) or on ion-pairs in non-aqueous solvents; for example in the phenol-chloroform mixtures which are used to purify corrinoids by extraction from the aqueous phase. This is partly because corrinoids containing a net positive or negative charge are relatively rare. The commonly studied cobalamins which contain a mono-basic anion are neutral; the charges on the cobalt(III) ion are balanced by the charges on the co-ordinated anion, the corrin ring and the phosphate of the nucleotide side-chain. Aquocobalamin does, of course, carry a positive charge, while dicyanocobalamin and sulphitocobalamin carry one negative charge. Even where the side-chains are carboxylic acids it appears that they may often remain undissociated in the solid state; see, for example, the corrinoid with six carboxylic acid side-chains (Hodgkin et al., 1959).

Some information is available on salts of aquocobalamin in the solid state. Smith, Ball and Ireland (1952a) prepared a sample of aquocobalamin by acidifying the aqueous solution with sulphuric acid labelled with ^{35}S and then adding acetone to induce crystallization. The activity of the product corresponded to one sulphate per two corrinoid molecules. One cannot, unfortunately, conclude from the infra-red spectrum (Dolphin and Johnson, 1965b) whether the sulphate is co-ordinated or not, but in view of the very low (and so far undetectable) formation constants for the co-ordination of simple oxy-anions by aquocobalamin (see Table 8.7) it seems very likely that the solid is the ionic salt aquocobalamin sulphate. It would seem likely that many analogous salts could be prepared depending on the anion present in the mother liquor (SO_4^{2-}, NO_3^{-}, Cl^{-}), provided, of course, that the formation constant for co-ordination of the anion is sufficiently low; and different samples of B_{12a} may differ in the anion they contain. The reflection spectrum of a sample of B_{12a} in the solid state has been studied (Firth et al., 1968d). The normal form shows the spectrum of aquocobalamin, but on drying the solid the spectrum changes reversibly to that of hydroxocobalamin. The simplest explanation would be that the "wet" form of B_{12a} is the ionic salt aquocobalamin hydroxide, which on drying is converted into the uncharged hydroxocobalamin, i.e.

$$[Co\!-\!OH_2]^+ + HO^- = [Co\!-\!OH]^0 + H_2O$$

But it is also possible that the counter-ion may be Cl^-, SO_4^{2-} etc. and that a more complicated equilibrium is involved, e.g.

$$[Co—OH_2]^+ + Cl^- + H_2O = [Co—OH]^0 + H_3O^+ + Cl^-$$

A similar but less complete change from the aquo to the hydroxo form is observed on drying cyanoaquocobinamide in the solid state (Firth *et al.*, 1968a).

A rather different type of salt is probably represented by the cobalamin-polypeptide complex isolated by Hedbom (1960). The absorption spectrum shows a band at 350 nm, which indicates the presence of aquocobalamin, although the co-ordination of a carboxylate from the polypeptide cannot be completely excluded; and the aquocobalamin and polypeptide are probably held together by hydrogen-bonds (Hill *et al.*, 1970b). The positive charge on the aquocobalamin may therefore be compensated by the negative charge of a carboxylate on the polypeptide, to give a type of inner salt involving both components of the complex. Similarly, Babior and Li (1969) have concluded from measurements of the circular dichroism spectra that when B_{12a} is bound by the protein ethanolamine deaminase it is present as the positively charged aquocobalamin. The binding of molecules by corrinoids through the formation of hydrogen-bonds is discussed in more detail in Chapter 6, Section II.

Smith, Ball and Ireland (1952a) used sodium salts labelled with ^{24}Na in an attempt to show that when sulphitocobalamin and dicyanocobalamin (both of which possess a single negative charge) are extracted from aqueous solution into phenol and benzyl alcohol respectively, they are accompanied by one sodium ion per cobalt. Both NaCN and Na_2SO_3 were, however, fairly readily extracted into the organic phase and after allowing for a large "blank", they could only conclude that sulphitocobalamin appeared to form a salt with one sodium ion. Similar experiments showed that nitrocobalamin (no net charge) formed no such salt.

Many organocobalamins will react rapidly with KCN when the two solids are ground together in the solid state (Firth *et al.*, 1968d). The products are the organocyanocobalamins, or rather the potassium salts of these anionic corrinoids. But the more interesting fact is that such reactions occur so readily in the solid state; the movement of ions is obviously facilitated by the large amount of water of crystallization in the lattice of the corrinoids. Cyanide does not, however, rapidly expel the 5-deoxyadenosyl ligand in the solid state as it does in aqueous solution, so that 5-deoxyadenosylcyanocorrinoids may be prepared and studied in the solid state (Firth *et al.*, 1968d).

The addition of soluble salts of Ag(I) or Zn(II) to aqueous solutions of dicyanocobalamin is reported to precipitate insoluble purple salts (Smith *et al.*, 1952a). No analytical data were given, but the purple colour clearly indicates the presence of a dicyanocorrinoid. A red silver salt of dithiocyanatocobalamin has also been reported (Smith *et al.*, 1952a), but in this case colour is no proof of the existence of a dithiocyanato corrinoid in the solid state.

A variety of other "adducts" or "compounds" have been reported from the reaction of, for example, B_{12} with gold, platinum, palladium and mercury salts or with heteropoly acids. The structures of none of these have been established. They probably involve the amide side-chains and are discussed in Chapter 10, Section II.

9

EQUILIBRIA INVOLVING THE CORRIN RING

Metal-free corrinoids, both naturally occurring and synthetic, have recently been obtained and it has become possible to examine the co-ordination and removal from co-ordination of several metal cations. The preparation, structure, acid-base equilibria and other properties of the metal-free corrinoids are dealt with in Section I. The co-ordination and removal of metal ions, together with evidence for the stability of the cobalt-corrin bond, are discussed in Section II. Little has yet been conclusively established about the acid-base properties of the corrin ring in the cobalt-containing corrinoids. However, B_{12} and other corrinoids dissolve in strong acids such as liquid HF and concentrated H_2SO_4 to give complexes of a type not observed in aqueous solution; and it appears that the corrin ring has been reversibly protonated under these conditions (see Section III). In strongly alkaline solution B_{12} and B_{12a} undergo a process of "self-reduction", probably initiated by the ionization of a proton from C_8, in which the cobalt ion is reduced at the expense of hydrogen atoms at the periphery of the molecule. The reversible loss of a proton from C_8, uncomplicated by the occurrence of any irreversible side-reaction, can be observed in the synthetic [7,7,12,12,19-pentamethyl, 15-cyano-corrin]-nickel-(II) cation (Bormann et al., 1967). These equilibria and reactions involving the loss of a proton from C_8 together with reactions involving hydrogen-deuterium exchange in the conjugated corrin ring (C_{10} only in the naturally occurring corrinoids, but C_5 and C_{15} as well in synthetic corrinoids) are dealt with in Chapter 15, Section I (electrophilic and nucleophilic attack at C_8 and C_{10}) and Chapter 11, Section II (self-reduction). Finally, the possible existence of isomers of the corrin ring (iso-corrinoids) and variations in the conformation of the corrin ring have already been mentioned in Chapter 6, Section I.

I. METAL-FREE CORRINOIDS

Toohey (1965) reported the isolation of certain orange-red cobalt-free corrinoids from a strain of the photosynthetic purple sulphur bacterium *Chromatium*. He subsequently examined various other micro-organisms, including representatives of all three classes of photosynthetic bacteria, for the occurrence of both coenzymes and cobalt-free corrinoids (Toohey, 1966). Of the photosynthetic bacteria the purple sulphur bacterium *Chromatiun* contains only cobalt-free corrinoids, while the purple non-sulphur bacterium *Rhodospirillum rubrum* contained the same cobalt-free corrinoids together with about 1% of a coenzyme and *Rhodopseudomonas palustris* yielded approximately equal amounts of cobalt-free corrinoids and coenzymes. The addition of cobalt to the medium had no effect on the relative proportions of the cobalt-free corrinoids to the coenzymes, showing that the former are not produced because of a deficiency of cobalt. The cobalt-free corrinoids appear to be unique but normal constituents of these photosynthetic bacteria. Both *Chromatium* and *R. rubrum* have yielded the same five cobalt-free corrinoids and in very similar proportions. These compounds differ in charge (three are positively charged, one neutral and one negatively charged in neutral solution) but are otherwise very similar in their spectra and chemical properties. The neutral compound contains 1 phosphate, 1 ribose and 1 aminopropanol per molecule, but has no heterocyclic base; while one of the positively charged compounds was found not to contain phosphate. They will all incorporate cobalt (e.g. on heating with 0.01 M $CoCl_2$ and 0.02 M NH_4OH at 100° for 2 minutes or at 22° for 10 hours) to give products with spectra identical to those of cobalt-containing cobinamides. The cobalt-containing products from the neutral and from one of the positively-charged compounds showed similar growth promoting activity (in assays with B_{12}-requiring bacteria) to those of cyanoaquocobamide and cyanoaquocobinamide respectively (Perlman and Toohey, 1966, 1968). This provides fairly good evidence for the identity of the corrinoid structures in both the metal-free and cobalt-containing forms, the charges in the metal-free forms being due to the presence of protons on two of the central nitrogen atoms of the corrin ring (Toohey, 1966).

A synthetic metal-free corrinoid was prepared by Fischli and Eschenmoser (1967). The corrin ring has so far only been synthesized in the form of a ligand co-ordinated to a metal by a "template" synthesis involving the cyclization of an open-chain tetradentate ligand occupying four co-ordination positions in a plane around the metal. In this case the metal ion used was zinc which, unlike cobalt and nickel, could be removed by the action of trifluoroacetic acid in acetonitrile; racemic 15-cyano-1,2,2,7,7,12,12-heptamethylcorrin was obtained in crystalline form as the hydrochloride (see Fig. 9.1). This free corrin ligand is a moderately strong base with a pK of 8.6 in dimethylcellosolve-water mixtures. There is no direct evidence as to which nitrogen atoms are protonated in either form of the compound. The absorption spectrum of the hydrochloride in ethanol is similar to that of Toohey's compounds in water at pH 7 except that the bands are slightly shifted to higher energy.

The absorption spectra of Toohey's orange-red metal-free corrinoids (see Fig. 9.2) are remarkably similar to those of, for example, B$_{12}$ itself, except that the intense band in the ultraviolet region occurs at higher energy in the cobalt-free corrinoid (329 nm) than in cyanocobalamin (361 nm). These spectra provide the evidence for concluding that the main absorption bands of the cobalt corrinoids are due to π–π^* transitions of the organic chromophore and are discussed in Chapter 5, Section II. All five of Toohey's compounds change colour from red to yellow in alkaline solution. Several changes are involved (see

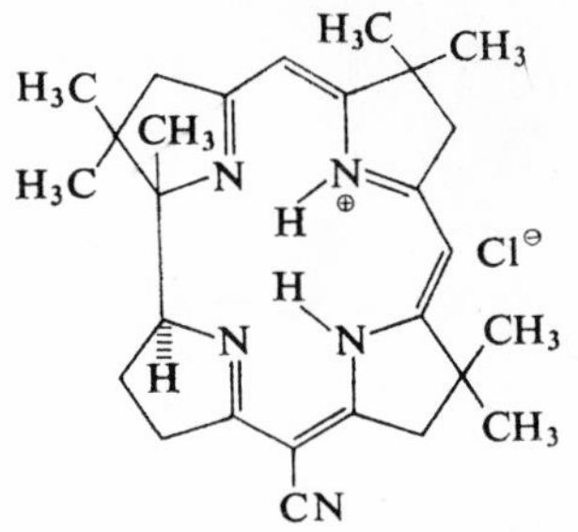

Fig. 9.1. The structure of Fischli and Eschenmoser's metal-free corrinoid, the hydrochloride of *rac.*-15-cyano-1,2,2,7,7,12,12-heptamethylcorrin. From Fischli and Eschenmoser (1967).

Fig. 9.2). If the pH is raised slowly the first change is accompanied by the disappearance of the bands at 524, 329 and 269 and the appearance of new bands at 482 and 288 nm; the change appears to be reversible when carried out in the absence of oxygen, but irreversible under normal conditions and shows a pK of 9.6. On raising the pH further a second and reversible change is observed with a pK of 11.2, the final product having an absorption band at 370 nm. Yet another compound is formed with a band at 385 nm if the cobalt-free corrinoid is added directly to 0.1 N NaOH; this is converted to the compound with the band at 370 nm on heating. The first, irreversible change is also brought about by the action of dilute HCl or by exposure to strong light. The variation of electrophoretic mobility with pH provides evidence for ionization with a p$K \geqslant 11$, but none in the range of pH 6–11 (Toohey, 1966). The structural changes accompanying these ionizations and reactions have not yet been established. But Thomson (1969) points out that the three compounds with bands at 524, 482 and 370 nm formed on gradually increasing the pH have absorption spectra typical of a symmetrical cyanine (i.e. a conjugated system containing an odd number of atoms, as in the corrin ring, and with the two protons symmetrically disposed either on N_{21} and N_{24} or on N_{22} and N_{23}), an unsymmetrical cyanine (only one nitrogen atom protonated) and a polyene

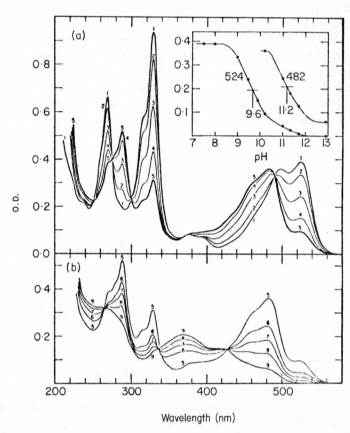

Fig. 9.2. Changes in the absorption spectrum of one of Toohey's metal-free corrinoids on raising the pH to show the presence of three different structures, represented by spectra 1, 5 and 9. The spectra correspond to the following pHs: 1, 7.5 and 8.0; 2, 9.0; 3, 9.4; 4, 9.9; 5, 10.2; 6, 11.0; 7, 11.3; 8, 11.7; 9, 12.9. From Toohey (1965).

respectively (i.e. an even number of atoms in the conjugated chain). He suggested that the ionization with a pK of 9.6 corresponded to the removal of a proton from one of the corrin nitrogen atoms and that the polyene structure of the third compound was formed by extension of the conjugated system to include C_1 or C_{19} through the loss of a proton from one of these carbon atoms.

II. THE CO-ORDINATION AND REMOVAL OF METAL IONS

All five of Toohey's metal-free corrinoids will incorporate cobalt when the reaction is carried out in alkaline solution (Toohey, 1966). The best conditions were reported to be: 0.01 M CoCl$_2$, 0.2 M NH$_4$OH and either 2 minutes at 100° or 10 hours at 22°. Ferric, manganese and nickel ions were not incorporated under similar conditions. Cobalt was not, however, incorporated when added to neutral solutions of the original orange-red compounds or to neutralized solutions of the yellow products formed by alkaline treatment (see preceding section). It seems reasonable that reaction occurs more readily when the ligand is neutral or carries a negative charge than when it carries a positive charge (i.e. at pH ⩽ 9).

Fischli and Eschenmoser's (1967) synthetic 15-cyano-1,2,2,7,7,12,12-heptamethylcorrin hydrochloride (see Fig. 9.1) will also incorporate cobalt when it is allowed to react with an excess of [Co^{II}(DMF)$_6$](ClO$_4$)$_2$ in acetonitrile for 2 hours at room temperature; reoxidation with air in a mixture of 1 N aqueous HCl and acetonitrile, followed by reaction with aqueous KCN gave crystalline racemic dicyano-[15-cyano-1,2,2,7,7,12,12-heptamethylcorrin]-cobalt(III) in over 90% yield.

No other metal ion has yet been incorporated into a metal-free corrinoid ligand, though nickel (Eschenmoser, 1963; Eschenmoser et al., 1965) and palladium (Yamada et al., 1969) and zinc (Fischli and Eschenmoser, 1967) as well as cobalt (Felner et al., 1967) corrinoids can be synthesized by reactions in which the metal cation is first co-ordinated by an open-chain tetradentate ligand which is subsequently cyclized to give the metal corrinoid. The only case in which the metal has been removed from the metal corrinoid is that of zinc; as described in the preceding section, this provides the method for the synthesis of a metal-free corrinoid (Fischli and Eschenmoser, 1967).

The cobalt ion is held extremely firmly by the corrinoid ligand. The stability of the cobalt-corrin bond is the main factor which has allowed the equilibria and reactions of cobalt corrinoids to be examined with such a wide range of reagents, e.g. with strong ligands such as cyanide (see Chapter 8, Section IV on formation constants with different ligands), strong acids such as liquid HF or concentrated H$_2$SO$_4$ (see next section), strongly alkaline solutions such as 30% NaOH at 120° (see Chapter 11, Section II on "self-reduction" in alkaline solution) and reducing agents (see Chapter 11, Section IV). The cobalt could not be removed by treating solid cobalamin-cobalt(II) with concentrated H$_2$SO$_4$ even at 80° (Diehl and Murie, 1952). The cobalt ion is, of course, liberated when the corrin ligand is completely destroyed; these reactions are discussed in Chapter 15. It certainly appears from the above qualitative observations that the corrinoid ligands may be compared with the phthalocyanine ligands in the firmness with which they bind transition metal ions.

7

III. COBALT CORRINOIDS IN STRONG ACIDS

The data of Table 8.7 and the equilibria discussed in Chapter 8, Section IV, show that when solutions of cobalamins are acidified, the Bzm is displaced from co-ordination and protonated, i.e.

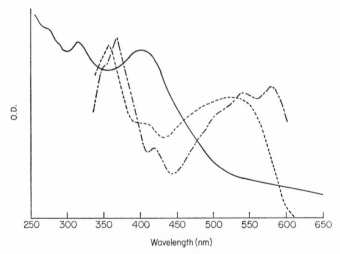

The pK depends on the nature of X and varies from p$K \sim 3$ for alkyl ligands to p$K \sim -3$ for $X = H_2O$, i.e. these equilibria are observed in very dilute to medium strong acid. Additional and so far unidentified equilibria and complexes have been observed under more strongly acidic conditions, namely in liquid HF and concentrated H_2SO_4.

Fig. 9.3. The absorption spectra of B_{12} in liquid HF (——) and of the recovered product after dissolution in water (– – – –) and the further addition of cyanide (–·–·–). From Katz (1954).

Katz (1954) reported that B_{12} dissolved in liquid HF to give an olive-green solution. The spectrum of this solution showed no change over 48 hours at 25°. Removal of HF under vacuum left a red solid which dissolved in water to give a red solution with an absorption spectrum which indicated the presence of a "modified cobalamin"; on adding KCN this gave the spectrum of B_{12} or dicyanocobalamin (see Fig. 9.3). Microbiological assay indicated that the major part of the product retained activity, i.e. the side-chains had not been attacked. The spectrum he shows of the "modified cobalamin" has a γ-band at $\lambda \geqslant 360$ nm and increased absorption around 480 nm; this is, in fact, the spectrum one would expect for B_{12} at pH $\sim$0, where some of the Bzm has been displaced and protonated and the spectrum will be intermediate between that of cyanocobalamin and cyanoaquocobinamide. We can probably conclude that when cyanocobalamin is dissolved in liquid HF the Co–CN bond, as well as the side-chains, remain intact. The spectrum of the olive-green solution in HF is unusual in showing absorption to beyond 650 nm; the first main absorption band occurs at $\sim$405 nm (see Fig. 9.3).

In 1962 it was reported (Hill *et al.*, 1962) that aquo- and cyano-cobalamin

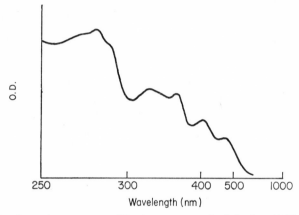

Fig. 9.4. The absorption spectrum of B_{12} in concentrated sulphuric acid. From Hill *et al.* (1962).

both dissolved in concentrated H_2SO_4 to give yellow solutions; the spectrum of cyanocobalamin in H_2SO_4 is given in Fig. 9.4. It was subsequently found that methylcobalamin also forms a new complex or complexes in H_2SO_4 (Pratt, 1964), that cobinamides behave similarly to cobalamins (Hayward *et al.*, 1965) and that 70% $HClO_4$ can be used as well as H_2SO_4 (Hayward *et al.*, 1965). Although the number and nature of these complexes have not yet been established, certain pieces of evidence have been obtained. The fact that the usual spectra of cyano- and methyl-cobalamin are regenerated when their solutions in concentrated H_2SO_4 are diluted with water shows that the Co—CN and Co—CH$_3$ remain intact (Pratt, 1964). Methyl- and cyano-cobalamin in H_2SO_4 are, however, both unstable towards light (Pratt, 1964). It has also been shown that cobalamins and cobinamides in sulphuric acid have identical absorption spectra above 300 nm, i.e. Bzm is not co-ordinated in the cobalamins (Hayward *et al.*, 1965), in contradiction to an earlier conclusion

(Hill *et al.*, 1962). It is puzzling that the first absorption band of the nucleotide benziminazole (whether free or bound in the cobalamins) occurs at 288 nm in alkaline solution, at 288.5 nm when co-ordinated to the cobalt and at 284 nm when carrying one proton (Beaven *et al.*, 1949, 1950) but at 288 nm again in concentrated sulphuric acid (Hayward *et al.*, 1965), presumably due to the addition of a second proton to the heterocycle. The identical position of the absorption band when co-ordinated and in concentrated H_2SO_4 was the reason for the original erroneous conclusion that Bzm was co-ordinated to the cobalt in cobalamins in H_2SO_4. The nature of the second axial ligand, if any, is not known. But since methylcobinamide appears to be mainly five-co-ordinate in aqueous solution (see Chapter 8, Section III) and since H_2SO_4 is a weaker donor than H_2O, it seems likely that the methylcorrinoids are five-co-ordinate in H_2SO_4. One may tentatively conclude, therefore, that the marked difference between the spectra in aqueous solution and in H_2SO_4 is caused by a change in the conjugated corrin ring, e.g. by protonation, which might occur at one of several different sites. Similar arguments about five-co-ordination cannot be made in the case of cyanocorrinoids in H_2SO_4, but it seems quite likely that the corrin ring may be protonated in this case too. The occurrence of acid-catalyzed hydrogen-exchange at C_{10} in the corrin ring of several corrinoids provides additional evidence for protonation of the ring (see Chapter 15, Section I). The relationship between the corrinoids observed in HF and in H_2SO_4 or $HClO_4$ is not yet clear.

It should also be mentioned that Alicino (1951) reported that when a solution of B_{12} in glacial acetic acid was titrated with $HClO_4$, the addition of more than eight equivalents of $HClO_4$ per molecule of B_{12} precipitated an amorphous orange-coloured solid of well-defined composition. Elemental analysis and titration of the acid in the solid agreed with its formulation as $B_{12}.6HClO_4$. The infrared spectrum of the solid showed that the cyanide had not been lost. When the solid was dissolved in water B_{12} was regenerated quantitatively as shown both by spectrophotometry and by microbiological assay. Since the solid is orange and not red in colour, some change has occurred in the axial ligands and/or the structure of the corrin ring. The Bzm has probably been displaced from co-ordination and protonated, since it is the most strongly basic part of the cobalamin molecule, to leave CN^- and H_2O or $CH_3CO_2^-$ as the axial ligands; this compound would, like cyanoaquocobinamide, be orange in colour. It is possible that the corrin ring has also been protonated and that Alicino's compound is analogous to those observed in solution in concentrated H_2SO_4 and $HClO_4$; the remaining protons would be accommodated by the phosphate of the nucleotide and by the amide side-chains.

There is clearly plenty of scope for the further study of corrinoids in strongly acid media, which could provide interesting information on structures and equilibria which are not observed in aqueous solutions.

10

EQUILIBRIA INVOLVING THE SIDE-CHAINS

The naturally occurring corrinoids possess side-chains which contain functional groups with weakly basic or acidic properties such as heterocyclic bases, amides, carboxylic acids, hydroxyl and phosphate groups. Equilibria involving the loss or gain of a proton from the side-chains are summarized in Section I and equilibria involving the co-ordination of metal ions in Section II. As indicated below, there is slight overlap with the subject matter of Chapter 8, since the heterocyclic base of a nucleotide side-chain can be treated either as part of the side-chain or, when co-ordinated to the cobalt, as an axial ligand.

The presence of basic and acidic groups in the side-chains also results in the formation of hydrogen-bonds, which play an important role in determining the properties of the corrinoids. The formation of hydrogen-bonds has been discussed in Chapter 6, Section II.

I. ACID-BASE PROPERTIES OF THE SIDE-CHAINS

The reversible loss or gain of a proton can occur at several places in the corrinoid molecule. In the case of the cobalamins the only functional groups which show equilibria in the range of pH 0–14 are Bzm, the phosphate and a hydroxyl group of the ribose, all of which form part of the nucleotide side-chain. In certain cases the second axial ligand may lose a proton (e.g. H_2O, imidazole) or gain a proton (e.g. the adenine portion of the 5-deoxyadenosyl ligand in the coenzymes); these equilibria are discussed elsewhere (see Chapter 8, Section IV). The amide side-chains can be protonated in more strongly acid solutions. Other acid-base equilibria may be observed in other groups of corrinoids, e.g. the dissociation of carboxylic acid side-chains or the protonation of other heterocyclic bases.

Of the three equilibria involving the nucleotide side-chain in the cobalamins quantitative measurements of the pK have been made only in the case of Bzm. This equilibrium involves the displacement of Bzm from co-ordination to the cobalt with simultaneous protonation, i.e.

The change in the absorption spectrum which accompanies this change in the axial ligands enables the pK to be determined by spectrophotometry. By contrast, the ionization of the phosphate and ribose groups (and carboxylic acids etc. in other classes of corrinoids) can only be studied by techniques such as potentiometric titration or the effect of pH on ionophoretic mobility. The pK of the free nucleoside 1-β-D-ribo-5,6-dimethylbenzimidazole has been determined as 4.7 (Davies et al., 1951). The base present in the side-chain of the cobalamins, however, has the α-link, but it is reasonable to assume that the pK of the base present in the cobalamins would also be 4.7, if it were not co-ordinated to the cobalt. Co-ordination to the cobalt stabilizes the unprotonated form and therefore lowers the observed pK. This pK is very dependent on the nature of the ligand in the *trans*-position (X), as can be seen from the following examples:

$$X = H_2O \qquad CN^- \qquad CH_3^- \qquad CH_3CO^-$$
$$pK = -2.4 \qquad +0.1 \qquad 2.7 \qquad \sim 4.5$$

Many such pKs have now been determined; for further examples and references see Table 8.7.

Evidence for the ionization of the phosphate and ribose hydroxyl groups is rather indirect. The pKs occur at ~ 1 and ~ 12.5 respectively in free nucleotides (Phillips, 1966). Very early work in 1949 on the potentiometric titration of aqueous solutions of B_{12} failed to reveal any ionization over the range of pH 2.40–11.45 (Fantes et al., 1949) or "in aqueous solution" (pH range not stated) (Brink et al., 1949). A subsequent study of the electrophoretic behaviour of B_{12} down to pH 1 revealed the uptake of a proton with p$K \leqslant 1$ (Ericson and Nihlén, 1953; Nihlén and Ericson, 1955). Ladd, Hogenkamp and Barker (1961) studied the acid-base properties of DBC and other coenzymes over the range of pH 2–12.5. They determined the pK for the displacement of Bzm (p$K \sim 3.5$) and for the protonation of the adenine part of the 5-deoxyadenosyl ligand (p$K = 3.5$). They also obtained evidence from potentiometric titration for another pK at the lower end of the range (p$K \approx 2$), which they ascribed to the phosphate, and from ionophoretic mobilities for an additional pK at the higher end of the range (p$K \approx 12$), which they did not comment upon, but which can probably be ascribed to the ionization of a hydroxyl group of the ribose.

Additional equilibria are observed under more acidic conditions. Potentiometric titration of B_{12} in glacial acetic acid showed it to be polybasic (Brink et al., 1949), while the addition of excess perchloric acid precipitated a solid of composition $B_{12} \cdot 6HClO_4$, a similar product also being obtained from B_{12a} (Alicino, 1951). Presumably both Bzm and some of the amide groups are protonated in these cases. When B_{12} is dissolved in concentrated H_2SO_4 it appears that Bzm carries a second proton and that the corrin ring itself is protonated; for a further discussion of the nature of corrinoids in strong acids see Chapter 9, Section III.

Some pKs have been reported for the dissociation of carboxylic acid side-chains; for example, the pK of Factor V_{1a} or cyanoaquo-[cobyric acid], in which the carboxylic acid is located on side-chain f, is 5.7 (Bernhauer et al., 1960c), while pKs of 3.1–3.9 have been reported for other corrinoids in which the carboxylic acid is situated on some other side-chain (Friedrich, 1966a). The effects of hydrogen-bonding between an ionized carboxylate anion and a co-ordinated H_2O are mentioned in the section on stereoisomerism involving the axial ligands (Chapter 8, Section II). The pK of the second dissociation constant of the primary phosphoric ester in cyanoaquo-[cobinamide-O-phosphoric acid] is reported as 6.9 (Bernhauer et al., 1960b). Finally, pKs have also been reported for the protonation of adenine in the nucleotide side-chain. The adenine in AC or 5′-deoxyadenosyl-[adenylcobamide] remains unco-ordinated in both acid and alkaline solution (Hill et al., 1970b) and its pK is approximately 3.4 (Ladd et al., 1961), while the adenine in ψ-B_{12} or cyano-adenine-[adenylcobamide] remains co-ordinated in both neutral and protonated forms, the pK being 2.3 and the proton probably being located on the —NH_2 group of the adenine (Hill et al., 1970b).

II. CO-ORDINATION OF METAL IONS BY THE SIDE-CHAINS

One would expect the corrinoid molecules, and in particular the cobalamins with their nucleotide side-chains, to act as good complexing agents for the binding of many metal cations, since the side-chains possess a large number of nitrogen and oxygen donor atoms and offer many possibilities for the formation of chelate rings. However, little or no systematic work has been done along these lines.

Diehl and co-workers (Brierly et al., 1955) reported that a red precipitate is formed when solutions of B_{12} and mercury(II) acetate in ethanol are made alkaline. Analysis of the solid gave the ratio Hg:Co = 2.82. The infrared spectrum was virtually identical with that of B_{12} except that the amide bands were considerably modified. They stated that "the formation of mercurated B$_{12}$ containing 2.8 mercury atoms per cobalt is about that expected for a material containing five amide groups"; in fact, B$_{12}$ is now known to contain six amide groups and the agreement is therefore better. Since Hg(II) ions are known to co-ordinate amide and imide anions (Sidgwick, 1950), it seems likely that each Hg(II) ion co-ordinates two amide anions of the side-chains (R.CO.NH$^-$), presumably to give a polymeric structure. It has also been shown that the presence of HgCl$_2$ reduces the solubility of B$_{12}$ in water, which may be due to some interaction of the same type (Havemeyer and Higuchi, 1960), but has little or no effect (at a concentration of 10^{-3} M) on the R_F values of B_{12} in chromatography using a sec-butanol-water mixture (Firth et al., 1968c). Havemeyer and Higuchi (1960) also studied the effect of eighteen other metal chloride salts and complexes on the solubility of B$_{12}$ in water. The majority (such as NaCl, CdCl$_2$, CoCl$_2$, etc.) slightly increased the solubility. However, PdCl$_2$, [PtCl$_6$]$^{4-}$ and [AuCl$_4$]$^-$ first slightly increased and then at higher concentration markedly decreased the solubility of B$_{12}$, indicating that some interaction occurred. In addition, PdCl$_2$ and [AuCl$_4$]$^-$ appeared to remove the co-ordinated cyanide from B$_{12}$. The authors quoted values for the ratio of metal to cobalt, but these values were determined by three indirect methods, which gave widely different results, and cannot be considered reliable. It is possible that the Pd(II), Pt(IV) and Au(III) ions act like Hg(II) in co-ordinating the amide anions of the side-chains, but this has yet to be established.

Havemeyer and Higuchi (1960) also used solubility studies to provide evidence for the interaction of B$_{12}$ with several heteropoly acids or anions such as phosphomolybdates and phosphotungstates. The nature of this interaction is not known; one could envisage the formation either of a salt between the heteropoly anion and a derivative of cyanocobalamin carrying one or more positive charges due to the protonation of Bzm and the side-chains (cf. the salt of B$_{12}$ with HClO$_4$ mentioned in Section I) or of a structure in which the uncharged cyanocobalamin and heteropoly acid were linked together by hydrogen-bonds (see Chapter 6, Section II).

It has also been reported that Bzm in the cobalamins may be displaced from co-ordination to the cobalt by complexing with Ag(I) and Hg(II) ions (Hill et al., 1970a).

There is other evidence for the complexing of transition metal cations by cobalamins. For example, Cavallini et al. (1968a,b) showed that ordinary samples of B$_{12a}$ contained traces of some impurity (probably copper) which catalyzed the reduction of B$_{12a}$ to B$_{12r}$ by thiols and which could only be removed by special purification using a chelating resin. The presence of impurities, which may be transition metal cations, has also been detected in samples of B$_{12}$ by magnetic susceptibility measurements (Wallman et al., 1951) and in samples of DBC by e.s.r. spectroscopy (Hogenkamp et al., 1963).

Section 4

Reactions

11

OXIDATION AND REDUCTION OF THE COBALT ION

Corrinoids may undergo oxidation and reduction due to either

1. a change in the valency of the cobalt ion or
2. reactions of the organic part of the molecule.

Oxidation and reduction of the cobalt usually occur rapidly and independently of any change in the organic part of the molecule. The valencies involved are I–III (see Chapter 7). No complexes of formally higher valency are known (analogous to the ferryl porphyrin complexes), unless we include the adducts of cobalt(II) corrinoids with O_2 (see Chapter 6, Section III). Electron transfer reactions between corrinoids of different valencies are discussed in Section I. By contrast, oxidation and reduction of the organic ring are slow and require more powerful reagents; these reactions are discussed in Chapter 15. There are, however, certain conditions under which oxidation and reduction of the cobalt must be considered in conjunction with the organic part of the molecule or with the environment (e.g. H_2O). In alkaline solution, for example, the Co(III) ion is reduced to Co(II) and eventually to Co(I) by the hydrogen atoms of the organic part of the molecule; this is termed "self-reduction" and is discussed in Section II. Secondly, B_{12s} is unstable below pH 5 and decomposes to give H_2 and B_{12r}; the evolution of H_2 and possible reactions involving the uptake of H_2 are discussed in Section III. Chemical reduction and oxidation are discussed in Sections IV and V respectively and redox reactions which are catalyzed by corrinoids in Section VI.

The term "redox reaction" is used for any oxidation or reduction reaction or sequence of such reactions, and "autoxidation" for the oxidation of a compound by O_2.

I. EQUILIBRIA BETWEEN THE DIFFERENT VALENCIES

The cobalt ion exhibits the valencies I–III in the corrinoid complexes and the following equilibrium is theoretically possible:

$$2Co^{II} \rightleftharpoons Co^{I} + Co^{III}$$

The polarographic half-wave potentials (see Chapter 7, Section VI) suggest that when Bzm and H_2O are the only axial ligands the equilibrium lies far to the left in aqueous solution. B_{12a} and B_{12s} do, in fact, react "instantaneously" and completely to give B_{12r} (Hill et al., 1962, unpublished work).

Attempts have been made to show the reverse disproportionation of Co(II) to Co(I) and Co(III) by removing either Co(I) by reaction with CH_3I or Co(III) by complexing. B_{12r} will, for example, react slowly with CH_3I to give methylcobalamin and B_{12a}. It was assumed that CH_3I can react only with Co(I) and that this reaction provides evidence for the disproportionation of Co(II); this assumption is not, however, justified since the pentacyanocobalt(II) complex can react directly with CH_3I. These reactions are discussed further in Chapter 13, Section I,D.

Schrauzer and Windgassen (1966b) reported that when KOH was added to a solution of B_{12r} in methanol, absorption bands characteristic of B_{12s} appeared in the spectrum, which they interpreted as evidence for the disproportionation of cobalt(II) to cobalt(I) and cobalt(III). This interpretation has been criticized by Yamada et al. (1968a), who pointed out that the authors had not excluded the possibility that the cobalt(I) complex was formed by self-reduction (see Section II).

It must be concluded that there is no direct evidence as yet for the disproportionation of cobalt(II) corrinoids.

II. SELF-REDUCTION OF CORRINOIDS

The hydrogen atoms of the organic part of the corrinoid molecule are potentially reducing agents and, under certain conditions, do in fact reduce the cobalt ion. Changes in the valency of the cobalt can be followed by the appearance of the very characteristic absorption spectra of the cobalt(II) and cobalt(I) corrinoids (see Chapter 7, Sections III and V). But the nature of the changes in the organic part of the molecule can only be established by comparison with compounds of known structure using chromatographic techniques.

Bonnett et al. (1957b) observed that when B_{12} is refluxed in strong alkali a brown solution is formed which turns red on cooling. The various products, in which one or more of the side-chains have been hydrolyzed to yield carboxylic acids, all contain a lactam ring formed by the fusion of the acetamide side-chain c on to C_8 with the elimination of two hydrogen atoms (see Fig. 2.1). They suggested (Bonnett et al., 1957a) that the colour change was due to the reduction of cobalt to the divalent stage with the concomitant formation of a radical at C_8.

It was subsequently shown that alkaline de-oxygenated solutions of B_{12a} turn brown even at room temperature and that the product has a spectrum very similar to that of B_{12r}, i.e. reduction of the cobalt has definitely occurred. The rate of reaction increased with pH; in 1 N NaOH at 9° the reaction followed first-order kinetics with $t_{1/2} \sim 8$ hours (Pratt, 1964). Yamada et al. (1964, 1966a) then reported that the heating of strongly alkaline solutions of B_{12} (30% NaOH, 120°, 1 hour) in the absence of air actually gave a spectrum very similar to that of B_{12s}. More recently it has been found that B_{12a} in 10 N KOH slowly gives the spectrum of a cobalt(I) corrinoid even at room temperature (Hill et al., unpublished work). The cobalt ion can obviously be reduced fairly readily to the cobalt(II) stage and with more difficulty to the cobalt(I) stage by a reaction involving some internal oxidation-reduction, which may be termed "self-reduction". The potential reducing power of the organic part of the corrinoid is only activated in alkaline solution, presumably due to the ionization of a proton and the formation of some active, negatively-charged organic functional group.

Yamada et al. (1964, 1966a) have tried to determine the changes in the organic part of the molecule which accompany reduction of the cobalt. Mild treatment (e.g. 10 minutes in 0.4% NaOH at 100°) of B_{12} gave a brown solution (i.e. cobalt(II)) which reacted slowly with methyl iodide to give a mixture of corrinoids with a methyl ligand on the cobalt (for the possible disproportionation of cobalt(II) to cobalt(III) and cobalt(I) and the reaction with methyl iodide see Chapter 13, Section I,D). The neutral compound isolated in 13% yield was identified as the methyl analogue of dehydrovitamin B_{12} i.e. methyl-Bzm-[8-amino-(5,6-dimethylbenzimidazolyl)cobamic acid-abdeg-penta-amide-c-lactam]. They also compared the rates of "self-reduction" to cobalt(II) of vitamin B_{12} and dehydrovitamin B_{12} and of the corresponding hydroxo complexes. In both cases the cobalamins underwent self-reduction much faster. These results suggest that the main source of reducing equivalents is represented by the hydrogen atoms on C_8 and the c side-chain, which are lost when the lactam ring is formed. Since the rate increases with pH, the initial stage is probably the ionization of a proton from C_8 to place an additional negative charge on the corrin ring. There is no evidence for the nature of the subsequent steps. Presumably two atoms of cobalt are reduced to the cobalt(II) stage for each mole of lactam formed, so that the product of self-reduction would be a mixture of the cobalt(II) cobalamin and cobalt(II)-"dehydrocobalamin". The self-reduction of the dehydrocobalamins shows that other hydrogen atoms, so far unidentified, can also act as reducing agents; one might, for example, expect C_3 and C_{13} to undergo reactions similar to that of C_8. All these self-reductions, because they take place in strongly alkaline solution, are accompanied by extensive hydrolysis of the side-chains.

As expected, the self-reduction of B_{12} is inhibited by the presence of excess cyanide (which would form dicyanocobalamin) and apparently by mercaptoacetate (which would itself reduce the cobalt ion) (Bonnett *et al.*, 1957a; Yamada *et al.*, 1966a). No quantitative comparison of the rate of self-reduction of B_{12} and B_{12a} has been made, but since only the latter has been reported to react at room temperature it is presumably the more reactive.

The essential changes involved in the reduction to cobalt(I) have not yet been established (Yamada *et al.*, 1964, 1966a). The more drastic treatment (e.g. 30% NaOH at 120° for 1 hour) leads to more extensive hydrolysis of the side-chains. The main product obtained after cyanocobalamin has undergone self-reduction to the cobalt(I) stage is a derivative of 8-amino-cobyrinic acid-c-lactam. Rather surprisingly, Yamada *et al.* found that the same methyl complex (apparently identical by absorption and i.r. spectra, paper chromatography and electro-phoresis) was formed by treating with methyl iodide the cobalt(I) complex formed from cyano-aquo-[8-amino-cobyrinic acid-c-lactam] by either (1) reduction with borohydride or (2) self-reduction on heating in alkali. They concluded that in the latter case reduction did not occur at the expense of the organic part of the molecule, but according to the following reaction:

$$[Co^{III}OH^-] + HO^- \rightarrow Co^I + H_2O + \tfrac{1}{2}O_2$$

The methyl complex was, however, obtained in only 39% yield. It cannot, therefore, be excluded that the reducing equivalents came from the corrinoids which were not isolated and there is no need to invoke the highly endothermic decomposition of H_2O or HO^- to oxygen and reducing equivalents.

Lee and Schrauzer (1968) reported that fresh solutions of B_{12a} show e.s.r. signals (at room temperature apparently), which they ascribe to a cobalt(II) complex (g-value not given) and to an organic radical ($g = 2.029$). It is difficult to judge the significance of these results, since no information is given to indicate the concentration of the cobalt(II) complex, the relation between the cobalt and organic signals and what changes are observed with time (i.e. whether reactions and/or equilibria are involved). It is conceivable that the observed signals are due to traces of a cobalt(II) corrinoid, in which a proton has been lost from C_8 to give a radical, in equilibrium with B_{12a} i.e.:

$$[Co^{III}(cobalamin)] \rightleftharpoons [Co^{II}(cobalamin-H)] + H^+$$

and that this compound then reduces another molecule of B_{12a} in the rate-determining step of self-reduction:

$$[Co^{II}(cobalamin-H)] + [Co^{III}(cobalamin)] \rightarrow$$
$$[Co^{II}(cobalamin-2H)] + [Co^{II}(cobalamin)] + H^+$$

Various yellow products are formed by the action of nitrogen-containing bases on B_{12a} in the presence of air. These reactions probably involve "self-reduction" catalyzed by the base, followed by reaction of the cobalt(II) corrinoids with O_2, which produces some stable yellow complex as a by-product. These reactions are discussed in Chapter 15, Section II.

III. HOMOGENEOUS REACTIONS INVOLVING H_2

Jaselskis and Diehl (1954) claimed that B_{12a} could be hydrogenated to B_{12r} without a catalyst, but no details of rates or conditions were given. Bayston and Winfield (1967) tried to repeat these results and observed a slight reduction of B_{12a} to B_{12r} by unpurified H_2, which could be ascribed to traces of CO. But Schrauzer and Windgassen (1967b) reported that B_{12} in methanol could be reduced by H_2 in the presence of a trace of B_{12r} as catalyst. Yamada et al. (1968a) found that when B_{12r} reacted with methyl iodide to form methylcobalamin, the yields were slightly higher in an atmosphere of hydrogen than in one of nitrogen, which suggested that H_2 could act as a reducing agent, albeit a very sluggish one. There is clearly a need for further work on the reactions of cobalt corrinoids with H_2.

Early qualitative observations suggested that both B_{12r} (Diehl and Murie, 1952; Hill et al., 1962) and B_{12s} (Hill et al., 1962) could liberate H_2 with simultaneous oxidation of the cobalt. It was later shown however that B_{12r}, in borate buffer at pH 9.3, was stable for over a month and B_{12r}, in 1 N H_2SO_4, was stable for at least 24 hours (Pratt, 1964). The liberation of H_2 by B_{12s}, on the other hand, has been confirmed and studied in more detail. Tackett, Collat and

Abbott (1963) studied the decomposition of B_{12s} over the range of pH 7–10. They identified H_2 and showed that at pH 9.6 the evolution of each mole of H_2 was accompanied by the oxidation of two mols of cobalt(I) to cobalt(II). The rate of decomposition shows a peculiar dependence on pH and under the conditions used approximately obeys the equation:

$$\text{rate} = 10^{0.38}[H^+]^{0.31} \text{ mol}^{-1} \text{ min}^{-1}$$

The half-life varies from 355 minutes at pH 10.0 to 87 minutes at pH 8.0. The rate of decomposition also depends on the nature of the buffer anion (EDTA, borate, phosphate) (Tackett *et al.*, 1963; Das *et al.*, 1968).

Finally, Schrauzer *et al.* (1968a) have reported that in the presence of a platinum catalyst B_{12s} is in equilibrium with B_{12r} and one atmosphere of H_2 at pH 9.9.

IV. CHEMICAL REDUCTION

Reduced corrinoids are known in which cobalt has the valencies II and I. The nature of these complexes and their potentials (mainly polarographic) have been discussed in Chapter 7. The products and rates of reducing the cobalt(III) corrinoids will obviously depend on both thermodynamic and kinetic factors. If we consider the cobalamins, where some of the relevant potentials are known (see Table 7.3), the potential for the Co(I)/Co(II) couple is very much more negative than that of the Co(II)/Co/III) couple and there will be a fairly sharp division between those reducing agents which can only produce Co(II) and those which can reduce the complex as far as Co(I). The most commonly used reducing agents for preparing Co(I) corrinoids are borohydride, zinc with NH_4Cl or acetic acid and Cr(II) complexes, while thiols in alkaline solution and catalytic hydrogenation are used to prepare Co(II) corrinoids. B_{12s} is thermodynamically and kinetically unstable in acid solution with respect to the liberation of H_2 and the formation of B_{12r} (see Section III) and can only be obtained in neutral or alkaline solution; the Cr(II) ion, for example, reduces B_{12} to B_{12s} at pH 9.5, but only gives B_{12r} at pH 3 (Beaven and Johnson, 1955). Since B_{12s} reacts very rapidly with B_{12a} to give B_{12r} (Hill *et al.*, 1962, unpublished work), the latter will always appear as an intermediate in the reduction of B_{12a} to B_{12s}. B_{12r} also appears as an intermediate in the reduction of B_{12}, but dicyanocobalamin (i.e. B_{12} in the presence of excess cyanide) is reduced directly to B_{12s} (Beaven and Johnson, 1955); this agrees with the relative potentials (see Table 7.3).

It is often difficult to decide from the literature whether a given reagent (X) acts as a reducing agent or not. If, for example, it is reported that a red solution of B_{12} turns yellow when treated with X this could be due to several causes other than reduction to B_{12r}.

1. Formation of a cobalt(II) corrinoid by "self-reduction" (see Section II); this may be the cause of the colour change observed on heating B_{12} in 90% aqueous ethanol (Beaven and Johnson, 1955).

2. The co-ordination of X to form a cobalt(III) cobalamin in which Bzm has been displaced from co-ordination to the cobalt (see below); this is probably the cause of the colour change observed on treating B_{12} with sulphite or dithionite (Schindler, 1951) or aquocobalamin with thiosulphate in acid (Brierly et al., 1953).

3. The formation of a "stable yellow" corrinoid (see Chapter 15, Section II), as in the catalytic hydrogenation of B_{12} in acid (Schmid et al., 1953).

On the other hand, reduction may also occur where no mention is made of any colour change; for example, HCN is liberated when B_{12} is heated with certain reducing agents (Boxer and Rickards, 1951), presumably through the intermediate formation of B_{12r}.

In the following list the reducing agents have been arranged into convenient, although sometimes rather arbitrary, groups. Reagents have only been included where there is reasonable evidence that they act as reducing agents or where there is some other point of interest. There are several examples of reagents which will reduce B_{12a} at room temperature, but B_{12} only on heating; and it can be assumed that a reagent which can reduce B_{12} will also be able to reduce B_{12a}.

A. CATALYTIC HYDROGENATION

B_{12} is reduced to B_{12r} by reduction at room temperature with one atmosphere of H_2 in the presence of platinum (Diehl and Murie, 1952; Kaczka et al., 1949; Schmid et al., 1953) or palladium catalyst (Beaven and Johnson, 1955; Schmid et al., 1953). B_{12s} can apparently also be formed under one atmosphere of H_2 above pH 9.9 (Schrauzer et al., 1968a). Complications arise in acid solution (Schmid et al., 1953). The cyanide is reduced to methylamine (CH_3NH_2) (Buhs et al., 1951; Ellingboe et al., 1955; Schmid et al., 1953).

B. METALS

B_{12} is reduced to B_{12s} by zinc in the presence of ammonium chloride (Schindler, 1951) or acetic acid (Müller and Müller, 1962b) or in alkaline solution (Collat and Abbott, 1964; Müller and Müller, 1962b). Zinc and HCl would merely give B_{12r} (see above). The rate of reduction by zinc and NH_4Cl is increased by the addition of metallic magnesium (Zagalak, 1963) or copper (Schrauzer, 1968).

C. METAL CATIONS AND COMPLEXES

B_{12} is reduced by $FeSO_4$ and $SnCl_2$ in acid at 100° with the evolution of HCN (Boxer and Rickards, 1951), by Cr(II) ions to B_{12s} in alkaline solution and to B_{12r} in acid solution (Beaven and Johnson, 1955; Boos et al., 1953) and by Ti(III) to B_{12r} (Bernhauer et al., 1961). Reduction of B_{12} by Ti(III) on a cellulose column has also been used for preparative purposes (B_{12a} and methylcobalamin) (Müller and Müller, 1962b). The rate of reduction of B_{12} to B_{12r} by Ti(III) in acid solution shows a first-order dependence on the concentrations of both, decreases with a rise in pH, and depends on the nature of other anions present (Cl^-, tartrate, citrate, oxalate, EDTA) (Pan and Hsu, 1967). B_{12a} is also reduced by $SnCl_2$ to B_{12r} in acid and to B_{12s} in very alkaline solution (Hill et al., 1962), and to B_{12r} by CuCl dissolved in KCl solution (Cavallini et al., 1968a,b).

D. ORGANIC COMPOUNDS

B_{12} is reduced by glucose, ascorbic acid, formaldehyde and formic acid at 100° with the evolution of HCN (Boxer and Rickards, 1951). B_{12a} is reduced to B_{12r} by formaldehyde, formic acid, ascorbic acid and hydroquinone at room temperature (Hill et al., unpublished work) and (? to B_{12r}) by various acyloins and keto-sugars (Schrauzer, 1968).

E. S-ANIONS

S-anions such as HS^-, thiols (RS^-), sulphite (SO_3^{2-}), thiosulphate ($S_2O_3^{2-}$), dithionite ($S_2O_4^{2-}$) and formaldehyde-sulphoxylate ($HOCH_2SO_2^-$), which are potentially both ligands and reducing agents, provide an interesting pattern, in which co-ordination and reduction, thermodynamic and kinetic factors can all be seen at work. Unless otherwise stated, the results mentioned here refer to the reaction with B_{12a}.

SO_3^{2-} and $S_2O_3^{2-}$ both act only as ligands, co-ordinated through the sulphur atom. In neutral solution they form the normal red cobalamin and in acid solution the yellow form, in which Bzm has been displaced and protonated (for equilibrium constants see Table 8.7); $S_2O_3^{2-}$, is of course, also decomposed by acid to give HSO_3^- and sulphur. The equilibrium constant for the displacement of co-ordinated H_2O by $S_2O_3^{2-}$ is only 7×10^3 M^{-1}, so that in alkaline solution (even in the presence of some excess $S_2O_3^{2-}$) it is decomposed to hydroxocobalamin and $S_2O_3^{2-}$. The formation constant for the binding of SO_3^{2-}, on the other hand, is 2×10^7 M^{-1} and sulphitocobalamin is therefore thermodynamically stable in alkaline solution in the presence of excess sulphite ion. The formation of sulphitocobalamin from hydroxocobalamin and SO_3^{2-} at pH 14 is, however, kinetically slow and probably proceeds through the intermediate formation of the O-bonded sulphitocobalamin, which then isomerizes to the stable S-bonded form (Firth et al., 1969). No formation of any cobalt(II) complex has been observed from either sulphitocobalamin or cobinamide, even at pH 14, though the latter undergoes some slow reaction whose nature is not known (Firth et al., 1969). Both sulphite complexes are decomposed by light in the presence of air to give sulphate, probably via the intermediate formation of B_{12r} and the anion radical SO_3^-, while thiosulphatocobalamin gives B_{12r} on photolysis under nitrogen (see Chapter 14, Section II).

Thiolate anions (RS^-) and sulphide (probably as HS^-) can act as both ligands and reducing agents. Kaczka et al. (1951) reported that when a slightly alkaline alcoholic solution of B_{12} was treated with H_2S the colour changed from red to brown, but turned red again on admitting air. B_{12r} was identified as the product of treating B_{12} with cysteine in alkaline solution by Beaven and Johnson (1955). Hill, Pratt and Williams (1962) found that sulphide, thioglycollate and cysteine could act as ligands to form red cobalamins which, like the cobalamins containing SO_3^{2-} and $S_2O_3^{2-}$, underwent a reversible change to a yellow form on acidification; reduction to B_{12r} occurred in alkaline solution. The identity of the thiolatocobalamins has subsequently been established quantitatively (see Chapter 8, Section IV). Thiols reported to reduce B_{12a} to B_{12r} include cysteine (Beaven and Johnson, 1955; Dubnoff, 1964; Hill et al., 1962; Pratt, 1964), homocysteine (Dubnoff, 1964), cysteamine (Cavallini et al., 1968a, b), thioglycollic acid (Hill et al., 1962; Smith, 1960), 2-mercaptoethanol (Dubnoff, 1964; Peel, 1963) and ethanethiol (Adler et al., 1966). Other thiols, which probably act as reducing agents, are mentioned in Dolphin and Johnson (1963) and Peel (1963). With most of these thiols there is evidence for the formation of the respective thiolatocobalamin, at least under certain conditions. The rate of reduction increases with pH (Cavallini et al., 1968a, b; Hill et al., 1962; Peel, 1963; Pratt, 1964) and the intermediate formation of the cobalamin may not be observed at high pH; see, for example, the reaction of B_{12a} with sulphide (Firth et al., 1969). Corrinoids are catalysts for the autoxidation of thiols (and presumably sulphide); these reactions are discussed in Section VI. It has recently been shown that cysteamine reacts with B_{12a} to form a cobalamin which does not undergo reduction to B_{12r} if either EDTA is added to the solution or the B_{12a} has been specially purified by passing through a chelating resin to remove trace metal impurities. Cysteamine will, however, reduce the purified B_{12a} on the addition of a trace of Cu(II); Fe(III), Co(II), Ni(II) and Zn(II) ions were ineffective. B_{12a} can also be reduced to B_{12r} by CuCl dissolved in aqueous KCl (Cavallini et al., 1968a, b). The evidence certainly suggests that the reduction by thiols is catalyzed by traces of copper. Glutathione appears to be unique among thiols in forming a cobalamin which undergoes reduction to B_{12r} only slowly or not at all (Dolphin and Johnson, 1965b; Dubnoff, 1964;

Wagner and Bernhauer, 1964); it seems quite likely that the amino-acid, carboxylate and two peptide groups of the co-ordinated glutathione could, like EDTA, tightly bind any Cu(II) ions which might otherwise catalyse the reduction. Thiols can also reduce B_{12a} to B_{12r} by a photochemical reaction (see Chapter 14, Section II). Side-reactions, which probably involve the corrin ring, are observed in the reaction of B_{12a} with sulphide and thiols (see Chapter 15, Section II).

B_{12} and B_{12a} both react rapidly with sodium dithionite ($S_2O_4^{2-}$) and slowly with sodium formaldehyde sulphoxylate ($HOCH_2SO_2^-$) to give the same yellow product, which is probably sulphoxylatocobalamin, in which Bzm is not co-ordinated (see Chapter 8, Section IV,G). At high pH B_{12a} reacts with dithionite to give the cobalamin as an intermediate, which then reacts further to form B_{12s}, while formaldehydesulphoxylate gives B_{12r} and then B_{12s} without the cobalamin being observed as an intermediate (Hill et al., unpublished work).

All the above mentioned S-anions can act as ligands, co-ordinated through the sulphur atom. They form three groups, depending on the occurrence of any subsequent reduction, as follows.

1. No reduction: SO_3^{2-}, $S_2O_3^{2-}$.
2. Reduction to B_{12r}; sulphide (HS^-), thiols (RS^-).
3. Reduction to B_{12s}: $S_2O_4^{2-}$, $HOCH_2SO_2^-$ (or probably SO_2^{2-}).

In both groups 2 and 3 the rate of reduction increases with pH, and at high pH the cobalamin may not be observed as an intermediate.

F. OTHER INORGANIC ANIONS

B_{12} is reduced by BH_4^- at room temperature (Beaven and Johnson, 1955) and by H_3PO_3 and H_3PO_2 at 100° with the liberation of HCN (Boxer and Rickards, 1951). B_{12a} is reduced by BH_4^- to B_{12s} in neutral or alkaline solution and to B_{12r} in acid solution (Hill et al., 1962). The reduction of B_{12} to B_{12s} by borohydride is catalyzed by the addition of copper, nickel or cobalt ions (Schrauzer, 1968).

G. SIMPLE GASES

For possible reactions with H_2 see Section III.

Bayston and Winfield (1967) discovered that B_{12a} can be reduced by CO; the reaction is extremely slow at room temperature but can be followed conveniently at 35° or above. Two mols of B_{12r} are produced for each mol of CO taken up and CO_2 was identified as the only gaseous product i.e.

$$2[Co^{III}.OH_2] + CO + 2H_2O \rightarrow 2[Co^{II}] + CO_2 + 2H_3O^+$$

First-order kinetics were observed and the rate depended linearly on the concentration of B_{12a} and the partial pressure of CO. The rate varied with pH, showing maxima at pH $\sim$ 6 and <1. The activation energy was determined to be 12.3 kcal/mol at pH 7.3. B_{12} and cyanoaquocobinamide were almost inert towards CO, while diaquocobinamide was twice as reactive as B_{12a}. They suggested that the rate-determining step for the reaction at pH 6 was

$$[Co^{III}OH_2] + CO \rightarrow [Co^{III}CO] + H_2O$$

followed by

$$[Co^{III}CO] + HO^- \rightarrow [Co^{III}.^-CO.OH]$$
$$[Co^{III}.^-CO.OH] + [Co^{III}.^-OH] \rightarrow 2[Co^{II}] + H_2CO_3$$

The reaction of CO has been confirmed by Lee and Schrauzer (1968), who studied the reduction of B_{12a}, cyanoaquocobinamide and the two corresponding lactams. The reactions followed first-order kinetics and showed no induction period. The rates were faster at pH 12.9 than at 5.6 (which appears to disagree with Bayston and Winfield), cyanoaquocobinamide reacts faster than B_{12a} (which again disagrees with Bayston and Winfield) and both these corrinoids reacted faster than the corresponding lactams. From this last observation they concluded that the C_8 position plays some part in the reaction and that CO reacts not with B_{12a}, but with the small quantity of a cobalt(II) corrinoid which exists in equilibrium with B_{12a} and which is formed by the ionization of the proton from C_8 followed by "self-reduction" (see Section II).

As can be seen from the above there is very little evidence about the mechanisms of reduction or even the relative rates, and it is now clear that simple and obvious interpretations may not be correct (e.g. the role of copper in the reduction by thiols, and the possible role of cobalt(II) corrinoids in the reduction by CO). In addition, one cannot decide from the observed formation of B_{12r} whether the initial step in reduction involves a one or two-electron change, since B_{12r} (the natural product of a one-electron reduction) could equally well be formed by the rapid reaction between B_{12a} and B_{12s} (formed by a two-electron reduction).

Very little has been reported on the reduction of corrinoids other than B_{12} and B_{12a}. The catalytic hydrogenation of methylcobalamin gives stoichiometric yields of B_{12r} and methane (Dolphin et al., 1964b). Most organo-cobalamins are very stable towards reduction by BH_4^-; exceptions are ethynyl-($HC\equiv C^-$), carboxymethyl-($HOOC.CH_2^-$), trifluoroethyl-($CF_3CH_2^-$) and sulphomethyl-cobalamins ($HO_3SCH_2^-$), of which carboxymethylcobalamin has been shown to yield acetic acid in almost quantitative yields (Firth et al., 1968d; Ljungdahl and Irion, 1966). Sulphitocobalamin is also readily reduced by borohydride (Dolphin and Johnson, 1965b). Cyanoaquocobinamide appears to behave similarly to B_{12} and B_{12a}. It is reduced to Co(I) by BH_4^- (Firth et al., 1968a) and by zinc and NH_4Cl (Müller and Müller, 1962b) and to Co(II) by BH_4^- and $SnCl_2$ at pH 0 (Hill *et al.*, unpublished work). It is an excellent catalyst for the autoxidation of thiols (see Section VI).

Reduction of the cobalt ion below the level of Co(I) or of the corrin ring appears to be very difficult except by catalytic hydrogen, which eventually yields colourless compounds (Beaven and Johnson, 1955; Schmid *et al.*, 1953).

V. CHEMICAL OXIDATION

Relatively little quantitative work has been reported on the oxidation of cobalt(I) and cobalt(II) corrinoids. As in Section IV, the reactions will be discussed according to the nature of the oxidizing agents, which are again arranged into rather arbitrary groups. For the reactions of more powerful oxidizing agents such as Cl_2, which attack the organic part of the corrinoid molecule, see Chapter 15.

A. O_2 AND H_2O_2

Cobalt(I) and cobalt(II) corrinoids are sensitive to oxygen. Green solutions of B_{12s}, for example, react virtually instantaneously with air to give yellow solutions of B_{12r}, which are then oxidized more slowly to red B_{12a}.

Cobalt(II) corrinoids will form adducts with O_2 at low temperature (Bayston *et al.*, 1969), i.e.

$$[Co^{II}] + O_2 \rightleftharpoons [Co^{II}O_2]$$

For further details see Chapter 6, Section III. These complexes are undoubtedly intermediates in the autoxidation of cobalt(II) corrinoids at room temperature, but the kinetic evidence to be discussed below shows that autoxidation is not a simple reaction.

It has been claimed that the quantitative oxidation of B_{12s} to B_{12a} requires 0.5 mols of O_2 (Dolphin *et al.*, 1964b), but this is at variance with the results of work on the autoxidation of B_{12r}. Earlier work concerned the oxidation of B_{12r}, which had been prepared by the catalytic hydrogenation of B_{12}, where complications could arise through the presence of methylamine (from the reduction of cyanide) (Buhs *et al.*, 1951; Ellingboe *et al.*, 1955; Schmid *et al.*, 1953) and reduction of the organic part of the molecule (Beaven and Johnson, 1955). More recent work has been done on B_{12r}, prepared either by the photolysis of organocobalamins under nitrogen or by controlled potential reduction; in the latter case no complications due to extraneous molecules are possible. Similar results have been obtained in all cases. When B_{12r} (prepared by c.p.r.) is oxidized by air, the spectrum shows the presence of a by-product absorbing at 460 nm in addition to B_{12a} (Hill *et al.*, unpublished work). The same by-product is obtained from the oxidation of B_{12r} prepared by the photolysis of DBC (Hogenkamp, 1964) or vinylcobalamin (Pratt, 1964) or by the catalytic hydrogenation of B_{12} (Smith, personal communication). In the first of these three cases B_{12a} was obtained in only 60–70% yield (Hogenkamp, 1964). The maximum yield of B_{12a} prepared by the catalytic hydrogenation of B_{12} followed by oxidation is also approximately 70% (Boos *et al.*, 1953). The nature of the yellow by-product which absorbs at 460 nm is discussed in Chapter 15, Section II; the corrin ring has probably been hydroxylated and its formation may be due to some reaction of H_2O_2 produced during the autoxidation of B_{12r}. The oxidation of B_{12r} should proceed according to the stoichiometry

$$4Co^{II} + O_2 + 2H_2O \rightarrow 4Co^{III} + 4HO^-$$

It was found, however, that 1.83 mols of O_2 were absorbed for each mol of B_{12r}, while 0.23 mols of CO and 0.60 mols of some unidentified gas were formed in addition to the expected 1 mol of hydroxide (Ellingboe *et al.*, 1955). The oxidation of B_{12r} is clearly not simple.

The kinetics of the autoxidation of B_{12r} are interesting. When B_{12r} is prepared in the absence of any additional reducing agents by the photolysis of vinylcobalamin under N_2 or by controlled potential reduction, oxidation by air at room temperature follows first-order kinetics with $t_{1/2} = 20$–30 minutes. Good isobestic points are observed during the formation of B_{12a} from B_{12r}, which indicates the absence of any significant concentration of a Co(II)-O_2 complex (Hill *et al.*, unpublished work; Pratt, 1964). The rate of autoxidation is greatly accelerated by the presence of certain reducing agents (usually $M/100$) such as thiols, quinol and pyrogallol, ascorbic acid, *m*- and *p*-phenylenediamine, phenylhydrazine and ferrocyanide; on the other hand NH_3, NH_2OH, N_2H_4, amines and aniline, heterocyclic bases such as pyridine, imidazole, quinoline and benziminazole, phenol and various other organic compounds containing sulphur were inactive. The spectrum showed that B_{12a} was formed by oxidation in the presence of quinol and ascorbic acid, while the presence of cysteine gave cysteinatocobalamin, which is known to be formed very rapidly by the reaction of cysteine with B_{12a}. In most cases the oxidation step was followed by slow reduction back to B_{12r} by the excess reducing agent. Small concentrations of the quinhydrone radical ($C_6H_4O_2^-$) could be detected by e.s.r. immediately after the oxidation of B_{12r} in the presence of quinol; no radical was formed under identical conditions in the absence of B_{12r} (Hill *et al.*, unpublished work; Pratt and Williams, 1968). These facts can be explained (Pratt and Williams, 1968) by postulating that O_2 cannot readily undergo a one-electron reduction, and that the oxidation of Co(II) occurs much more rapidly if the O_2 simultaneously receives one or two electrons from another molecule (HA), i.e.

$$[Co^{II}] + O_2 \rightleftharpoons [Co^{II}O_2]$$

followed by

$$[Co^{II}O_2] + HA \rightarrow [Co^{III}O_2H^-] + A\cdot$$
$$[Co^{II}O_2H^-] + H_2O \rightarrow [Co^{III}OH_2] + HO_2{}^-$$

It is interesting that the "catalysts" are compounds which are known to undergo one-electron oxidations very easily and that a free radical was detected in the case of quinol.

The probable reason for this behaviour can be understood by reference to the redox potentials for the reduction of O_2 at pH 7 (George, 1964).

$$O_2\text{---------}O_2{}^-\text{---------}H_2O_2\text{---------}HO^{\cdot}\text{---------}H_2O$$

$$
\begin{array}{ccccc}
& -0.45 & +0.98 & & +0.38 & +2.33 \\
& & +0.27 & & & +1.35
\end{array}
$$

In other words, although O_2 is a powerful oxidizing agent when it can accept two or more electrons, it is a very poor oxidizing agent when only one electron is available; hence the requirement for an additional reducing agent to convert the endothermic one-electron reduction of O_2 by Co(II) alone into an exothermic two (or three) electron reduction. The analogy between the autoxidation of thiols etc. by B_{12a} and the autoxidation of thiols, ascorbic acid and p-phenylenediamine by cytochrome oxidase and cytochrome c has been pointed out (Pratt and Williams, 1968).

H_2O_2 oxidizes B_{12r} much more rapidly than O_2 and produces very much larger amounts of the yellow product which absorbs at 460 nm (Hill et al., unpublished work). B_{12r} is also rapidly oxidized by a compound, probably the methylperoxy radical, which is produced during the photolysis of methylcobalamin in air (Pratt, 1964).

B. OTHER SIMPLE INORGANIC COMPOUNDS

I_2 oxidizes B_{12r} stoichiometrically (Brierly et al., 1953). $BrO_3{}^-$ does not oxidize B_{12r} (Boos et al., 1953). N_2O oxidizes B_{12s} to B_{12r} according to the equation:

$$2Co^I + N_2O \rightarrow 2Co^{II} + N_2$$

This was one of the first reactions of N_2O with a transition metal complex to be discovered (Banks et al., 1968). No reaction was observed between NO and B_{12r} (Firth et al., 1969).

C. METAL CATIONS AND COMPLEXES

Ferricyanide $[Fe(CN)_6]^{3-}$ oxidizes B_{12r} stoichiometrically (Diehl and Murie, 1952).

D. ORGANIC COMPOUNDS

Excess of cyanide apparently converts B_{12r} fairly rapidly (Diehl and Murie, 1952; Hill *et al.*, 1962) and B_{12s} very slowly (Yamada *et al.*, 1968b) to dicyanocobalamin even in the absence of oxygen. Traces of some compound which reacted with Nessler's reagent were detected in the latter case and the product assumed to be NH_3 (Yamada *et al.*, 1968b). It could also have been methylamine CH_3NH_2, since the pentacyanocobaltate(II) ion is known to be able to reduce cyanide to methylamine (Iguchi, 1942). Flavins and triphenyl tetrazolium chloride will apparently oxidize B_{12r} (Aronovitch and Grossowicz, 1962).

Many organic nucleophiles such as acetylene and alkyl halides react with Co(I) corrinoids to form organocorrinoids; methyl radicals react with B_{12r} to give methylcobalamin. These reactions are discussed in Chapter 13, Section I. Crotonic acid ($CH_3CH{=}CH.COOH$) oxidizes B_{12s} to B_{12r} (Smith *et al.*, 1964), perhaps via the intermediate formation of an organocobalamin.

E. OTHER ELECTROPHILES

B_{12s} reacts with protons to liberate H_2 and form B_{12r} (see Section III). B_{12s} also reacts with the acid chlorides of certain sulphur-containing oxy-acids such as SO_2Cl_2 and RSO_2Cl to form cobalamins with a Co—S bond (see Chapter 13, Section III) and with trialkyltin halides and dialkylarsenic halides to give very air-sensitive compounds, which have not been isolated or characterized, but which probably contain Co—Sn and Co—As bonds (Schrauzer and Kratel, 1965).

VI. CATALYTIC REACTIONS

Corrinoids can obviously act as catalysts for the interaction of oxidizing agents (O) and reducing agents (R) where O is known to be able to oxidize the reduced corrinoid alone and R to reduce the oxidized form alone. Examples which have been specifically mentioned or studied as catalytic reactions are: the oxidation of thiols and iodide by O_2 (discussed in more detail below); the oxidation of CO by O_2, which probably proceeds via the formation of cobalt(II) (Bayston and Winfield, 1967) (see Section IV,G); the reduction of

N_2O by BH_4^-, which proceeds via the formation of cobalt(I) (Banks et al., 1968) (see also Section V,B); the reduction of flavins, triphenyltetrazolium chloride and viologen dyes by thiols (Aronovitch and Grossowicz, 1962; Schrauzer et al., 1968b); the reduction of methylene blue by thiols, sulphide, ascorbic acid, triose reductone, hydrazine and phenylhydrazine (Schrauzer et al., 1968b) (see also below); the electrolysis of water to give hydrogen (Das et al., 1968); and the reductive methylation of aniline, N-methylaniline and thiols to N-methylaniline, N,N-dimethylaniline and methylthioethers by formaldehyde and H_2 according to the equations

$$Ar.NHR + HCHO + H_2 \rightarrow Ar.NR.CH_3 + H_2O \ (R = H \text{ or } CH_3)$$
$$RSH + HCHO + H_2 \rightarrow RSCH_3 + H_2O$$

which is catalyzed by B_{12r} in aqueous methanol at room temperature (Schrauzer and Windgassen, 1967a,b).

Many of these reactions are catalyzed by other groups of cobalt complexes; for example, the autoxidation of thiols is catalyzed by the bis-DMG (Schrauzer and Windgassen, 1967b) and phthalocyaninetetrasulphonate complexes (Kundo and Keyer, 1968), the reduction of N_2O by BH_4^- by the bis-DMG and tris(bipyridyl) complexes (Banks et al., 1968), reductive methylation by the bis-DMG complexes (Schrauzer and Windgassen, 1967a), and the reduction of methylene blue and benzylviologen by several other cobalt complexes (Schrauzer et al., 1968b). There appears to be nothing unique about the catalytic activity of cobalt corrinoids in vitro and many more parallels will doubtless be discovered in the future.

Corrinoids appear to catalyze the reduction of disulphides (RSSR) to thiols (RSH) in cells; see, for example, Dubnoff (1950). But neither the direct reduction of a disulphide by a cobalt(I) or cobalt(II) corrinoid nor the reduction of disulphides catalyzed by corrinoids have yet been reported. The bis-DMG complexes, however, catalyze the reduction of disulphides to thiols by hydrogen (Schrauzer and Windgassen, 1967b).

A. AUTOXIDATION OF THIOLS

Dubnoff (1950) was the first to report that B_{12} catalyzed the oxidation of thiols (glutathione and homocysteine) by air. These reactions have been studied in more detail by Peel (1962a,b, 1963) and by Aronovitch and Grossowicz (1962) (hereafter referred to as A and G). The simple reduction of corrinoids by thiols has already been discussed in Section IV, E. A and G (1962) reported that four sylphydryl groups were oxidized for every mol of O_2 consumed and identified cystine and homocystine as the oxidation products of cysteine and homocysteine respectively. Peel (1963) also found that the uptake of O_2 corresponded (within 96%) to that expected for the oxidation of mercaptoethanol to the disulphide. The stoichiometry of these reactions is therefore:

$$4RSH + O_2 \rightarrow 2RSSR + 2H_2O$$

The rate of the catalytic reaction depends in a complex manner on a large number of factors. Peel found that when high concentrations (0.2 M) of mercaptoethanol were used the rate of uptake of O_2 in the presence of either cyanoaquocobinamide or B_{12a} decreased with time, due probably to the occurrence of some side-reaction which poisoned the catalyst. In the presence of B_{12}, however, the rate was initially lower and increased with time, obviously due to the slow removal of cyanide to form the catalytically more active B_{12a}. When lower concentrations of thiol (3×10^{-2} M) were used and the rate of oxygen consumption measured polarographically, the rate was found to be constant until the partial pressure of O_2 had fallen to about one fifth of the original level. The rate of autoxidation of mercaptoethanol varied linearly with the concentration of cyanoaquocobinamide over the range studied (up to 1.8×10^{-8} M); and the rate increased with the concentration of the thiol (studied up to 1.5×10^{-2} M), but showed a saturation effect, the half maximal rate being observed with 0.3×10^{-2} M thiol (Peel, 1963). A and G stated that the rate was directly proportional to the concentration of the thiol and of the corrinoid, but in fact the data presented in Table 1 of their paper for the effect of varying the concentration of the corrinoid on the rate of oxygen uptake show a very marked saturation effect. The cause of this discrepancy may be that A and G used much higher concentrations (up to 10^{-5} M cyanoaquocobinamide and 2×10^{-4} M B_{12}) than Peel. The variation of the rate of autoxidation of mercaptoethanol with pH in the presence of cyanoaquocobinamide is sigmoid, rising from virtually zero at pH 5 to a plateau at pH ~ 8 with a point of inflection at pH ~ 7.2 (Peel, 1963). A and G reported similar results in the autoxidation of homocysteine. The relative catalytic activity of different corrinoids in the autoxidation of mercaptoethanol was reported as: DBC 0.3, B_{12} 1.0, B_{12a} 10, various cobalamins with altered side-chains 7–50, Factor D (structure unknown) 2500, cyanoaquocobinamide 4000 (Peel, 1963). A and G also observed the order cyanoaquocobinamide $> B_{12a} > B_{12}$ for the autoxidation of homocysteine at pH 8, but reported that DBC was almost as active as B_{12a} (1962); they did not, however, state whether they took precautions to prevent the photolysis of DBC, which would rapidly convert it into B_{12a}. Peel (1963) found that the rate of oxygen uptake in the presence of cyanoaquocobinamide at pH 7.1 varied with the nature of the thiol in the following order (relative rates taken from Table 2 and corrected to correspond to a concentration of 3×10^{-2} M): glutathione 12, cysteine 20, thioglycollate 30, 2-mercaptoethanol 100, 2,3-dimercaptopropanol 156, dihydro-6-thioctic acid amide 2040.

A and G (1962), on the other hand, state that glutathione, cysteine, mercapto-ethanol and dimercaptopropanol are all oxidized at approximately equal rates in the presence of B$_{12a}$ or cyanoaquocobinamide; again it may be that the higher concentration of corrinoid leads to different kinetics. To give an example of the catalytic affect of cyanoaquocobinamide one can use the data given by Peel (1963) in Table 2 and Fig. 5 of that work. The rate of autoxidation of 3×10^{-2} M mercaptoethanol at pH 7.1 is increased over a hundred-fold from about 5.6 μl O$_2$ (or 1.0×10^{-6} equivs) to about 700 μl O$_2$ (or 1.3×10^{-4} equivs) per minute per litre of solution by the presence of 1.8×10^{-8} M cyano-aquocobinamide (N.B. Peel quotes results for 8 ml of solution).

The question arises as to which cobalamin and which cobinamide are the catalytically active complexes. The dicyano complexes are inert, since the catalytic activity can be completely suppressed by the presence of 10^{-4} M KCN (Aronovitch and Grossowicz, 1962; Peel, 1963), and it has been shown that dicyanocobinamide is not attacked by thiols (Peel, 1963). B$_{12a}$ (see Section IV,E) and cyanoaquocobinamide (Firth et al., 1969), on the other hand, both react instantaneously with thiols to give thiolate complexes, which then react further. B$_{12}$ is presumably attacked by thiols directly but at a much slower rate than B$_{12a}$; during the steady-state a proportion of the total cobalamin will be present as B$_{12}$, the amount depending on kinetic and thermodynamic factors such as the relative formation constants of the cyanide and thiolate complexes. Cyanoaquocobinamide will also produce a steady-state mixture of cobalt(III) cobinamides containing the ligands H$_2$O, HO$^-$, CN$^-$ and RS$^-$ in addition to Co(II) complexes. It is a pity that the catalytic activity of pure diaquocobinamide has not been studied. The sensitivity of the system to poisoning by cyanide is indicated by the fact that the rate of autoxidation of 3×10^{-2} M mercaptoethanol in the presence of 9×10^{-9} M cyanoaquocobin-amide at pH 7.1 is reduced by 50% by the presence of between 10^{-7} and 10^{-8} M free cyanide (calculated from the amount of KCN added and the pK_a of HCN) (Peel, 1963).

The mechanism of these reactions is undoubtedly complex and different paths may be involved in neutral solution, where kinetic studies have been made, and in alkaline solution, where only qualitative observations have been made. Peel (1963) observed that mercaptoethanol reacted with B$_{12a}$ at pH 11 to form the brown B$_{12r}$; shaking in air temporarily restored the red colour (Co^{III}), which then changed back to brown (Co^{II}). However, if B$_{12a}$ is treated with mercaptoethanol at pH 7.1, the red solution (H$_2$O $\rightarrow$ Co^{III}) immediately becomes violet (RS$^-$ $\rightarrow$ Co^{III}) and then more slowly yellow-brown. The spectrum of this brown compound was apparently similar to that of B$_{12r}$ but lacked the intense band at 313 nm (other details not given) and, furthermore, the colour did not change back to pink on shaking in air (Peel, 1963). A and G made similar observations. When B$_{12a}$ or cyanoaquocobinamide is allowed to react with homocysteine or mercaptoethanol (? at pH 8) the spectrum changes rapidly. The compound formed from cyanoaquocobinamide has a spectrum (shown in Fig. 2 of their paper) which is similar to, but not identical with, that of cobinamide-cobalt(II) (see Table 7.1); the first band occurs at 475 nm, but the band at 315 nm is much less intense than in cobinamide-cobalt(II). They also report that this compound is not converted to a cobalt(III) complex by O_2, H_2O_2 or cyanide (Aronovitch and Grossowicz, 1962). The nature of the brown intermediate in neutral solution remains unknown, and it cannot be assumed that the catalytic oxidation in neutral solution proceeds via the formation of B_{12r}; cf. the oxidation of iodide (see next section). In addition, it is now known that the reduction of B_{12a} by thiols may be catalyzed by traces of copper (see Section IV,E) and that the autoxidation of B_{12r} is greatly accelerated by the presence of thiols (see Section V,A); though it should be mentioned in this connection that Peel (1963) found that the autoxidation of mercaptoethanol at pH 7.1 in the presence of cyanoaquocobinamide was neither inhibited by the presence of 10^{-3} M EDTA nor accelerated by the addition of 10^{-5} M $CuSO_4$. In view of the uncertainties in the steps involved it is hardly worth speculating on the nature of the rate-determining step. But it seems clear from the variation of the rate of the catalytic reaction with the concentration of corrinoid, of thiol and of O_2 that there are two (or more) reactions with similar rates. The point of inflection at pH 7.2 in the variation of rate with pH corresponds neither to the pK_a of mercaptoethanol, which Peel (1963) determined to be 9.5, nor to the formation of cyanohydroxocobinamide ($pK_a = 11$, see Table 8.7).

B. AUTOXIDATION OF IODIDE

The catalytic effect of B_{12a} on the oxidation of iodide by O_2 in acid was discovered by Brierly, Ellingboe and Diehl (1953). The overall reaction is (assumed to be)

$$4I^- + 4H^+ + O_2 \rightarrow 2I_2 + 2H_2O$$

They studied the effect of varying the concentration of B_{12a}, I^- and H_2SO_4 (pH 0.5–2) on the rate of formation of iodine in air at 27° and determined the amount of iodine liberated by potentiometric titration with thiosulphate. The rate rises, but decreasingly so, as the concentration of B_{12a} is increased; they attributed the fall-off at higher concentrations to the supply of O_2 being inadequate to support the maximum possible rate. The rate also rises with increasing concentration of I^- or H_2SO_4 (but is still noticeable at a pH as high as 4 (Pratt and Thorp, 1966)) and again shows a saturation effect. They analyzed their kinetic data by the methods used for enzyme kinetics, i.e. plots of (rate)$^{-1}$ versus (concentration)$^{-1}$, and showed that they could be interpreted in terms of intermediates containing one I^- and one H^+ with the following dissociation constants: for the $B_{12a}-I^-$ complex $K_{diss} = 0.40$ M, for the $B_{12a}-H^+$ complex $K_{diss} = 0.43$ M. The association or formation constants are the reciprocals, viz. 2.5 M^{-1} for $B_{12a} + I^-$ and 2.3 M^{-1} for $B_{12a} + H^+$; the latter corresponds to a pK of 0.4. They found that B_{12} had virtually no catalytic activity and that the activity of B_{12a} was not enhanced by the addition of histidine or certain proteins. They also noted that B_{12r} was stoichiometrically oxidized by I_2 to B_{12a} in acid solution and that no B_{12r} was formed from B_{12a} and I^- (Brierly *et al.*, 1953).

No other kinetic studies on this reaction have been reported, but Pratt and Thorp (1966) have studied the equilibria exhibited by B_{12a}, I^- and acid under nitrogen. B_{12a} reacts with I^- to give iodocobalamin; the formation constant in 0.5 N KNO_3 is 32 M^{-1}. On acidification, the Bzm is protonated and displaced; the pK lies between 0 and 1. No formation of B_{12r} was observed. These values are the same, within an order of magnitude, as the values obtained from kinetic studies (see last paragraph). This suggests that the reactive intermediate is iodo-[cobalamin(BzmH$^+$)]; this may be a five-co-ordinate complex (see Chapter 8, Section III). The O_2 presumably attacks this complex directly, since there is no evidence for the formation of B_{12r}; one possibility is that the O_2 becomes co-ordinated in the position *trans*- to I^- and that the redox reaction occurs by the transfer of electrons from I^- to O_2 through the cobalt ion.

C. REDUCTION OF METHYLENE BLUE BY THIOLS

In studying the reduction of methylene blue by thiols, catalyzed by cobalt corrinoids, Schrauzer and Sibert (1969) found that the rate increased with the concentration of the corrinoid (and with the nature of the complex in the order cyanoaquocobinamide > B_{12a} > B_{12}), with the concentration of the thiol (and mercaptoethanol > thioglycollic acid > thiomalic acid), with the pH and, at low concentrations only, with the concentration of methylene blue. They suggested that the rate-determining step was the conversion of the thiolato-cobalt(III) corrinoid into the cobalt(II) complex, i.e.

$$[RS^- \rightarrow Co^{III}] \rightarrow [Co^{II}] + RS\cdot$$

12

LIGAND SUBSTITUTION REACTIONS

Ligand substitution reactions of the cobalt corrinoids concern mainly the cobalt(III) complexes. No ligands have yet been found which co-ordinate reversibly to the cobalt(I) ion (see Chapter 7, Section V), though irreversible reactions may occur with nucleophiles such as CH_3I (see Chapter 13, Section I). A few ligands are known which co-ordinate reversibly to the cobalt(II) ion (see Chapter 6, Section III and Chapter 7, Section III) but no kinetic data have yet been reported; these reactions are probably very fast. The range of ligands which can co-ordinate to the cobalt(III) ion, on the other hand, is very large (see Table 8.7). Only a few quantitative kinetic studies have so far been reported, but qualitative observations provide some additional information.

Some general features of ligand substitution reactions observed in simple cobalt(III) complexes are described in Section I as a background to the discussion of ligand substitution in cobalt(III) corrinoids in Section II.

I. COBALT(III) COMPLEXES IN GENERAL

Most kinetic studies of ligand substitution reactions have been carried out on octahedral cobalt(III) and square planar platinum(II) complexes. Work on the platinum(II) complexes revealed a regular pattern of reactivity, which included first- and second-order kinetics and a strong influence of the ligand in the *trans*-position—the so-called "*trans*-effect". By contrast, no real pattern could be detected in the large amount of experimental data accumulated on cobalt-(III) complexes, mainly ammine and bisethylenediamine complexes, up to 1960s; for reviews of this work see Chan and Miller (1965), Tobe (1966), Basolo and Pearson (1967) and Pratt and Thorp (1969). The situation has changed completely within the last decade due to the study of cobalt(III) complexes with other ligands, and a brief survey of the more recent and relevant work on substitution reactions of cobalt(III) complexes will provide a useful background for a discussion of the corrinoids. See also the review in Pratt and Thorp (1969).

Kinetic studies provide information of two kinds:

1. the order of the reaction, which may provide evidence for the mechanism of reaction and
2. the rate constants, which one attempts to interpret in terms of electronic theories of the complex.

By analogy with mechanisms established for substitution reactions in organic chemistry we can distinguish two extreme types of mechanism for the substitution of one ligand Y by another Z in octahedral cobalt(III) (and other transition metal) complexes; these are designated S_{N1} and S_{N2} (substitution, nucleophilic, unimolecular and bimolecular respectively). In the S_{N1} mechanism the initial step is the breaking of the Co—Y bond to give a five-co-ordinate intermediate, which then picks up the new ligand Z. The configuration of the S_{N1} intermediate may be approximately square pyramidal or trigonal bipyramidal; in the case of the cobalamins, however, the geometry of the corrin ring can allow only the square pyramidal type of intermediate. In the S_{N2} mechanism the initial step is the formation of the new Co—Z bond to give a seven-co-ordinate intermediate, which then loses the ligand Y. The incoming ligand Z could attack on the same side as the leaving ligand Y or on the opposite side; again the presence of the corrin ring allows only the front-side attack. Whether the mechanism approximates to S_{N1} or S_{N2} will depend on the degree of interaction between the attacking and leaving ligands and there need be no hard and fast distinction between them.

Two kinetic rate equations are observed experimentally for ligand substitution reactions of cobalt(III) complexes: first-order, where the rate depends only on the concentration of the initial cobalt complex (here designated CoL_5Y), i.e.

$$\text{Rate} = K_1[CoL_5Y]^1$$

and second-order, where the rate also depends on the concentration of the attacking ligand Z, i.e.

$$\text{Rate} = K_2[CoL_5Y]^1[Z]^1$$

When Z is a solvent molecule (e.g. H_2O), its concentration dependence cannot be studied experimentally and first-order kinetics are observed. A dependence on pH, i.e. on $[H^+]^1$ or $[HO^-]^1$, is frequently observed due to the ionization of a co-ordinated or attacking ligand (e.g. H_2O/HO^-, NH_3/NH_2^-, NH_4^+/NH_3, HN_3°/N_3^-). A good example is shown in Fig. 12.1. A few reactions show a change from second-order kinetics at low concentrations of attacking ligand Z to first-order kinetics at higher concentration (see below).

It is not always easy to deduce the mechanism and molecularity of the reaction from the kinetic order of the reaction. First-order kinetics do indicate a unimolecular reaction except when Z is a solvent molecule or when some unimolecular rearrangement of the complex precedes the bimolecular step. But second-order kinetics could be observed for any of the following reaction mechanisms:

1. True bimolecular reaction (S_{N2}), i.e.

$$[CoL_5Y] + Z \rightarrow [CoL_5YZ] \rightarrow [CoL_5Z] + Y$$

2. Extremely rapid and reversible formation of the five-co-ordinate intermediate, followed by a relatively slow uptake of Z, i.e. S_{N1}

$$[CoL_5Y] + Z \rightleftharpoons [CoL_5] + Y + Z \rightarrow [CoL_5Z] + Y$$

Increasing the concentration of Z and hence the rate of the second step may in certain cases lead to a change to first-order kinetics; this is called a "limiting S_{N1} mechanism".

3. The formation of an ion-pair which then liberates Y by an unimolecular reaction, followed by the incorporation of Z, i.e.

$$[CoL_5Y] + Z \rightleftharpoons [CoL_5Y]Z \rightarrow [CoL_5]Z + Y \rightarrow [CoL_5Z] + Y$$

The base-catalyzed hydrolysis of ammine and bisethylenediamine complexes is probably a more complicated example of (3), in which the HO^- first forms an ion pair and then removes a proton, for example from NH_3 to give co-ordinated NH_2^-; the presence of NH_2^- then labilizes the complex to undergo a unimolecular elimination of Y.

No S_{N2} mechanism has yet been conclusively established for any cobalt(III) complex. But in the following cases there is fairly definite evidence for an S_{N1} mechanism:

1. Kinetic studies have established the S_{N1} mechanism for five groups of complexes (charges omitted):

(a) $[Co(CN)_5H_2O] + Z \rightleftharpoons [Co(CN)_5Z] + H_2O$
where Z is H_2O, HO^-, Cl^-, Br^-, I^-, I_3^-, NCS^-, N_3^- and HN_3° (Haim et al., 1965; Grassi et al., 1967)

(b) $[Co(CN)_4SO_3H_2O] + CN^- \rightarrow [Co(CN)_5SO_3] + H_2O$ (Tewari et al., 1967)

(c) $[Co(NH_3)_4SO_3Y] + Z \rightleftharpoons [Co(NH_3)_4SO_3Z] + Y$
where Y and Z are HO^-, NH_3, NO_2^-, NCS^- and CN^- (Halpern et al., 1966)

(d) diaquo[haematoporphyrin]-cobalt(III) + NCS^- and the hydroxoaquo analogue + CN^- (Fleischer et al., 1968)

(e) substitution of H_2O by imidazole, benzimidazole and PPh_3 in complexes of the type $[R . Co\{(DOH)(DO)pn\}H_2O]^+$, where R is an organo-ligand and $\{(DOH)(DO)pn\}$ is the 1,3-bis(biacetylmonoximeimino)-propanato ligand (Costa $et\ al.$, 1970)

2. Competition studies have shown the presence of a common S_{N1} inter-mediate in certain aquation reactions of pentammine complexes; for example, the Hg(II)-catalyzed hydrolysis of the chloro and bromo com-plexes in water containing O^{16} and O^{18} gives the same isotopic ratio in both reactions, indicating the occurrence of some common intermediate, which must therefore be the five-co-ordinate intermediate of the S_{N1} reaction (Dolbear and Taube, 1967). The ratios of cis- and $trans$-isomers produced in the base-catalyzed hydrolysis of the complexes $[Co.en_2XY]$ is virtually independent of the nature of the leaving group Y, which again suggests the occurrence of a common S_{N1} intermediate (Jordan and Sargeson, 1965).
3. Evidence has also been obtained for the existence of five-co-ordinate BAE (Costa $et\ al.$, 1966), salen (Costa $et\ al.$, 1967) and corrinoid complexes (see Chapter 8, Section III) when one of the axial ligands is an alkyl group. The observation of a five-co-ordinate complex under certain conditions is, of course, no proof that ligand substitution reactions occur by an S_{N1} mecha-nism under other conditions or with other ligands, but is nevertheless suggestive.

The second important point which has been established recently is the strong labilizing effect of S-bonded sulphite and of organo-ligands (compared to H_2O, Cl^-, NH_3, etc.). The effect of sulphite has been observed in the tetrammine (Halpern $et\ al.$, 1966), tetracyano (Chen $et\ al.$, 1966; Tewari $et\ al.$, 1967) and bis-DMG complexes (Tsiang and Wilmarth, 1968). The effect of organo-ligands has been established in complexes of the type $[R . Co\{(DOH)(DO)pn\}-H_2O]^+$ where $\{(DOH)(DO)pn\}$ is the 1,3-bis(biacetylmonoximeimino)pro-panato ligand; the $trans$-labilizing effect of the organo-ligands appears to increase in the order $\phi < Me < \phi CH_2 \sim Et < n$-Pr ? $<$ iso-Pr (Costa $et\ al.$, 1970). Qualitative observations suggest that an alkyl ligand also has a strong labilizing effect in $[RCo(CN)_5]^{3-}$ (Johnson $et\ al.$, 1967), bis-DMG (Schrauzer and Windgassen, 1966), BAE and salen complexes (Costa $et\ al.$, 1966, 1967). It is not yet known whether these strong labilizing ligands exert their effect predominantly on the $trans$-position or not; see the discussion in Pratt and Thorp (1969). The nature of the cis-ligands may also have a very marked effect on the rate, as will be discussed in Section II.

There are several other points of general interest with respect to cobalt(III) complexes. Kinetic studies have revealed that undissociated acids such as HN_3° (Haim $et\ al.$, 1965) and HNO_2° (Hague and Halpern, 1967) and even protonated bases such as $N_2H_5^+$ (Barca $et\ al.$, 1967) can act as nucleophiles, as well as the more familiar Cl^-, N_3^-, NH_3 etc. pH can affect the rates and equilibria in several other ways due to equilibria involving either the ligand which is to be replaced or other ligands within the complex. Ionization of co-ordinated H_2O, for example, gives the hydroxo ligand, which is kinetically far more inert towards substitution (Haim et al., 1965), while the addition of a proton assists the removal of co-ordinated anions of weak acids such as F^-, CO_3^{2-}, NO_2^- and SO_3^{2-}, as well as N_3^-, through the formation of co-ordinated $HF°$, etc. Alkali catalyzes the reactions of complexes containing NH_3 or ethylenediamine through the formation of co-ordinated NH_2^- etc. which has a strong labilizing effect on other ligands in the complex (Basolo and Pearson, 1967). I_2 also catalyzes the reversible reaction of $[Co(CN)_5H_2O]$ with I^- through the formation of the more reactive I_3^- (Grassi et al., 1967). Cl^-, Br^- and I^- are removed by ions such as Ag(I), Hg(II) and Tl(III) (Posey and Taube, 1957), while $HgCl_2$ reacts with $[Co(CN)_5CH_3]^{3-}$ to give CH_3HgCl (Halpern and Maher, 1964). The formation of ion-pairs between the charged complexes and other ions in solution also affects the rates, especially in the case of ammine and bis-ethylenediamine complexes.

Information on the ligand substitution reactions of cobalt(III) complexes can therefore be summarized as follows. The mechanism has been established as S_{N1} in certain cases, but in the majority of reactions the mechanism remains unknown. The rates of reaction depend on the nature of the leaving (Y) and entering nucleophile (Z), on the other ligands present in the complex and on external agents, as well as temperature and solvent. The ligand substitution reactions of the corrinoids can now be discussed against this background.

II. COBALT(III) CORRINOIDS

Very little quantitative kinetic work has yet been reported on corrinoids and virtually all of this relates to cobalamins. Randall and Alberty (1966, 1967) used stopped-flow and temperature-jump techniques to study the association and dissociation rate constants for the substitution of co-ordinated H_2O in aquocobalamin by NCS^-, N_3^-, NCO^- and imidazole in buffered solutions of pH 1–10 and a total ionic strength of 0.054 at 25°. These reactions all showed the kinetics expected for the simple reactions:

$$[Co\text{—}OH_2] + Z \xrightleftharpoons[K_1]{K_2} [Co\text{—}Z] + H_2O$$

i.e. second order for the association (K_2) and first order for the dissociation (K_1). The rate constants are summarized in Table 12.1. For reasons given in Section I the kinetics cannot decide between S_{N1} and S_{N2} mechanisms. Randall and Alberty favoured an S_{N2} mechanism (1966, 1967), but since corrinoids which are almost certainly five-co-ordinate can actually be observed

8

Table 12.1. *Kinetic data for ligand substitution reactions of certain cobalt(III) complexes*

$$\text{Trans-}[Co \cdot L_4 \cdot X \cdot H_2O] + Z \underset{K_1}{\overset{K_2}{\rightleftharpoons}} \text{trans-}[Co \cdot L_4 \cdot X \cdot Z] + H_2O$$

Cis-ligands(L_4)	X	Z	Temp. (°C)	K_2 ($M^{-1}\,sec^{-1}$)	K_1 (sec^{-1})	References
Corrin	Bzm	N_3^-	25	1.7×10^3	0.03	Randall and Alberty, 1967
		HN_3°		1.0×10^2	0.7	
		NCO^-		7.3×10^2	0.95	
		NCS^-		7.1×10^3	1.8	
		$imid^0$		27	6×10^{-4}	
		CN^-		$\sim1.5 \times 10^3$	$<10^{-9a}$	
$(CN)_4$	CN^{-b}	H_2O	40	8.0×10^{-5}	1.47×10^{-3}	Grassi *et al.*, 1967
		N_3^-			5.5×10^{-7}	Haim *et al.*, 1965
		$HN_3^{\circ -}$			3.2×10^{-3}	
		NCS^-			3.7×10^{-7}	
		Cl^-			4.5×10^{-4}	Grassi *et al.*, 1967
		Br^-			1.7×10^{-4}	
		I^-			7.5×10^{-6}	
		NH_3		2.06×10^{-4}		Barca *et al.*, 1967
		py		5.2×10^{-4}		
		N_2H_4		1.00×10^{-4}		
		$N_2H_5^+$		1.47×10^{-4}		
$(DMG)_2$	H_2O	Cl^-	25		1.0×10^{-4}	Ablov and Sychev, 1959
		Br^-			0.7×10^{-4}	
	Cl^-	Cl^-			2.7×10^{-4}	Ablov and Palade, 1962
	NO_2^-	Cl^-			1.03×10^{-4}	
		Br			1.15×10^{-4}	
	NO_2^-	N_3^-	25	5.7×10^{-4}		Hague and Halpern, 1967

Complex	Ligand	Ligand			Temp.	Reference
I⁻	NCS⁻		5.8 × 10⁻⁴	1.2 × 10⁻⁴		Hague and Halpern, 1967
	Cl⁻		0.8 × 10⁻⁴	1.2 × 10⁻⁴		
	Br⁻		1.6 × 10⁻⁴			
	NCS⁻		1.2 × 10⁻³	0.6 × 10⁻⁴		
	Cl⁻		2.3 × 10⁻⁴	0.7 × 10⁻⁴		
	Br⁻		3.0 × 10⁻⁴			
en₂	H₂O	Cl⁻		2.5 × 10⁻⁶	25	Chan, 1963
	Cl⁻	Cl⁻		3.5 × 10⁻⁵	25	Baldwin et al., 1961
	NO₂⁻	Br⁻		1.12 × 10⁻⁴	25	Chan and Tobe, 1963b
		Cl⁻		1 × 10⁻³	25	Ašperger and Ingold, 1956
		Br⁻		4.3 × 10⁻³	25	Langford and Tobe, 1963
	NH₃	Cl⁻		2.9 × 10⁻⁵	63	Tobe, 1959
		Br⁻		~9.5 × 10⁻⁵	60	
	CN⁻	Cl⁻		8.3 × 10⁻⁵	25	Chan and Tobe, 1963a
(NH₃)₄	Cl⁻	Cl⁻		1.8 × 10⁻³	25	Pearson et al., 1955
	NH₃	N₃⁻		2.1 × 10⁻⁹	25	Lalor and Moelwyn-Hughes, 1963
Haemato-porphyrin[c]	H₂O	NCS⁻	≥300		25	Fleischer et al., 1968
	HO⁻	CN⁻	≥40		25	

[a] Corrected for the minimum value of the equilibrium constant given in Hayward et al. (1965).

[b] The forward reactions where $Z = H_2O$ to I^- inclusive proceed by a limiting S_{N1} mechanism and the authors give values for the ratio of the rates of reaction of the five-co-ordinate intermediate with Z and with H_2O. The apparent second-order rate constant K_2 observed for $Z = N_3^-$ as $[N_3^-] \to 0$ has been included for comparison.

[c] Both reactions occur by a limiting S_{N1} mechanism. Apparent second-order rate constants as $[Z] \to 0$ have been calculated from the data in Table 1 from Fleischer et al. (1968) and included in the above table. Ionic strength various; for details consult the original papers.

when the axial ligand is SO_3^{2-} or an alkyl group (see Chapter 8, Section III), it seems likely that the cobalamins react via a five-co-ordinate transition state or at least by a mechanism that approximates to S_{N1}, and that the rate of breaking the Co—OH$_2$ bond is so great that it never becomes the rate-determining step even at the highest concentrations of Z.

Thusius (1968) also studied the reaction between aquocobalamin and thiocyanate by the temperature-jump method at 25° and $\mu = 0.5$ M. He observed

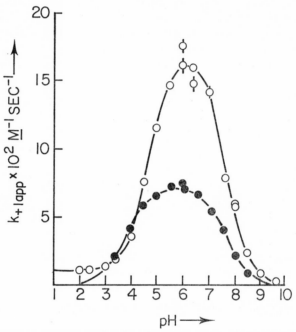

Fig. 12.1. Plots of the apparent association rate constants (k_{+1app}) *vs* pH for the binding of azide (o) and cyanate (●) to aquocobalamin at 25°. From Randall and Alberty (1967).

relaxation rates which could be attributed to the binding of thiocyanate to cobalt and to the isomerization of the ligand, i.e.

$$[Co—OH_2] + NCS^- \underset{K_{21}}{\overset{K_{12}}{\rightleftharpoons}} [Co—SCN] \underset{K_{32}}{\overset{K_{23}}{\rightleftharpoons}} [Co—NCS]$$
$$+ H_2O$$

with the following rate constants: $K_{12} = 2.0 \times 10^3$ M^{-1} sec^{-1}, $K_{21} = 2$, $K_{23} \sim 4$, $K_{32} = 36$ sec^{-1}. K_{21} agrees well with the value obtained by Randall and Alberty, while K_{12} is considerably less.

The apparent rate constants are affected by pH in several ways. The experimental profile of apparent rate constant versus pH observed for the reactions of aquocobalamin with azide and cyanate are shown in Fig. 12.1. The rates fall on increasing the pH above 6 because the kinetically labile aquocobalamin is converted into the (relatively) inert hydroxocobalamin. The rates also fall on decreasing the pH as the strongly nucleophilic azide and cyanate ions are protonated to form the far less reactive and HN_3 HOCN. The uncharged HN_3 can, however, act as an attacking nucleophile, as shown by the low, pH-independent value of the rate constant observed in the case of azide at pH < 3. Conn and Wartman (1952) also found when studying the binding of cyanide by hydroxocobalamin in 0.1 M borate buffer at 25° that at pHs greater than the pK of HCN the apparent rate constant decreased as the pH rose and concluded that CN^- reacted only with aquocobalamin.

From the existence of a pronounced thermodynamic *trans*-effect in the corrinoids (see Chapter 8, Section V) one would also expect to observe a kinetic *trans*-effect, i.e. that any given ligand substitution reaction would increase in rate as the ligand in the *trans*-position was changed in the order H_2O < Bzm < CN^- < CH_3^-, etc. The main difficulty in the way of observing such a kinetic *trans*-effect is that the majority of ligand substitution reactions of corrinoids are too rapid to be studied by conventional techniques. Pseudo-first-order rate constants have, however, been reported for the substitution of co-ordinated NH_3 by H_2O at 30° with the following ligands in the *trans*-position: H_2O 1.4×10^{-5} sec^{-1}, Bzm 8.6×10^{-5} sec^{-1}; CN^-, SO_3^{2-} and CH_3^-, all $\geqslant 3 \times 10^{-1}$ (Hayward *et al.*, 1971). This order of ligands observed for the kinetic *trans*-effect (H_2O < Bzm < CN^-, SO_3^{2-}, CH_3^-) parallels that observed for the thermodynamic *trans*-effect. The substitution of H_2O by Bzm also increases the rate of removal of the vinyl, methyl and ethyl anions by mercury(II) ions (see Chapter 13, Section II,D).

This *trans*-effect order is also supported by some qualitative observations. Firstly, when solutions of cobalamins are acidified, Bzm is displaced from co-ordination by H_2O and is protonated; the equilibrium between the complexes with co-ordinated Bzm and H_2O is established "instantaneously" in every case so far reported except that of aquocobalamin in sulphuric acid-water mixtures, where the reaction is slow (Hayward *et al.*, 1965). In this case the ligands may be HSO_4^- rather than H_2O, but the result does suggest the *trans*-labilizing order H_2O (or HSO_4^-) < CN^-, CH_3^-, SO_3^{2-} etc. Secondly, cyanide is readily displaced by H_2O when the *trans*-ligand is cyanide (George *et al.*, 1960), vinyl, methyl, ethyl (Firth *et al.*, 1968d) or sulphite (Firth *et al.*, 1969). In cyano-aquocobinamide and cyanocobalamin, however, the cyanide is completely inert towards substitution by H_2O in the dark in aqueous acid (photoaquation occurs in light). The formation constants are not known accurately, but are very high (see Table 8.7). The presence of 0.1 M $HgCl_2$, which binds cyanide very strongly, does not remove the cyanide from cyanoaquocobinamide, but does prevent the reverse reaction after photolysis (Firth *et al.*, 1968c). This suggests that under these conditions cyanoaquocobinamide is thermodynamically unstable with respect to substitution of co-ordinated CN^- by H_2O, and that the stability of the complex must be ascribed to kinetic inertness. The cobalt-cyanide bond remains unbroken even in concentrated sulphuric acid (Pratt, 1964); it is hardly conceivable that the cyanide complex is thermodynamically stable under these conditions and the stability must again be ascribed to kinetic inertness.

Many other ligand substitution reactions can of course be observed which do not, at least in the overall reaction, involve co-ordinated H_2O, e.g. the reversible substitution of Bzm by cyanide in various cobalamins (Hayward et al., 1965) or by thiocyanate (Pratt, 1964) and the reaction of cyanoaquocobinamide with sulphite to give sulphitocobinamide (Firth et al., 1968c). In the last reaction the Co—CN bond is presumably broken through the intermediate formation of cyanosulphitocobinamide, in which the strong trans-effect of the sulphite ligand would labilize the Co—CN bond.

Ligand isomerization reactions have also been observed or postulated. As mentioned above, Thusius (1968) obtained evidence from temperature-jump studies for the isomerization of co-ordinated thiocyanate in the cobalamin

$$[\text{Co—SCN}] \underset{K_{-1}}{\overset{K_1}{\rightleftharpoons}} [\text{Co—NCS}]$$

and reported the rate constants $K_1 \sim 4$ and $K_{-1} = 36\ \text{sec}^{-1}$ at 25°. Hydroxocobalamin reacts rapidly with sulphite ion at pH 14 to give an intermediate which then very slowly gives sulphitocobalamin, in which the sulphite is known to be co-ordinated through the sulphur atom (Co—SO_3); it was suggested that the intermediate might be the O-bonded isomer (Co—OSO_2), which slowly isomerizes to the stable S-bonded from (Firth et al., 1969).

Lower limits have also been obtained for the interconversion of certain five- and six-co-ordinate corrinoids. Solutions of ethylcobalamin, vinylcobinamide and methylcobinamide which appear to exist as mixtures of the five- and six-co-ordinate complexes (with and without co-ordinated Bzm in the first case, with and without co-ordinated H_2O in the other two), showed only a single proton magnetic resonance due to H-10 of the corrin ring. This places an upper limit of 10^{-2} seconds for $t_{1/2}$ at room temperature in D_2O in the case of ethylcobalamin and at $-50°$ in CD_3OD in the case of the other two (Hill et al., 1968a; Firth et al., 1968a).

Examples are known in which the displacement of an inert ligand is assisted by a Lewis acid. Such reactions are, of course, most readily observed when the bond to cobalt is normally rather inert. Sulphite is displaced on acidifying solutions of sulphitocobalamin (Dolphin et al., 1963b), presumably through the intermediate formation of co-ordinated SO_3H^- with a lower thermodynamic stability. The cyanide ion can be removed from cyanocobalamin by the action of silver(I) ions (Hill et al., 1970a) and probably also palladium(II) and gold(III) complexes (Havemeyer and Higuchi, 1960). The removal of various organo-ligands can be assisted by protons and by mercury(II) ions (see Chapter 13, Section II).

Most of the features of ligand substitution reactions shown by the corrinoids find parallels amongst the reactions of other cobalt(III) complexes, viz. the inertness of the hydroxo- compared to the aquo-complex, the strong labilizing effect of S-bonded SO_3^{2-} and alkyl groups, the reaction with HN_3° as well as N_3^- and the removal of co-ordinated SO_3^{2-} by H^+ and of CH_3^- by $HgCl_2$. There is, however, a striking difference in the general rates of reaction. There are, unfortunately, no cases where X, Y and Z all remain the same and one can compare directly the *cis*-effects of corrin, $(DMG)_2$, $(NH_3)_4$ etc. A selection of kinetic data has therefore been presented in Table 12.1, from which the general pattern of reactivity can be seen. There is no doubt that the corrin ring has a very marked labilizing effect and that when X, Y and Z are roughly comparable the corrin ring appears to accelerate reactions by a factor of approximately 10^7 compared to the *cis*-ligands $(DMG)_2$, $(CN)_4$ and $(NH_3)_4$. The only other ligands so far discovered which exert a comparable labilizing effect are the porphyrins. Ligand substitution reactions of cobalt(III) porphyrins appear to be very fast or "instantaneous", though many have been studied in non-aqueous solvents and are therefore not strictly comparable. The cobalt(III) haematoporphyrin complexes, however, present a clearcut case. McConnel *et al.* (1953) made the qualitative observation that the substitution of H_2O by cyanide or pyridine in aqueous solution is "instantaneous". Subsequently Fleischer *et al.* (1968) have quantitatively studied the kinetics of the reaction of the diaquo-[haematoporphyrin]-cobalt(III) complex with thiocyanate to give the dithiocyanate complex and of the hydroxoaquo complex with cyanide to give the dicyanide complex and concluded that substitution proceeds by a limiting S_{N1} mechanism; the apparent second-order rate constants are given in Table 12.1. It is a pity that no kinetic data are available for cobalt(III) phthalocyanine complexes.

It is hoped that the above survey will stimulate interest in the wider range of problems presented by the ligand substitution reactions of corrinoids, both on the experimental side (application of techniques for the study of fast reactions, further data on the kinetic *trans*-effect) and on the theoretical side (e.g. the reason for the strong labilizing effect of the corrin and porphyrin rings).

13

FORMATION AND CLEAVAGE OF Co—C AND Co—S BONDS

As explained in the introduction to Chapter 8, the axial ligands can be divided into two groups. Ligands of the first group can exist free in aqueous solution (e.g. NH_3, CN^-) and the complex may be formed by the displacement of, for example, co-ordinated water; the equilibrium constants and rates of these ligand substitution reactions have been treated in Chapters 8 and 12 respectively. Ligands of the second group cannot exist free in aqueous solution (e.g. CH_3^-) and the complex must be prepared by an indirect route (e.g. $Co^I + CH_3I \rightarrow Co—CH_3 + I^-$); the formation and reactions of cobalt corrinoids with axial ligands of this type form the subject of this Chapter. The largest and most important group are the organo-ligands, which are treated in Sections I and II. Ligands co-ordinated through a sulphur atom show analogies to the organo-ligands, and there are several examples of the formation and cleavage of the Co—S bond by reactions which do not involve a free S-anion; these are discussed in Section III. It has also been reported that B_{12s} reacts with trialkyltin and dialkylarsenic halides to give very unstable and un-characterized products which probably contain Co—Sn and Co—As bonds (Schrauzer and Kratel, 1965). There are obviously many corrinoids of this type waiting to be synthesized and characterized.

The study of the organocorrinoids can be traced back to Lenhert and Hodgkin (1961), who showed that the naturally occurring 5'-deoxyadenosyl-cobalamin or DBC (for the structure of the ligand see Fig. 1.3) contained a cobalt-carbon bond. It was subsequently shown that DBC was diamagnetic and could be regarded as a cobalt(III) complex with a co-ordinated carbanion (Hill, J. A. *et al.*, 1962, 1964). DBC was, in fact, the first naturally occurring organometallic complex to be discovered. It is now known, however, that methyl-corrinoids also occur in nature and there is some evidence for the occurrence of a carboxymethylcorrinoid (Co—CH_2COOH) (see Chapter 3). It should be mentioned that all known organocorrinoids are diamagnetic and can be re-garded as cobalt(III) complexes with a co-ordinated carbanion (see Chapter 7, Section II). The characterization of DBC soon led to the synthesis of a wide range of other organocorrinoids (see Table 13.3) and other (non-corrinoid) organo-cobalt(III) complexes, such as the pentacyanides $[RCo(CN)_5]^{3-}$ (Halpern and Maher, 1965), bis-DMG (Schrauzer, 1968) and salen complexes (Costa *et al.*, 1967).

The important contribution made by the organocorrinoids to the develop-ment of the co-ordination chemistry of the corrinoids and, together with non-corrinoid organo-cobalt(III) complexes, to our understanding of co-ordina-tion chemistry in general has been emphasized elsewhere (see Chapter 1, Section I, Chapter 8, Section I and Chapter 18). Two aspects deserve special mention. Firstly, the very striking difference between the typical organo-ligands (such as CH_3^-) and the ligands more commonly studied by co-ordina-ion chemists (such as NH_3 and CN^-) in their effects on the rest of the complex and in their reactions, together with the existence of a series of carbanions (NC^-, $HC{\equiv}C^-$, $CH_2{=}CH^-$, $CH_3CH_2^-$), in which one can see a regular and gradual change in these effects, has provided the basis for the study of *cis*- and *trans*-effects; this aspect is not considered here (see summary in Chapter 18). Secondly, a greater range of σ-bonded organo-ligands have been placed on the metal in cobalt corrinoids than in any other comparable group of metal com-plexes, and possibly also a greater range of their reactions studied. This aspect covers most of the material of this Chapter. As will be shown, the Co—C bond may be formed or broken by reactions, in which the transition state may correspond to

1. Co(III) + R^- (carbanion),
2. Co(II) + R· (radical) or
3. Co(I) + R^+ (carbonium ion).

In addition, the organo-ligand R may be reversibly or irreversibly modified to R'. These reaction types can be shown schematically as follows:

$$Co-R'$$

$$Co^I + R^+ \;\rightleftharpoons\; Co-R \;\rightleftharpoons\; Co^{III} + R^-$$

$$Co^{II} + R\cdot$$

Reactions leading to the formation of the Co—C bond are considered in Section I, all other (thermal) reactions in Section II. Photochemical reactions, which initially lead to the formation of a cobalt(II) complex and a free radical, are discussed in the next Chapter (see especially Chapter 14, Section III).

I. FORMATION OF THE Co—C BOND

Corrinoids which possess a Co—C bond can be formed by several methods. By far the most common and widely applicable method is the reaction of Co(I) corrinoids with electrophilic reagents (Section I,A). Reactions of Co(II) complexes with radicals and of Co(III) complexes with nucleophilic reagents are mentioned in Sections I,B and I,C respectively; the Co—CN bond is, of course, usually formed by the reaction of free cyanide ion with the Co(III) ion. Other reactions of unknown mechanism are discussed in Section I,D.

A. ELECTROPHILES AND Co(I)

There are three basic mechanisms for the formation of Co—C bonds from Co(I) corrinoids, which can be represented by the following examples:

(A) Substitution, e.g. $Co(I) + CH_3I \rightarrow [Co-CH_3] + I^-$

(B) Ring-opening, e.g. $Co(I) + CH_2\overset{O}{\overset{/\backslash}{-}}CH_2 + H^+ \rightarrow [Co-CH_2CH_2OH]$

(C) Addition, e.g. $Co(I) + HC\equiv CH + H^+ \rightarrow [Co-CH=CH_2]$

It was at one time considered that B_{12s} was a cobalt(III) hydride, i.e. hydrido-cobalamin, because it was able to add to multiple bonds as in (C) and to react with diazomethane to give methylcobalamin. But it is now known that B_{12s} is simply cobalamin-cobalt(I) over the pH range 5–15 (see Chapter 7, Section V). If the addition reactions (C) occurred via the intermediate formation of the cobalt(III) hydride, the rate of addition would increase rapidly with a fall in pH. No pH dependence has yet been reported for any of these reactions, and it seems safe to conclude that the reactions A–C all involve the Co(I) complex and that the rate-determining step is the formation of the Co—C bond, followed (in B and C) by the very rapid uptake of a proton.

Schrauzer and co-workers (Schrauzer and Deutsch, 1969; Schrauzer et al., 1968a) have studied the kinetics of alkylation of B_{12s} and certain other cobalt(I) complexes by alkyl halides according to the equation

$$Co^I + RX \rightarrow Co-R + X^-$$

Table 13.1. *Second-order rate constants for the reaction of B_{12s} with alkyl halides (RX)*

$Co^I + RX \rightarrow Co-R + X^-$	
RX	$K \, (\text{mol}^{-1} \, \text{sec}^{-1})$
CH_3Cl	5.0
CH_3CH_2Cl	4.7×10^{-2}
$CH_3(CH_2)_2Cl$	3.7×10^{-2}
$CH_3(CH_2)_3Cl$	2.8×10^{-2}
$CH_3(CH_2)_4Cl$	2.5×10^{-2}
$CH_3(CH_2)_5Cl$	2.6×10^{-2}
$(CH_3)_2CHCH_2Cl$	4.1×10^{-3}
CH_3Br	1.6×10^3
CH_3CH_2Br	3.1×10^1
$CH_3(CH_2)_2Br$	1.4×10^1
$(CH_3)_2CHBr$	1.8
$(CH_3)_2CHCH_2Br$	2.1
$(CH_3)_3CCH_2Br$	9.6×10^{-2}
$(CH_3)_2CH(CH_2)_2Br$	5.2
CH_3I	3.4×10^4
$(CH_3)_2CHI$	2.3×10^2

2nd order

Data from Schrauzer and Deutsch (1969). Conditions: methanol, 0.10 F in NaOH, 25°.

The reactions all followed second-order kinetics; their rate constants for the alkylation of B_{12s} are given in Table 13.1. From the observation of second-order kinetics and the effects of R and X on the rate constants they concluded that the alkylation of B_{12s} (and other cobalt(I) complexes) occurred by a classical S_{N2} mechanism. The reactivity of the cobalt(I) ion in B_{12s} can be compared with other nucleophiles by using the nucleophilic reactivity constant (n_{CH_3I}), which is defined as

$$n_{CH_3I} = \log(K_Y/K_{CH_3OH})$$

where K_Y and K_{CH_3OH} are the second-order rate constants for the reaction of CH_3I in methanol at 25° with the nucleophile Y and with methanol (i.e. solvolysis) respectively (Pearson et al., 1968). Table 13.2 lists the values of

n_{CH_3I} determined by Schrauzer and co-workers (1968a) for B_{12s} and three bis-DMG-cobalt(I) complexes together with the values of certain other nucleophiles selected by them for comparison from Pearson *et al.* (1968). The data show quite clearly that the cobalt(I) complexes are some of the most powerful nucleophiles known. One slightly unexpected finding was that variation in R caused the same relative change in the rates with B_{12s}, with bis-DMG-cobalt(I) and with iodide, i.e. the reactions with B_{12s} are not subject to any greater steric hindrance (Schrauzer and Deutsch, 1969). They also found that solvent had only a small effect on the rate of reaction of B_{12s} with CH_3Cl (ratio of rate in

Table 13.2. *Nucleophilic Reactivity Constants towards* CH_3I (n_{CH_3I})

Nucleophile	n_{CH_3I}
CH_3OH	0.00
Cl^-	4.37
NH_3	5.50
Br^-	5.79
I^-	7.42
$P(n\text{-}C_4H_9)_3$	8.69
$S_2O_3^{2-}$	8.95
$(C_6H_5)_3Sn^-$	~11.5
$(C_6H_5)_3Ge^-$	~12
$[Co^I(DMG)_2.P(n\text{-}C_4H_9)_3]$	13.3
$[Co^I(DMG)_2.py]$	13.8
$[Co^I(DMG)_2.H_2O]$	14.3
Cobalamin-Co(I)	14.4

Data taken from Schrauzer *et al.* (1968a).

H_2O to that in MeOH 6.2) and that cobalamin-cobalt(I) (B_{12s}) alone or in the presence of excess pyridine, 4-cyanopyridine, cyclohexylisocyanide, tributylphosphine or dimethylsulphide, and cobinamide-cobalt(I) all gave essentially the same rate constants (Schrauzer and Deutsch, 1969). The similarity between cobinamide- and cobalamin-cobalt(I) agrees with the fact that Bzm is not co-ordinated in the latter (see Chapter 7, Section V).

The synthesis of organocorrinoids is usually carried out by reducing an aqueous solution of the (red) cobalt(III) corrinoid (e.g. B_{12}, B_{12a}, cyanoaquo-cobinamide) with a reagent such as borohydride, Cr(II) or Zn with acetic acid or NH_4Cl, which is powerful enough to form the green Co(I) complex. This solution is then treated in the presence of excess reducing agent with the required alkylating agent. In most cases alkylation occurs very rapidly and can be seen as a change in colour from green to red (cobalamins) or yellow (cobinamides). For details consult the original papers.

Yields are often almost quantitative, but may be low in a few cases due to the occurrence of further reactions such as the following. Certain ligands such as ethinyl (HC≡C—), trifluoroethyl (CF$_3$CH$_2$—) and sulphomethyl (HO$_3$SCH$_2$—) are readily cleaved by borohydride (Firth *et al.*, 1968d); in these cases B$_{12s}$ should be prepared by the use of other reducing reagents such as Cr(II) (Johnson *et al.*, 1963a). Crotonic acid (CH$_3$CH=CH.COOH) oxidizes B$_{12s}$ to B$_{12r}$ and is itself reduced (Smith *et al.*, 1964), presumably to butyric acid, i.e. B$_{12s}$ appears to catalyze the reduction of the intended alkylating agent. Complications may also arise from three other sources: alkylation of cobalt on the lower side (where Bzm is normally co-ordinated in the cobalamins) to produce the l-isomer instead of the usual u-isomer, alkylation of other atoms in the organic part of the molecule and the possibility of the electrophilic reagent reacting in more than one way. Friedrich and Nordmeyer (1968) have studied the methylation of B$_{12s}$ in detail; their results are discussed more fully in Chapter 8, Section II,C. The main product is the u-isomer of methylcobalamin, while the l-isomer together with the analogues in which Bzm has also been methylated and cannot therefore co-ordinate to the cobalt are formed in small quantities; the ratios depend on the nature of the methylating agent (MeI, Me$_2$SO$_4$). Bromoacetylene is a good example of an electrophile which can react with B$_{12s}$ in two ways. One product shows a band at 1996 cm^{-1}, which can be ascribed to co-ordinated ethinyl (i.e. HC≡C—Co), while the other product is identical with the product from the reaction of B$_{12s}$ with 1,2,-dibromoethylene and must therefore be bromovinyl-cobalamin (BrCH=CH—Co) (Johnson *et al.*, 1963). Smith and co-workers (1964) have obtained "acetylcobalamin" in a yellow form as well as the usual red form and found that the yellow form is slowly converted into the red form in solution; its nature is not known. Zagalak (1963) finds that the use of borohydride in EDTA buffer at pH 9.5 to form cobinamide-cobalt(I) for the preparation of alkylcobinamides produces some unidentified by-products and recommends the use of zinc and ammonium chloride with the addition of magnesium to increase the rate of reduction.

The characterization of organocorrinoids by standard techniques is difficult. Micro-analysis, for example, is of little use in principle for determining one additional methyl group in the presence of the large amount of organic material in the corrinoid part of the complex and inconsistent results are often obtained in practice, presumably due to the presence of cobalt and phosphorus (Johnson *et al.*, 1963a). The usual procedure in the organocorrinoid field is, firstly, to show the purity of the complex by chromatographic techniques and, then, merely to infer the structure by analogy with other known complexes and, in the ultimate analysis, with DBC. Synthetic DBC, prepared via the alkylation of B$_{12s}$, has been shown to be identical with the naturally occurring DBC of known structure by chromatographic techniques, electrophoresis and

Table 13.3. *Reagents for the formation of Co—C bonds by reaction with Co(I) corrinoids*

(A) Substitution

Reagent	Product	References
RX (R = CH_3—$C_{10}H_{21}$; X = Cl, Br, I)	—R	Bernhauer et al. (1962a); Müller and Müller (1962b); Johnson et al. (1963a); Schrauzer and Deutsch (1969); Smith et al. (1962); Zagalak (1963)
iso-propyl chloride	—$CHMe_2$	Firth et al. (1968d)
cyclohexyl iodide	—cyclohexyl	Brodie (1969)
sec-butyl Br/I	—$CHMeEt$	Brodie (1969)
tert-butyl Br/I	—[a]	Johnson et al. (1963a); Smith et al. (1964)
CH_2=CH.CH_2Br	—CH_2.CH=CH_2	Friedrich et al. (1964)
ϕBr	—[a]	Smith et al. (1964)
ϕCH_2Cl	—$CH_2\phi$	Smith et al. (1962, 1964)
XCH_2.CH_2.OH (X = Cl, Br)	—CH_2.CH_2OH	Johnson et al. (1963a); Müller and Müller (1963); Smith et al. (1962)
$BrCH_2$.CHOH.CH_3	—CH_2.CHOH.CH_3	Yamada et al. (1965)
$ClCH_2$.CHOH.CH_2OH	—CH_2.CHOH.CH_2OH	Yamada et al. (1965)
$Br(CH_2)_2Br$	—[a]	Smith et al. (1964)
$Cl(CH_2)_3Br$	+[b]	Smith et al. (1964)
$Br(CH_2)_4Br$	Co—$(CH_2)_4$—Co dimer and some Co—$(CH_2)_4$Br	Smith et al. (1964)
3-bromobutylcobalamin $(Br(CH_2)_4$—Co)	Co—$(CH_2)_4$—Co dimer	Smith et al. (1964)
$X(CH_2)_n$.COOR (X = Cl, Br; n = 1, 2; R = H, CH_3)	—$(CH_2)_n$—COOR	Hogenkamp et al. (1965); Johnson et al. (1963a); Müller and Müller (1962b); Smith et al. (1962)
$ClCH_2$.CH_2CN	—CH_2.CH_2CN	Hogenkamp et al. (1965)
ICH_2.CF_3	—CH_2.CF_3	Firth et al. (1968d)
ICH_2SO_3H	—CH_2SO_3H	Firth et al. (1968d)
$BrCH=CH_2$	—CH=CH_2	Johnson et al. (1963)
$BrCH=CHBr$	—CH=CHBr	Johnson et al. (1963a)

Compound	Group	References
$BrC{\equiv}CH$	$-C{\equiv}CH$ and $-CH{=}CHBr$	Johnson et al. (1963a)
$BrC{\equiv}N$	$-C{\equiv}N$	Johnson et al. (1963a)
CH_2Cl_2	$-CH_2Cl$	Wood et al. (1968a)
CHF_3	$-$[a]	Wood et al. (1968a)
CHX_3 (X = Cl, Br, I)	$-CHX_2$	Wood et al. (1968a)
CCl_4	$-CCl_3$	Wood et al. (1968a)
CCl_2F_2	$-CClF_2$	Wood et al. (1968a)
$CH_3.COCl$	$-CO.CH_3$	Bernhauer and Irion (1964b); Johnson et al. (1963a); Smith et al. (1962, 1964)
$RNHCH_2.CO.Cl$ (R = H and $CH_3.CO{-}$)	$-CO.CH_2NHR$	Bernhauer and Irion (1964b)
ClCOOEt	$-COOEt$	Müller and Müller (1963); Zagalak (1963)
$COCl_2$	$+$	Müller and Müller (1963)
$(CH_3CO)_2O$	$-CO.CH_3$	Müller and Müller (1962b); Johnson et al. (1963a); Smith et al. (1964)
$H.CO.O.CO.CH_3$	$-$[a]	Müller and Müller (1963)
MeOOC.COOMe	$-CH_3$	Smith et al. (1964)
R_2SO_4 (R = Me, Et)	$-R$	Bernhauer et al. (1962a); Friedrich et al. (1964); Johnson et al. (1963a); Müller and Müller (1962b); Smith et al. (1962); Zagalak (1963)
Et_3PO_4	$-Et$	Johnson et al. (1963a)
Adenosine Triphosphate (ATP)	$-$[a]	Johnson et al. (1963a); Müller and Müller (1963)
$RSO_3.C_6H_4.CH_3$ (p-tosylates) (R = Me, Et, $MeO{-}CH_2{-}CH_2{-}CH_2{-}$) (R = adenosyl, etc.)	$-R$	Bernhauer et al. (1962a); Hogenkamp et al. (1965); Johnson et al. (1963a); Müller and Müller (1962b)
ROH (R = Me, Et)	$+$[b]	see text
R_2O (R = Me, Et)	$-$[a]	Pratt, unpublished work
p-methoxyphenol	$+$[b]	Pratt, unpublished work
$NMe_4^+Cl^-$	$-$[a]	Pratt, unpublished work
$^+Me_3N.CH_2.CO_2^-$	$-$[a]	Pratt, unpublished work
$Me_3S^+ClO_4^-$	$+$[b]	Pratt, unpublished work
S-methylmethionine(I)	$-CH_3$	Müller and Müller (1963)
S-adenosylmethionine	$-CH_3$	Friedrich and König (1962)
CH_2N_2	$-CH_3$	Johnson et al. (1963a); Müller and Müller (1962b)

Table 13.3 (continued)

Reagent	Product	References
	(B) Ring-opening	
Ethylene oxide	—CH$_2$.CH$_2$OH	Johnson et al. (1963a); Müller and Müller (1963)
Ethylene imine	—CH$_2$.CH$_2$.NH$_2$	Friedrich et al. (1964); Hogenkamp (1966b)
Cyclopropane	—[a]	Pratt, unpublished work
Tetrahydrofuran	—(CH$_2$)$_4$OH	Müller and Müller (1963)
Propylenesulphide	+[b]	Pratt, unpublished work
β-propiolactone(II)	+[b]	Pratt, unpublished work
2,5-Diketopiperazine(III)	+[b]	Bernhauer and Irion (1964b)
	(C) Addition	
HC≡CH	—CH=CH$_2$	Johnson et al. (1963a)
HC≡C.COOH	—CH=CH.COOH	Johnson et al. (1963a)
φC≡C.COOH	—[a]	Johnson et al. (1963a)
HC≡CBr.	—CH=CHBr and —C≡CH	Johnson et al. (1963a)
CH$_2$=CH$_2$	—[a]	Johnson et al. (1963a)
φCH=CH$_2$	—[a]	Johnson et al. (1963a)
CH$_2$=CH.COOH	—CH$_2$.CH$_2$.COOH	Johnson et al. (1963a)
CH$_3$.CH=CH.COOH	(→ B$_{12r}$)	Smith et al. (1964)
CF$_2$=CF$_2$.	—CF$_2$.CF$_2$H	Mays and Wilkinson (1964)

[a] — = no organo-corrinoid observed (but see text).
[b] + = organo-corrinoid observed, but not identified.

(I) (CH$_3$)$_2$·$^+$SCH$_2$CH$_2$CHNH$_2$COOH

(II) CH$_2$—O   (III) NH—CO
    | | CH$_2$ CH$_2$
   CH$_2$—CO   CO—NH

absorption spectra in neutral and acid solution (Bernhauer et al., 1962a; Johnson et al., 1963a; Smith et al., 1962). Many other organocorrinoids can be prepared by exactly analogous reactions and show similar absorption spectra, charge, chromatographic behaviour, photosensitivity, reversible change in spectra on acidification, reaction with cyanide etc.; they clearly have analogous structures. Only in a few cases is additional evidence available, e.g. the i.r. band of $HC \equiv C$—Co (mentioned above). Where the ligand could react in more than one way, the identity of the complex can usually be established by preparation via another route (see the example in the previous paragraph). The question as to the identity of the two possible isomers of the alkylcobinamides is discussed in Chapter 8, Section II,C; the u-isomer is almost always formed.

The reagents which react with Co(I) corrinoids to form a Co—C bond are listed in Table 13.3 and are grouped according to the reaction mechanisms A–C; diazomethane (CH_2N_2) is included in group A. Most work has been done on the cobalamins and all the reagents listed except for allyl bromide and ethyleneimine have been used with B_{12s}. The little work done on cobinamides (see, in particular, Zagalak (1963) and Firth et al. (1968d) suggests that there are few differences in behaviour between cobinamide- and cobalamin-cobalt(I) and the same probably applies to other corrinoids. Some reagents are reported not to react, but it is often not clear whether this means simply that no organocorrinoid could be isolated or even detected or whether it means that no reaction of any sort (reduction, elimination of HX etc.) occurs. These reagents are identified by the sign – in the product column of the Table. Organocobalamins which have been reported without mention of the alkylating agent include those with the ligands —$C \equiv C$—CN and —CH=CH—CN (Smith et al., 1964) and —$CH_2CH_2NMe_3^+$ (Hogenkamp, 1966). Certain unspecified amines failed to react with B_{12s} (Schrauzer and Windgassen, 1967b). Certain reagents of interest mainly to biochemists and organic chemists have been omitted from the Table; for example, certain complex halogen-containing molecules which are important biological alkylating agents, e.g. chlorambucil or p-N,N-di(β-chloroethyl)-aminophenylbutyric acid (Gupta and Huennekens, 1964). Biologically important molecules which apparently do not react with B_{12s} include FAD, DPN, DPNH and TPN (Müller and Müller, 1963) and N^5-methyltetrahydrofolic acid (Guest et al., 1964; Schrauzer and Windgassen, 1967b) in addition to ATP (adenosine triphosphate) (Müller and Müller, 1963; Johnson et al., 1963a). ATP will, however, react with B_{12s} in the presence of an enzyme and magnesium ions to form DBC (Vitols et al., 1964).

The original and most important goal of these alkylation reactions was the partial synthesis of DBC, i.e. the placing of the 5-deoxyadenosyl ligand on the cobalt. This was accomplished independently and almost simultaneously by Bernhauer, Müller and Müller (1962a) and by Smith, Mervyn, Johnson and

Shaw (1962) by the reaction of B_{12s} with 2',3'-O-isopropylidene-5'-O-p-toluenesulphonyladenosine and 2',3'-O-diacetyl-5'-O-p-toluenesulphonyladenosine, the protecting groups (isopropylidene and acetyl) being removed by hydrolysis after formation of the cobalamin. Other methods have been used subsequently (Yurkevich *et al.*, 1969) and various analogues containing nucleosides which differ from adenosine in either or both of the sugar and the heterocyclic base have been synthesized by similar methods (Müller and Müller, 1962a; Johnson *et al.*, 1963a; Hogenkamp and Oikawa, 1964; Zagalak and Pawełkiewicz, 1965a).

Several comments can be made about the reagents and products listed in Table 13.3. Firstly, the ligands produced are all carbanions; there is no evidence for the formation of π-bonded olefin complexes. The high charge of the Co(III) cation clearly favours the anionic form of the ligand ($CH_2{=}CH^-$ or $HC{\equiv}C^-$) compared to the uncharged hydrocarbon ($CH_2{=}CH_2$ or $HC{\equiv}CH$). Secondly, the ligands represent a far wider range of carbanions than is known for any other group of transitional metal complexes and includes ligands in which the co-ordinated carbon atom may be tetrahedral, trigonal (Co—$CR{=}CR_2$, Co—CO.R, Co—CO.OR) or linear (Co—$C{\equiv}CR$). The ligand derived from chlorambucil and that present in DBC must rank as some of the most unwieldy organo-ligands ever to be placed on a metal.

The classification of reagents by mechanism has some relevance to the nature of the ligand which can be placed on the cobalt. Reactions of type (A) provide the simplest means of adding ligands which do not contain another strongly nucleophilic group (such as —SH or —NH_2). The latter are best prepared by the ring-opening reactions of type (B). Olefinic ligands are best prepared by route (C).

Group (A) includes a wide range of alkylating and acylating reagents where the leaving group is Cl^-, Br^-, I^- or oxy-anions such as carboxylate, sulphate and tosylate, together with the uncharged N_2 (in CH_2N_2) and R_2S. No reaction is observed with tert-butyl halides, obviously because there is too must steric hindrance, or with bromobenzene, due presumably to the kinetic inertness of the aryl bromide. The unreactivity of fluorocarbons (e.g. CHF_3), alcohols, ethers, amines and tetraalkylammonium salts may be due to either or both of thermodynamic stability or kinetic inertness of the reagent.

The driving force in most of the ring-opening reactions (B) is presumably the release of strain in the small sized rings. It is perhaps surprising that tetrahydrofuran acts as an alkylating agent, since the five-membered ring is relatively free from strain, and that cyclopropane does not. This type of reaction offers interesting potentialities, which have hardly yet been explored.

Olefins will react with Co(I) if activated by substituents as in $CF_2{=}CF_2$ or $CH_2{=}CH.COOH$. Acetylenes, on the other hand, will react directly with

Co(I), while reaction is prevented by the presence of bulky substituents at both ends (e.g. $C_6H_5.C\equiv COOH$); the same effect would presumably operate in the olefins.

B. RADICALS AND Co(II)

Schrauzer and co-workers (1968b) found that the photolysis of methyl-cobaloxime under nitrogen in the presence of B_{12r} produced some methyl-cobalamin. Since methyl radicals are produced by photolysis under these conditions (see Chapter 14, Section III,A) this is evidence for the occurrence of the reaction:

$$CH_3 \cdot + Co^{II} \rightarrow CH_3—Co$$

Friedrich and co-workers (Friedrich and Nordmeyer, 1968; Friedrich and Messerschmidt, 1969) report that the u- and l-isomers of certain methyl-corrinoids can be isomerized by heating the solutions in an atmosphere of carbon monoxide or by photolysis, presumably through the formation of Co(II) and methyl radicals (see Chapter 8, Section II,C).

C. NUCLEOPHILES AND Co(III)

Wagner and Bernhauer (1964) report that when dicyano-[cobyrinic acid heptamethyl ester] is treated with an excess of methyl magnesium iodie (? in ether/tetrahydrofuran) a methyl group is placed on the cobalt and the ester side-chains are converted into tertiary alcohol groups. Direct alkylation of the cobalt atom could also be achieved by the use of lithium alkyls. This reaction can be written in the generalized form ($R = CH_3$ or other alkyl radical)

$$[Co^{III}CN^-] + R^-(Li^+, MgI^+) \rightarrow [Co^{III}R^-] + CN^-$$

The reaction can probably be carried out with any corrinoids which are soluble in solvents which do not decompose the Grignard reagents and lithium alkyls. CN^- will, of course, react readily with most cobalt(III) corrinoids.

D. OTHER REACTIONS

There have been several reports that B_{12r} (Bayston and Winfield, 1967; Yamada et al., 1968a) and other cobalt(II) corrinoids (Yamada et al., 1964, 1966a; Lee and Schrauzer, 1968) react slowly with methyl iodide to give methyl-cobalt(III) corrinoids in the absence of complicating factors such as the presence of thiols (see below). Yamada, Shimizu and Fukui (1968a) found that the reaction of B_{12r} with methyl iodide requires the addition of some electrolyte (e.g. 1 M NaCl), but even then is fairly slow and was allowed to proceed overnight. No reaction was observed in the absence of electrolyte with cobalt(II) concentrations of $2\text{--}3 \times 10^{-4}$ M, but some reaction occurred in saturated solutions of cobalamin-cobalt(II). One product was identified as methylcobalamin and isolated in $43\text{--}46\%$ yield, the other (after extraction and exposure to air) as aquocobalamin. The overall reaction is therefore

$$2[Co^{II}] + CH_3I + H_2O \rightarrow [Co^{III}OH_2] + [Co^{III}CH_3^-] + I^-$$

Reactions were also observed between B_{12r} and the monohaloacetates (XCH_2COOH). The problem is the mechanism of this reaction, and whether it involves the formation of cobalt(I) by disproportionation. No cobalamin-cobalt(I) could be detected spectroscopically even in the presence of the sodium chloride required to catalyze the reaction.

There are two possible mechanisms:

(A) Since cobalamin-cobalt(I) reacts very rapidly with methyl iodide (see Chapter 13, Section I,A), the reaction could involve disproportionation, i.e.

$$2Co^{II} \rightarrow Co^{I} + Co^{III}$$

followed by the reaction of cobalt(I)

$$Co^{I} + CH_3I \rightarrow [Co^{III}CH_3^-] + I^-$$

This is the mechanism suggested by Yamada et al. (1968a).

(B) The pentacyanocobalt(II) ion also reacts with alkyl halides (RX) according to the stoichiometry

$$2[Co^{II}(CN)_5] + RX \rightarrow [Co^{III}(CN)_5R] + [Co^{III}(CN)_5X]$$

The kinetics and the dependence of the rate on the nature of R and X support the following mechanism

$$[Co^{II}(CN)_5] + RX \rightarrow [Co^{III}(CN)_5X] + R\cdot$$
$$[Co^{II}(CN)_5] + R\cdot \rightarrow [Co^{III}(CN)_5R]$$

in which the first step is rate-determining (Halpern and Maher, 1965). The reaction of B_{12r} with methyl iodide could proceed by an analogous mechanism or conversely by the initial abstraction of a methyl radical to leave an iodine atom.

The methyl radical is known to react with cobalamin-cobalt(II) to form methylcobalamin (Schrauzer et al., 1968b), while iodine, and presumably iodine atoms, will also oxidize the cobalt(II) (Brierly et al., 1953). One cannot at present decide between the two mechanisms, but kinetic studies might provide the answer; a first-order dependence of the rate on the concentration of B_{12r} would support mechanism (B), a second-order dependence mechanism (A).

The situation becomes more complicated when thiols are present. Dolphin and Johnson reported in a note (1963) that methyl iodide will react with B_{12a}

in the presence of thiols or sulphide to give methylcobalamin; some experimental details were given in a subsequent paper (1965b). Wagner and Bernhauer also found that the cobalt can be alkylated by treating B_{12a} with alkylating agents in the presence of excess glutathione (Wagner and Bernhauer, 1964; Bernhauer et al., 1963), but gave no experimental details. Dolphin and Johnson added CH_3I to solutions of B_{12a} and thiols in a buffer of pH 2.5, which contained the purple thiolatocobalamins, and allowed the mixture to stand for 24 hours. The thiols used were glutathione, 2-mercaptoethanol, thioglycollic acid, cysteine, homocysteine, ethanethiol and ω-mercaptotoluene. Methylcobalamin was formed in each case. No reaction was observed in the presence of other sulphur-anions such as sulphite, p-toluene-sulphonate or thiocyanate (Dolphin and Johnson, 1965b). The interesting question is, of course, whether the reaction proceeds via the formation of B_{12r}. Thiols reduce B_{12a} to B_{12r} at a rate increasing with pH (see Chapter 11, Section IV,E). The reactions under discussion are obviously fairly slow, and the rate-determining step could be the formation of B_{12r}. Methylation occurred much more rapidly (within 5 minutes) in the presence of sulphide; in this case Na_2S was added to an unbuffered solution of B_{12a} in water and B_{12r} was formed rapidly (4 minutes). The alkylating agents used were methyl and ethyl iodide, propyl chloride, bromide and iodide, methyl p-toluenesulphonate and chloracetic acid. The reaction is markedly faster if B_{12a} and sulphide are allowed to react to produce B_{12r} before CH_3I is added, i.e. the reaction appears to involve B_{12r}; but B_{12r}, prepared by some other method, will not react in the absence of sulphide. Dolphin and Johnson refer to the "brown compound or intermediate", but it is not clear whether this is identical with B_{12r} or not. They suggest the following mechanism for the reaction, without specifying the role of HS^- or the nature of the oxidation step (Dolphin and Johnson, 1963):

$$[Co^{II}SH^-] \xrightarrow{CH_3I} [Co^{II}CH_3^-] \rightarrow [Co^{III}CH_3^-]$$

Another possibility is that CH_3I reacts with B_{12r} to form a small quantity of methylcobalamin and iodine atoms (or iodocobalamin and methyl radicals) in equilibrium with the starting materials, i.e.

$$Co^{II} + CH_3I \rightleftharpoons [Co^{III}CH_3^-] + I\cdot$$

and that the role of HS^- or H_2S is to remove the radical (e.g. by reducing iodine atoms to I^- with the concomitant formation of sulphur or H_2S_2) and drive the reaction to completion. It seems likely that thiols would behave similarly to sulphide, but further experiments are needed before one can usefully make suggestions about the mechanism.

Some unusual reaction appears to take place when corrinoids are reduced in the presence of adenine. Pawełkiewicz and co-workers (1960) reported that the reduction of cyanoaquocobinamide ("corphinamide" in their paper) with dithionite ($S_2O_4^{2-}$) in the presence of adenine gave a compound whose absorption spectrum and certain other (unspecified) properties were identical to those of 5-deoxyadenosylcobinamide ("SB_{12p}"). Bernhauer and co-workers (1960a) also found that the catalytic hydrogenation of B_{12a} in the presence of adenine produced a compound, which had a spectrum like that of B_{12r}, but which was stable to oxygen in the dark (and therefore presumably photosensitive, though this was not stated explicitly). Brady and Barker (1961), on the other hand, observed no reaction between B_{12r} and either adenine or adenosine (in the absence of the platinum catalyst) and Johnson *et al.* (1963a) also reported failure, but mentioned neither the starting material nor the reducing agent; neither of these results can be considered to contradict the original observations of Pawełkiewicz and Bernhauer.

II. REACTIONS OF ORGANOCORRINOIDS

The wide range of available organo-ligands R provides an interesting spectrum of reactivity. The general pattern of reactions has already been indicated schematically in the introduction to this Chapter. The Co—C bond may remain intact and the organo-ligand undergo reversible changes (e.g. dissociation of Co—CH_2COOH or the co-ordination of Ag(I) ions to Co—CH=CH_2) or irreversible reactions (e.g. the conversion of Co—C≡CH to Co—$COCH_3$ in acid). The Co—C bond can be broken to give a Co(I), Co(II) or Co(III) corrinoid. Homolytic dissociation into Co(II) and a free radical is mechanistically the simplest reaction. This occurs readily under the influence of light (see Chapter 14). Thermal reactions leading to Co(II) are much less common; these are discussed in Section II,A. Heterolytic fission of the Co—C bond to give Co(I) or another Co(III) complex can occur by transfer of a carbonium ion, a carbanion or a related ion to the attacking agent, or by the loss of H^+, HO^- etc. from R under the influence of the attacking reagent. With the exception of a very few organocorrinoids which appear to decompose slowly even in neutral aqueous solution (see Section II,B), heterolytic fission of the Co—C bond is brought about by the deliberate addition of nucleophiles or electrophiles. These reactions have been classified broadly according to the nature of the attacking agent. All reactions observed in neutral, acid or alkaline solution in the absence of other reagents are discussed in Section II,B, followed by reactions involving cyanide (Section II,C). Reactions with other nucleophiles and electrophiles, including the interesting transfer reactions (e.g., of CH_3 and $COCH_3$), are considered in Section II,D. The reduction of organocorrinoids by borohydride and by catalytic hydrogenation, however, have been mentioned in Chapter 11, Section IV. Most work has been done on the organocobalamins; certain differences have been noted between the cobalamins and the cobinamides, and it cannot be assumed that the two groups of organo-corrinoids will behave similarly.

The equilibria and/or reactions observed on treating an organocorrinoid with a particular reagent may be quite complicated, since there are several points of attack in the molecule, viz:

1. The organo-ligand. Electrophiles can add to a lone pair of electrons (e.g. $Co—CH_2CH_2OH + H^+$) or to a double bond (e.g. $Co—CH{=}CH_2 + Ag(I)$), replace a proton (perhaps in $Co—C{\equiv}CH + Ag(I)$) or attack the co-ordinated carbon atom in a transfer reaction (e.g. the transfer of CH_3^- to I_2 or Hg(II) ions). A similar range of reactions can be envisaged for nucleophiles.

2. The cobalt ion. A nucleophile such as CN^- may co-ordinate to the cobalt ion either to form a stable complex, as in the case of methylcyanocobinamide, or to labilize the Co—C bond, as in the decomposition of DBC to dicyanocobalamin.

3. Bzm. The N_3 atom may be protonated or become co-ordinated by ions such as Ag(I) and Hg(II), which may simultaneously attack the organo-ligand.

A. HOMOLYTIC FISSION OF THE Co—C BOND

One can discuss together several reactions involving the hypothetical equilibrium

$$Co—R \rightleftharpoons Co^{II} + R\cdot$$

The photolysis of methylcobaloxime (cobaloxime = bis-DMG) in the presence of cobalamin-cobalt(II) produces some methylcobalamin, which can be taken as evidence for the reaction of Co(II) with methyl radicals to form the Co—C bond (Schrauzer et al., 1968b). The photochemistry of methylcobalamin can be interpreted in terms of an initial homolysis to give Co(II) and methyl radicals, followed by the reaction of the latter with O_2 etc. or, if carried out under nitrogen, by rapid reformation of methylcobalamin (see Chapter 14, Section III,A). The position of the above equilibrium clearly lies far over to the left, and the equilibrium will only be displaced to the right if energy is supplied in the form of heat or light to overcome the endothermic nature of the homo-lysis and if one or other of the products are removed by further reactions. The u- and l-isomers of certain methylcorrinoids can be isomerized by heating the solutions under CO or by photolysis (Friedrich and Nordmeyer, 1968; Friedrich and Messerschmidt, 1969); the reaction presumably involves the formation of Co(II) and methyl radicals, which then react together again (see Chapter 8, Section II,C).

Solid alkylcobalamins will decompose on heating. Methylcobalamin in an atmosphere of nitrogen will decompose at 215–225° to yield roughly equal amounts of methane and ethane, ethylcobalamin gives 99% ethylene with traces of ethane and butane, while *n*-propylcobalamin gives only propylene (Schrauzer *et al.*, 1968b). The nature of the corrinoid produced was not recorded; but the relative amounts of the organic products formed by pyrolysis of the solid were very similar to those observed on photolysis of the solutions and the initial step in pyrolysis can therefore be considered to be the homolytic fission of the Co—C bond to give the Co(II) complex and the alkyl radical. The pyrolysis of other organo-cobalt(III) complexes has also been studied under nitrogen and the products found to be similar to those from photolysis of the solutions (Schrauzer *et al.*, 1968b; Schrauzer and Windgassen, 1966a) and in the case of the salen complexes the cobalt(II) complex was identified as the product both of photolysis of the solution and of pyrolysis of the solid under nitrogen (Costa and Mestroni, 1967).

The breaking of the Co—C bond in ethylcobalamin by cyanide (see Section II,C) requires the presence of oxygen and shows an inductoin period, which suggests that free radicals may be involved. Homolytic fission of the Co—C bond due to attack by a radical on the organo-ligand is clearly a possibility, but there is no direct evidence yet for the mechanism of this reaction.

There is also some evidence for the homolytic fission of the Co—C bond in DBC, when associated with an enzyme in the presence of substrate (Foster *et al.*, 1970) (see also Chapter 17).

B. REACTIONS IN ACID AND ALKALINE SOLUTION

The Co—C bond of both cobalamins and cobinamides is very stable in neutral aqueous solution in the dark. For example, none of the coenzymes (AC, BC or DBC) show any decomposition on storing for several months in dilute neutral solution at −10° or on heating for 20 minutes at 100° in 0.01 M sodium acetate buffer pH 6.0 (Barker *et al.*, 1960a,b), while ethinylcobalamin shows no change in spectrum after one month at 20° in a borate buffer pH 9.3 (Pratt, 1964). The Co—C bond does, however, appear to be broken fairly easily in the isopropyl complexes (Firth *et al.*, 1968a); the Co—C bond is probably labilized by steric compression involving the secondary alkyl ligand (see Section II, D).

The Co—C bond may be broken or the organo-ligand irreversibly modified by the action of acid or alkali; these reactions are summarized in Table 13.4. Additional notes (rates, conditions etc.) on these and related reactions are given below. Although most organocorrinoids are fairly stable towards dilute alkali, several have been reported to decompose in 1 N NaOH; see, for example, methyl- (Pailes and Hogenkamp, 1968), ethyl- and vinyl-cobinamide

Table 13.4. *Reactions of organocobalamins in acid and alkaline solution which involve the organo-ligand*

Ligand	H+	References	HO⁻	References
—CN	—	b	—[a]	g
—C≡CH	Co—CO.CH₃	b	—[a]	b
—CH=CH₂	Co³ + ?CH₂=CH₂	b,c	—[a]	b
—CH₃	—	c	—[a]	b,c
—CH₂CH₃	Co³ + CH₂=CH₂	d,c		g,d,c
—CH₂CH₂OH	Co³ + CH₂=CH₂	d,c		d
—CH₂CH₂OCH₃	Co³ + CH₂=CHR			d
5'-deoxyadenosyl (DBC)	(See text)	a		
—CH₂CH₂NH₂	+	e		d
—CH₂CH₂NMe₃⁺	—	a	—	
—CH₂CH₂CN	—	c	?Co¹ + CH₂=CHCN	h,d
—CH₂CH₂COOH	—	c	—	d
—CH₂CH₂COOMe	—	c	+	d
—CH₂COOH	—	c	—	c
—CH₂COOMe	—	c		
—COCH₃	—	f	Co¹ + CH₃COOH	f,i

The reaction products are indicated where known; Co³ is B₁₂ₐ and Co¹ is B₁₂ₛ.
+ indicates that a reaction was observed, but the products were not stated.
— no reaction observed.
[a] No reaction observed during the determination of formation constants for the displacement of Bzm by cyanide in alkaline solution.

References:
b Hayward et al., 1965.
c Hogenkamp et al., 1965.
d Hogenkamp, 1966.
e Wagner, 1966.
f Bernhauer and Irion, 1964b.
g Firth et al., 1968d.
h Barnett et al., 1966.
i Yamada et al., 1968b.

(Firth *et al.*, 1968d). The nature of these reactions is not known. Few organo-corrinoids have been studied in very strong acid; the Co—CH_3 bond is, however, stable even in concentrated sulphuric acid at room temperature (Pratt, 1964).

Acid and alkali may also cause the reversible displacement of an acid-base equilibrium, e.g. Co—CH_2COOH (see Chapter 8, Section IV,I), the phosphate ($pK \sim 1$) and ribose hydroxyl ($pK \sim 12.5$) of the nucleotide side-chain (see Chapter 10, Section I), the protonation of Bzm with simultaneous displacement from co-ordination (see Chapter 8, Section IV and Table 8.7) and the protonation of the adenine moiety of the 5'-deoxyadenosyl ligand (see Chapter 8, Section IV,I). The protonation and displacement of Bzm will, of course, affect the reactions of the Co—C bond by changing the nature of the ligand in the *trans*-position. Strongly acid or alkaline solutions will also hydrolyze the side-chains to give a variety of products (see Chapter 16). Some of these complicating factors are mentioned below when discussing the decomposition of the coenzymes by acid.

Historically the first reaction of this type to be discovered was the decomposition of the coenzymes by heating in acid (Barker *et al.*, 1958; Weissbach *et al.*, 1959). But it is more convenient to discuss the reactions of simpler organo-ligands first.

Cobalamins containing the ligands R = —CH_2CH_2OH and —CH_2CH_2 OCH_3 react with acid to give ethylene and B_{12a}. The reactions apparently show first-order kinetics and the following rate constants have been reported for decomposition in 10^{-2} M HCl at 100°: R = —CH_2CH_2OH, $k = 16 \times 10^{-3}$ sec^{-1}; —$CH_2CH_2OCH_3$, 4×10^{-3} sec^{-1}. The mechanism proposed involves protonation (presumably reversible) of the oxygen atom, followed by a concerted elimination (Hogenkamp, 1966b):

$$\text{Co—}\overset{\overset{\displaystyle H}{|}}{\underset{\underset{\displaystyle H}{|}}{C}}\text{—}\overset{\overset{\displaystyle H}{|}}{\underset{\underset{\displaystyle H}{|}}{C}}\text{—OR} + H^+ \rightleftharpoons \text{Co—}\overset{\overset{\displaystyle H}{|}}{\underset{\underset{\displaystyle H}{|}}{C}}\text{—}\overset{\overset{\displaystyle H}{|}}{\underset{\underset{\displaystyle H}{|}}{C}}\text{—}\overset{\oplus}{\underset{\underset{\displaystyle H}{|}}{O}}\text{—R} \rightarrow Co^{III} + CH_2 = CH_2 + ROH$$

Ethylene is also assumed to be the product of the decomposition of vinyl-cobalamin in acid, and it was suggested that the reaction involved the intermediate formation of the π-ethylene complex:

$$\text{Co—CH=CH}_2 + H^+ \rightleftharpoons \left[Co^{III} \leftarrow \overset{\displaystyle CH_2}{\underset{\displaystyle CH_2}{\|}} \right] \rightarrow Co^{III} + CH_2{=}CH_2$$

This reaction is fairly slow at room temperature ($t_{1/2} \sim 45$ minutes in 10 N H_2SO_4) (Hayward *et al.*, 1965). A similar mechanism, involving the intermediate formation of the π-ethylene complex could also be put forward for the acid-catalyzed decomposition of the above-mentioned β-hydroxy- and methoxy-ethyl-cobalamins:

$$Co—CH_2—CH_2—OR + H^+ \rightleftharpoons \left[Co^{III} \leftarrow \begin{matrix} CH_2 \\ \| \\ CH_2 \end{matrix} \right] + ROH \rightarrow Co^{III} + CH_2{=}CH_2 + ROH$$

The hydration of ethinylcobalamin to acetylcobalamin in acid solution, i.e.

$$Co—C{\equiv}CH + H_2O \rightarrow Co—CO—CH_3$$

parallels the hydration of acetylenes to aldehydes catalyzed by Hg(II) salts in sulphuric acid (Coates and Wade, 1967) and is the only example so far known of a reaction involving the co-ordinated carbon atom of an organocorrinoid without breaking the Co—C bond. The reaction is fairly fast at room temperature ($t_{1/2} \sim 10$ minutes in 1 N H_2SO_4) (Hayward et al., 1965).

The decomposition of organocorrinoids in alkaline solution appears to involve heterolysis to give the Co(I) ion. Barnett, Hogenkamp and Abeles (1966) studied the decomposition of β-cyanoethylcobalamin in the presence and absence of air. The decomposition at 25° in the presence of air is first-order in both hydroxide and cobalamin and independent of the nature of the buffer anion, i.e. rate $= K_2[\text{cobalamin}][\text{HO}^-]$, where $k_2 = 230$ M^{-1} min^{-1} or 3.8 M^{-1} sec^{-1}. Decomposition in the absence of air was carried out in order to identify the products. Acrylonitrile ($CH_2{=}CH.CN$) was obtained in almost stoichiometric yields. The spectrum showed that B_{12r} was the cobalamin produced, but when the reaction was carried out in the presence of methyl iodide some methylcobalamin (yield not stated) was formed, which the authors took as evidence for the intermediate formation of B_{12s}. They concluded that the overall reaction is

$$Co—CH_2CH_2CN + HO^- \rightarrow Co^I + CH_2{=}CH.CN + H_2O$$

followed by the reaction of Co(I) with O_2 or methyl iodide. Hogenkamp later suggested (1966) that the initial step is the removal of a proton from the β-carbon atom by HO$^-$, followed by the elimination of the Co(I) ion. Since β-cyanoethylcobalamin can be formed by the reaction of B_{12s} with acrylonitrile they further concluded that the above reaction is reversible. One hopes, however, that more direct evidence for the formation of B_{12s} and for the reversibility of this reaction can be obtained. They also showed by quantitative comparison of the rates that the previously reported decomposition of β-cyanoethylcobalamin by cyanide was due almost entirely to attack by HO$^-$.

Yamada et al. (1968b) have demonstrated the formation of B_{12s} when acetylcobalamin decomposes in alkaline solution. This type of reaction was, in fact, discovered by Bernhauer and Irion (1964b), who found that acetylcobalamin was decomposed by, for example, aqueous ammonia, but they established neither the nature of the attacking reagent (HO$^-$ or NH$_3$) nor the nature of the product(s); these reactions are discussed again in Section II,D. Yamada et $al.$ followed the reaction of acetylcobalamin in $\sim$0.05 N NaOH in the absence of oxygen by spectrophotometry, and showed that acetylcobalamin initially gave B_{12s} ($t_{1/2} \geqslant 15$ minutes from the data in Fig. 3), which is then replaced by B_{12r} ($t_{1/2} \geqslant 2$ hours). Acetic acid was identified as a product of the reaction. The reaction can therefore be written

$$Co—COCH_3 + HO^- \rightarrow Co^I + CH_3COOH$$

although the stoichiometry has not been established quantitatively. In view of the fact that the decomposition of acetylcobalamin in the presence of aqueous hydroxylamine (NH_2OH) gives acetylhydroxamic acid ($CH_3CONHOH$), the above reaction can probably be written as an attack by the nucleophile on the co-ordinated carbon atom (Bernhauer and Irion, 1964b) i.e.

$$\overset{HO^-_{}}{\underset{Co—CO.CH_3}{}} \longrightarrow Co^I + HO.CO.CH_3$$

Yamada et $al.$ also detected B_{12s} as an intermediate in the decomposition of acetylcobalamin by 0.05 N KCN, and they concluded that decomposition under these conditions was entirely due to HO^-, though no study was in fact made of the effect of cyanide ion on the rate at constant pH.

The decomposition of the coenzymes on heating in acid is rather more complex (Barker et $al.$, 1958; Weissbach et $al.$, 1959). At least three hydrolytic reactions occur under similar conditions.

1. Cleavage of the Co—C bond and splitting of the deoxyadenosyl ligand into the component sugar and adenine.
2. Hydrolysis of the amide side-chains to carboxylic acids; one of these, probably the amide group on the e side-chain, is hydrolyzed much more rapidly than the others.
3. Cleavage of the bond between the heterocyclic base and the ribose in the nucleotide side-chain.

In DBC the order of reaction is 2, 1, 3, while in AC the order is 3, then 1 (and presumably 2 before 1). Morley, Blakley and Hogenkamp (1968) have studied the hydrolysis of DBC in 0.5 N HCl at 38°. They showed that the first product (I) differed from DBC only in that one side-chain had been hydrolyzed to a carboxylic acid; by analogy with work on the acid hydrolysis of cyano-cobalamin, they assumed this to be the e side-chain. I then lost the deoxy-adenosyl ligand to give the analogous aquo complex (II). They studied the rates of formation of I and II from DBC under these conditions. The data in Fig. 2 of Morley et $al.$'s paper show that the concentration of DBC decreases exponentially ($t_{1/2} \sim 2\frac{1}{2}$ hours), while that of I rises and then falls, reaching a maximum corresponding to 30% of the total corrinoids at 3 hours, and the concentration of II rises in a sigmoid fashion (50% formed after $\sim 4\frac{1}{2}$ hours). Earlier work had shown that when DBC is treated with, for example, 0.1 N HCl at 100° for 90 minutes it yields adenine (Weissbach *et al.*, 1959; Barker *et al.*, 1960a) and the unsaturated sugar D-erythro-2,3-dihydroxypent-4-enal (Hogenkamp and Barker, 1961), which is also produced in the decomposition of DBC by cyanide (Johnson and Shaw, 1962). The rate of cleavage of the Co—C bond of DBC in 0.1 N HCl at 100° gives a half-time of approximately 20 minutes (from Fig. 2 of Hogenkamp and Oikawa, 1964). The ribose and 5,6-dimethylbenzimidazole are released only under more vigorous conditions (Barker *et al.*, 1960a; Ladd *et al.*, 1960; Weissbach *et al.*, 1959). Hogenkamp and Oikawa (1964) suggest that the decomposition of DBC is initiated by protonation of the ring oxygen of the sugar, followed by the elimination of the oxygen atom and the Co(III) ion from the β and α carbon atoms respectively to give the unsaturated sugar:

No comparison has been made of HCl with $HClO_4$ etc. so that the possibility cannot be excluded that Cl^- catalyzes the reaction by acting as a good nucleophile to the Co(III) ion.

AC differs from DBC and BC in that the adenine of the ribonucleotide side-chain is split off before the Co—C bond is broken (Weissbach *et al.*, 1960). When AC is heated in 0.07 N HCl for 10 minutes at 85°, for example, two yellow corrinoids are produced, whose spectra are identical and also very similar to that of AC above 300 nm (i.e. the Co—C bond has remained unbroken). It was shown that the adenine of the nucleotide side-chain had been lost from the main yellow component, but neither the point of rupture of the side-chain nor the difference between the two yellow corrinoids were established; the products may differ in whether an amide side-chain has been hydrolyzed or not (cf. DBC). The Co—C bond is destroyed by more vigorous treatment, e.g. by heating AC in 1 N HCl for 1 hour at 100°; the additional adenine, but not the sugar, has been identified as a product of this reaction. One may assume, however, that the cleavage of the Co—C proceeds similarly in DBC and in the derivative of AC with the incomplete side-chain.

Other 5'-deoxyadenosylcorrinoids presumably behave similarly, except for the varying rate of hydrolysis of the nucleotide side-chain. Toohey, Perlman and Barker (1961) have used biosynthetic methods to prepare 5'-deoxyadenosylcorrinoids which differ in the nature of the base in the nucleotide side-chain and commented on the differing conditions required to split off the heterocyclic base. The purines adenine and 2,6-diaminopurine both required relatively mild conditions (e.g. 1 hour in 0.1 N HCl at 100°) while all the benzimidazole derivatives (5-methyl-, 5-nitro-, 5-amino- and 4-trifluoro-methylbenzimidazole) required much more vigorous conditions (e.g. heating with 6 N HCl in a sealed tube at 150° for 20 hours). The liberation of benzimidazole from BC also requires these conditions (Weissbach et al., 1959).

Hogenkamp and Oikawa (1964) have also studied the hydrolysis of 2',5'-dideoxyadenosylcobalamin (DDAC) and 5'-deoxythymidylcobalamin (DTC) in 0.1 N HCl at 100°. The half-times for hydrolysis under these conditions (from Fig. 2 of Hogenkamp and Oikawa's paper) were: DDAC ~ 2 minutes, DBC ~ 20 minutes, DTC ~ 30 minutes. Adenine and thymine were isolated as the products from DDAC and DTC respectively, while the sugar originally present in the organo-ligand was isolated as trans-2,4-pentadiene-1-al (CH_2=CH.CH=CH.CHO) in both cases. They concluded that the rate of acid hydrolysis was determined by the susceptibility of the nucleoside glycosyl linkage to acid.

C. REACTION WITH CYANIDE

When treated with cyanide, the majority of organocorrinoids retain the Co—R bond intact and reversibly co-ordinate the cyanide ion in the trans-position (with the displacement of H_2O, Bzm etc.); the amount of the cyano complex formed will depend on the concentration of cyanide, pH and relevant formation constants, which are listed in Table 8.7. All organocorrinoids are light-sensitive and, at least in the case of the alkylcorrinoids, become extremely sensitive in the presence of cyanide (see Chapter 14, Section III). This sensitivity to light probably accounts for discrepancies in the earlier work on the interaction of alkylcorrinoids with cyanide. Alkylcorrinoids do, however, undergo a thermal (dark) reaction with high concentrations of cyanide in the presence of oxygen, which probably involves homolytic fission of the Co—R bond (see the last paragraph of this Section).

Cobalamins reported to be easily decomposed by cyanide include those where R is 5-deoxyadenosyl and related nucleosides (see below), —CH_2COOCH_3 (Hogenkamp et al., 1965), —$CH_2CH_2NMe_3^+$ (Hogenkamp, 1966), —CH_2CF_3 (Firth et al., 1968d) and cyclohexyl (Brodie, 1969). Those where R is —$COCH_3$ (Yamada et al., 1968b), —CH_2CH_2CN (Barnett et al., 1966), —$CH_2CH_2COOCH_3$ (Hogenkamp, 1966) and —$CH_2CH_2COOCH_2CH_3$ (Dolphin et al., 1964a) are also decomposed by adding cyanide to the solution, but in these cases it has been shown that the decomposition is due to attack by HO^- and not by CN^-. In fact, the only cases where it has been shown that decomposition is caused by CN^-, and not by HO^-, are those where R is 5-deoxyadenosyl and —$CH_2CH_2NMe_3^+$. Cobalamins reported to be stable (except for the reaction at very high concentrations of cyanide which involves oxygen) include those where R is an n-alkyl ligand (Müller and Müller, 1962b; Hogenkamp et al., 1965), —CH_2COOH (Müller and Müller, 1962b; Hogenkamp et. al., 1965), —CH_2CH_2COOH (Hogenkamp et al., 1965), —CH_2CH_2OH (Müller and Müller, 1963; Hogenkamp et. al. 1965), —$CH_2CH_2OCH_3$ (Hogenkamp et al., 1965) —$CH_2CH_2NH_2$ (Hogenkamp, 1966), and —$CH_2CH_2CH_2OH$ (Müller and Müller, 1963). Less work has been done on organocobinamides, but they seem to behave similarly to the organocobalamins; those where R is an n-alkyl group are stable towards cyanide (Müller and Müller, 1962b, 1963; Zagalak, 1963) while those where R is 5′-deoxyadenosyl or a related ligand are decomposed (see below). Carbethoxycobinamide (R = —COOEt) is also decomposed by cyanide (Zagalak, 1963).

The sensitivity of the coenzymes (DBC, BC and AC) to cyanide was noted soon after their isolation; treatment with cyanide gives the corresponding dicyano complex and adenine was isolated as one of the organic products in the ratio of 1 mol per atom of cobalt (Barker et al., 1958; Weissbach et al., 1959). The other organic product was later identified as the cyanhydrin of the sugar D-erythro-2,3-dihydroxypent-4-enal (Johnson and Shaw, 1962) and the reaction involves two eliminations as shown on page 246.

Barker and co-workers found that the rate of decomposition of the coenzymes increased with pH and with the total amount of KCN added, as expected if the rate-determining step involves attack by the cyanide anion (Barker, 1962; Weissbach et al., 1960). From the kinetic data given in Fig. 2 from Weissbach et al. (1960), it appears that the rate of decomposition of AC in unbuffered solutions containing 0.01 N KCN follows first-order kinetics with $t_{1/2} \sim 1\frac{3}{4}$ minutes and that the rate also shows a first-order dependence on the cyanide concentration (0.01–0.1 N KCN). The spectra observed during the decomposition of DBC show excellent isosbestic points, i.e. there is no detectable intermediate between DBC and dicyanocobalamin (Hayward et al.,

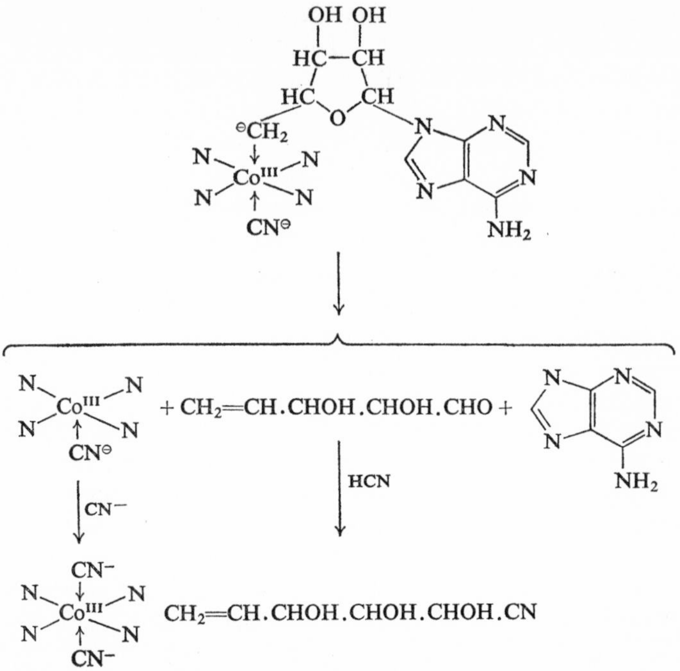

$$\underset{\text{CN}^\ominus}{\overset{\text{OH OH}}{\underset{N\diagdown\overset{\ominus CH_2}{\underset{N\diagup}{\overset{\downarrow}{Co^{III}}}}\diagup N}{\overset{HC-CH}{\underset{HC\diagdown O\diagup CH}{}}}}$$

(purine/adenine ring with NH_2)

$$\downarrow$$

$$\underset{CN^\ominus}{\overset{N\diagdown\quad\diagup N}{\underset{N\diagup\overset{\uparrow}{Co^{III}}\diagdown N}{}}} + CH_2{=}CH.CHOH.CHOH.CHO + \text{(adenine, } NH_2)$$

$$\Big\downarrow CN^- \qquad\qquad \Big\downarrow HCN$$

$$\underset{CN^-}{\overset{CN^-}{\underset{N\diagup\overset{\uparrow}{Co^{III}}\diagdown N}{\overset{N\diagdown\overset{\downarrow}{}\diagup N}{}}}} \qquad CH_2{=}CH.CHOH.CHOH.CHOH.CN$$

1965). The decomposition of DBC by cyanide is unaffected by the presence or absence of oxygen (Bernhauer and Müller, 1961).

Toohey, Perlman and Barker (1961) prepared coenzymes containing a variety of purine and benzimidazole derivatives in the nucleotide side-chain by biosynthesis and reported their spectra and reactions with cyanide. The coenzymes containing the purine bases (adenine and 5,6-diaminopurine) both had absorption spectra which showed that the base was not co-ordinated to the cobalt, i.e. the ligand *trans* to the organo-ligand is H_2O or is absent (see Chapter 8, Section III), and decomposed rapidly in 0.1 N KCN at room temperature (from Fig. 3 of the paper by Toohey *et al.* $t_{1/2} = 40$–60 seconds). The coenzymes containing benzimidazole bases (5-methyl-, 5-nitro-, 5-amino- and 4-trifluoro- as well as 5,6-dimethyl-benzimidazole), on the other hand, all had spectra which indicated that the bases were (at least partly) co-ordinated and decomposed much more slowly in 0.1 N KCN (from Fig. 3 of Toohey *et al.*'s paper $t_{1/2} \sim 2$ minutes for the 5-aminobenzimidazole derivative and 6–8 minutes for all the others). AC decomposes, therefore, about ten times faster than DBC. 5′-deoxyadenosylcobinamide, in which the *trans*-ligand is either H_2O or absent as in AC, also decomposes faster than DBC (Müller and Müller, 1962b). Since DBC exists in solution as a mixture containing about 10% of the form in which the base is not co-ordinated (Firth *et al.*, 1968a) (see also Chapter 8, Section III), the formation constant for the binding of any ligand (such as CN^-) in the position *trans* to the organo-ligand will be about ten times smaller for DBC than for AC. There is, therefore, a good agreement between the ratio of the rates of decomposition and the ratio of the formation constants for the binding of cyanide in the *trans*-position, and one can conclude that the first step in the reaction is the co-ordination of cyanide to form an organocyano-corrinoid. Because of the higher *trans*-effect of CN^- compared to H_2O or Bzm more negative charge is placed on the co-ordinated carbon atom of the organo-ligand and the Co—R bond is labilized. The organo-ligand can then be eliminated by an E_1 or E_2 mechanism. This differs from the mechanisms proposed previously (Johnson and Shaw, 1962; Hogenkamp *et al.*, 1965), in which cyanide attacks the cobalt ion in DBC on the same side as the organo-ligand, i.e. there is a direct substitution of R^- by CN^- without the formation of any intermediate.

The rate of decomposition of DBC and trifluoroethylcobalamin by cyanide is much slower in dimethylsulphoxide than in aqueous solution and under these conditions the complex containing both the organo-ligand and co-ordinated cyanide can be observed (Firth *et al.*, 1968d). Further work in non-aqueous solvents might yield interesting results.

Various analogues of the coenzymes have been synthesized, in which the organo-ligand consists of a sugar (or derivative) and a heterocyclic base (adenine, hypoxanthine, guanine, uracil, thymine). All of these analogues so far reported are decomposed by cyanide (Bernhauer *et al.*, 1960a; Hogenkamp and Oikawa, 1964; Johnson *et al.*, 1963a; Müller and Müller, 1962a,b, 1963; Zagalak and Pawełkiewicz, 1965a). Comparison of their rates of decomposition shows that factors other than the *trans*-labilizing effect of cyanide are involved. Müller and Müller (1962b) found the following order for the rate of decomposition in unbuffered solutions containing 0.01 M KCN: 5'-deoxyadenosyl cobalamin (12% decomposed after 10 minutes) > 2',3'-isopropylidene-5'-deoxyadenosylcobalamin (4% decomposed). Hogenkamp and Oikawa (1964) found that the rates of decomposition in phosphate buffers at pH 11.6 containing 0.1 N KCN fell in the order: 5'-deoxyadenosyl- (80% decomposed after 60 minutes) > 2',5'-dideoxyadenosyl- (40%) > 5'-deoxythymidylcobalamin (10%). It is rather surprising that the nature of groups situated so far from the cobalt can have such an effect on the rate of reaction. A change from one base to another can hardly affect the electron density of the ligand carbon atom, which would be one of the main factors influencing the rate of an E_1 elimination reaction. Change of base could, however, affect the hydrogen-bonds involving the oxygen atom on the β-carbon atom and affect its leaving tendency, which could thereby have an important influence on the rate of an E_2 elimination reaction.

To summarize, the effect of the nature of the *trans*-ligand is strong evidence
9

that the reactive intermediate contains cyanide co-ordinated in the position *trans-* to the organo-ligand, while the effect of small changes in the nature of the organo-ligand provides some evidence for the simultaneous elimination of cobalt and the oxygen atom, i.e.

The nature of the organic products produced by the decomposition of the cobalamin with $R = -CH_2CH_2NMe_3{}^+$ by cyanide has not been reported; by analogy with DBC one would expect the products to be ethylene and trimethylamine. The pseudo-first order rate constant for decomposition in 3.3×10^{-2} M KCN (unbuffered solution, ? room temperature) is 6.65×10^{-3} $\sec^{-1}$ (Hogenkamp, 1966).

Organocorrinoids with simple alkyl ligands are decomposed by cyanide only under certain conditions. Dolphin, Johnson and Rodrigo (1964a) reported that methylcobalamin is slowly decomposed in the dark in the presence of air and 1 N HCN, although it is stable in the absence of oxygen or in solutions of KCN. It was later found that high concentrations of cyanide will cause decomposition even at pH 11.4 of ethylcobinamide and more slowly of methyl-cobinamide, while vinylcobinamide was stable (Firth *et al.*, 1968d). Further unpublished work confirmed that the decomposition of ethylcobinamide under these conditions required the presence of oxygen and showed that the rate of reaction was rather variable and was autocatalytic over the first part of the reaction (Pratt and Thorp, unpublished work). All these features suggest that the reaction may involve free radicals, but there is no other evidence bearing on the mechanism. There are obvious parallels between the thermal and photolytic cleavage of the Co—C bond in that both are promoted by the presence of cyanide and oxygen.

D. OTHER NUCLEOPHILES AND ELECTROPHILES

The occurrence of corrinoid-dependent enzymatic reactions involving the transfer of a methyl group (see Chapter 17) has stimulated interest in discovering and studying analogous transfer reactions which occur in the absence of any enzyme.

The first reaction of this type was discovered by Woods and co-workers, who studied the transfer of the methyl group from methylcobalamin to homocysteine ($HS(CH_2)_2CHNH_2COOH$) to form methionine ($CH_3S(CH_2)_2$ $CHNH_2COOH$) both in the presence and the absence of an enzyme (Guest et al., 1962, 1964). Most of the reactions were carried out at 37° under an atmosphere of hydrogen in a phosphate buffer of pH 7.8, which also contained mercaptoethanol (apparently to protect the homocysteine from oxidation). Under these conditions methylcobalamin reacts slowly but spontaneously with DL-homocysteine to produce L-methionine, and the rate is enhanced by the addition of an enzyme fraction. Methylcobinamide showed the same activity as methylcobalamin in both the spontaneous and enzymatic reactions (Guest et al., 1964).

Schrauzer and Windgassen (1967b) have subsequently done further work on the transfer of methyl groups from methylcobalamin and bis-DMG complexes to thiols. When methylcobalamin in alcohol containing NaOH and CH_3SH is allowed to stand for 48 hours under nitrogen the formation of dimethylsulphide and B_{12s} is observed, i.e.

$$Co—CH_3 + CH_3SH \rightarrow Co^I + CH_3SCH_3$$

It is stated in a later paper (Schrauzer and Sibert, 1969) that DBC is less stable towards thiols than methylcobalamin.

Several other reactions involving the transfer of a methyl group to a nucleophile, which can be written schematically

$$[Co—CH_3] + X^- \rightarrow Co^I + CH_3X$$

have been discovered with other classes of cobalt complexes. The methyl-bis-DMG complex (methylcobaloxime) undergoes the reaction when $X^- = CN^-$ or NR_2^- as well as RS^- (Schrauzer, 1968), while the methyl-cobalt-salen complex reacts with CH_3MgI (i.e. $R^- = CH_3^-$) to give ethane as well as methane and hydrogen (Floriani et al., 1968).

Bernhauer and Irion (1964b) reported the occurrence of reactions involving the transfer of an acyl group from the cobalt atom to an attacking nucleophile, which could be written in the form:

$$[Co—CO.R] + X^-(or HX) \rightarrow R.CO.X + Co^I$$

where R is $—CH_3$ (i.e. acetylcobalamin), $—CH_2NH_2$ (glycyl) or $—CH_2NHCOCH_3$ (acetylglycyl). They studied the decomposition of these compounds in 0.25% aqueous ammonia and in aqueous hydroxylamine (NH_2OH) and claimed that the attacking nucleophile could be HO^-, NH_3 or NH_2OH. They identified acylhydroxamic acids ($R.CO.NHOH$) as products from the reaction of acylcobalamins with a slight excess of hydroxylamine for 3–5 hours in the dark. But in the decomposition of acetyl- and acetylglycyl-cobalamin by aqueous ammonia, no evidence was presented either for the nature of the attacking nucleophile (HO$^-$ or NH$_3$) or for the nature of the products (CH$_3$COOH, CH$_3$CONH$_2$ etc.). Glycylcobalamin, however, gave glycine, glycylglycine and oligopeptides, i.e. both HO$^-$ and glycine can be nucleophiles in this reaction. They also obtained indirect evidence for the formation of B$_{12s}$ by showing that when the decomposition of acetylcobalamin was carried out under nitrogen and in the presence of methyl iodide methylcobalamin was obtained in 40% yield (+60% hydroxocobalamin). Yamada *et al.* (1968b) subsequently obtained spectroscopic evidence for the formation of B$_{12s}$ during the decomposition of acetylcobalamin in ~0.05 N NaOH and also identified acetic acid as a product (see also Section II,B). In these acyl transfer reactions, therefore, the nucleophile can be HO$^-$, NH$_2$OH or glycine (HOOC.CH$_2$.NH$_2$), but there is as yet no experimental evidence for NH$_3$.

Bernhauer and Irion (1964a) also reported the first examples of electrophilic attack on the co-ordinated carbon atom of organocorrinoids. Iodine (in water or methanol) and iodine monochloride (in methanol) both attack DBC to give 5′-iodo-5′-deoxyadenosine. They claimed that the cobalamin produced in methanol was iodocobalamin, but in fact the spectrum quoted is that of hydroxo- and not iodocobalamin (cf. Table 5.1). Iodine monochloride attacked the corrin ring as well as the organo-ligand. Other organocorrinoids were also decomposed by iodine, the rates of reaction with ~0.03% I$_2$ in aqueous methanol falling in the order: methyl- and ethyl-cobalamin (reaction complete in 6 hours) > DBC and 5′-deoxyadenosylcobinamide (~3 days) > 2′,3′-isopropylidene-5′-deoxyadenosyl-cobalamin (~10 days). The last compound gave 2′,3′-isopropylidene-5′-iodo,5′-deoxyadenosine together with another product derived from cyclization with the elimination of iodine. The products from methyl- and ethyl-cobalamin were not identified. The reaction can be written schematically

$$[\text{Co—R}] + \text{I}_2 \text{ (or ICl)} \rightarrow [\text{Co}^{\text{III}}] + \text{RI} + \text{I}^- \text{ (or Cl}^-)$$

Mercury(II) ions form a second group of electrophilic reagents which can remove the organo-ligands, and these reactions have been studied in order to elucidate some of the steric and electronic factors involved in the reactions of organo-ligands (Hill *et al.*, 1970a). The second-order rate constants determined for the decomposition of various organo-cobalamins and cobinamides by mercury(II) acetate in aqueous solution at 30° are given in Table 13.5. In calculating the rate constants, allowance was made for the displacement of Bzm from co-ordination to the cobalt by complexing with the mercury. All these reactions produced the corresponding aquo-complex. The reaction of methylcobalamin with mercury(II) ions was shown by mass-spectrometry to give the methylmercuric ion, i.e. the overall reaction is

$$\text{Co—CH}_3 + \text{Hg}^{2+} + \text{H}_2\text{O} \rightarrow \text{Co}^{\text{III}}\text{OH}_2 + \text{CH}_3\text{Hg}^+$$

It was assumed that the other reactions also involved the electrophilic attack of Hg(II) ions on the organo-ligand. The experimental data revealed the following points:

1. Hg^{II} is a better electrophile towards co-ordinated methyl than I_2, not to mention the proton.

2. The substitution of one H in Me to give Et, Pr_n etc. stabilizes the ligand, presumably by sterically hindering the approach of Hg^{II} to the co-ordinated carbon atom.

Table 13.5. *Second-order rate constants for the removal of organo-ligands by Hg(II) ions*

| | K_2 (mol^{-1} sec^{-1}) | |
R	X = H$_2$O or absent	X = Bzm
—C≡CH	+	
—CH=CH$_2$	1.75×10^{-1}	7.05×10^{-1}
—CH$_3$	1.2×10^{-1}	3.7×10^{2}
—CH$_2$Me	$<10^{-5}$	2×10^{-1}
—CH$_2$CH$_2$Me	$<10^{-5}$	
—CHMe$_2$	3.8×10^{-3}	
5′-deoxyadenosyl	$<10^{-5}$	$<10^{-5}$

Data taken from Hill *et al.* (1970a). Conditions: mercury(II) acetate in aqueous solution, 30°.
+ Reaction observed, but rate constant not determined.

3. The substitution of a second H in Me, however, to give Pr^i labilizes the ligand. The change from a primary to a secondary alkyl ligand will, of course, change both the electron density and the electronic structure of the Co—C unit, but the most important factor in labilizing the Co—C bond is probably weakening by steric compression within the secondary alkyl ligand and between it and the corrin ring.

4. Bzm exerts a *trans*-labilizing effect compared to H$_2$O (and/or no ligand) in all three cases where comparisons are possible (R = vinyl, methyl and ethyl). This agrees with the order of *trans*-labilizing effect observed for the substitution of NH$_3$ by H$_2$O, viz. H$_2$O < Bzm < CN$^-$, CH$_3^-$, SO$_3^{2-}$ (see Chapter 12, Section II).

The reactivity of AgNO$_3$ was also studied (Hill *et al.*, 1970a). Ag(I) and Hg(II) ions form an interesting contrast. Ag(I) removes CN$^-$ (from cyano-cobalamin), but not organo-ligands, while Hg(II) removes organo-ligands, but not CN$^-$. Ag(I) ions are, however, involved in equilibria with the ethinyl and vinyl ligands, which were ascribed to the formation of, for example,

$Co-C\equiv C-Ag$ and $Co-CH\underset{CH_2}{\overset{Ag^+}{\diagdown}}$. The removal of ethinyl and vinyl ligands

by Hg(II) ions may proceed through the formation of similar intermediates.

III. FORMATION AND CLEAVAGE OF THE Co—S BOND

A large number of ligands are known which co-ordinate to the cobalt(III) ion in the corrinoids through a sulphur atom, e.g. sulphite SO_3^{2-}, thiosulphate $S_2O_3^{2-}$, probably sulphoxylate SO_2^{2-}, thiolates RS^-, sulphide probably in the form of hydrosulphide HS^-, sulphinates RSO_2^- (where R may be methyl, phenyl, p-tolyl etc.), thiocyanate NCS^- (it appears that both the N- and S-bonded isomers occur) and probably thiourea $SC(NH_2)_2$. No corrinoid complexes have yet been prepared containing thioethers R_2S. For full details of these complexes and, where known, their formation constants see Chapter 8, Section IV. N.B. Ligands co-ordinated through sulphur are here designated X_s. Names such as cobalamin-sulphonate and tosyl-cobalamin have been used by organic chemists for sulphito- and p-toluenesulphinatocobalamin respectively.

The Co—S bond in these corrinoid complexes may be formed in several different ways:

A. A cobalt(III) corrinoid such as aquocobalamin may react with the free ligand X_s. Cobalamins have been prepared by this method with all the X_s mentioned in the previous paragraph except SO_2^{2-}. The known equilibrium constants are given in Table 8.7. The Co—SCN and probably the Co—SO_3 bond may also be formed by isomerization of the Co—NCS (Thusius, 1968) and Co—OSO_2 forms (Firth et al., 1969) respectively.

B. Cobalt(III) corrinoids react with dithionite ($S_2O_4^{2-}$) or formaldehyde-sulphoxylate ($HOCH_2SO_2^-$) to give a complex in which the ligand is probably sulphoxylate SO_2^{2-} (see Chapter 8, Section IV,G). Since the sulphoxylate ion does not exist free in solution the reactions probably involve transfer of the SO_2^{2-} group, i.e.

$$[Co^{III}] + S_2O_4^{2-} \rightarrow [Co^{III}SO_2^{2-}] + SO_2$$
$$[Co^{III}] + HOCH_2SO_2^- \rightarrow [Co^{III}SO_2^{2-}] + H^+ + HCHO$$

C. Just as alkyl and acyl halides will react with Co(I) corrinoids to form a Co—C bond, so will the acid chlorides of certain sulphur oxy-acids. The following reactions have been reported:

(a) $[Co^I] + SO_2Cl_2 \rightarrow [Co^{III}SO_3^{2-}]$

for both cobalamins and cobinamides (Bernhauer and Wagner, 1963)

(b) $[Co^I] + RSO_2Cl \rightarrow [Co^{III}RSO_2^-]$

where R may be methyl (cobalamin only reported) (Smith *et al.*, 1964), phenyl (cobinamide only) (Bernhauer and Wagner, 1963) or *p*-tolyl (cobalamin and cobinamide) (Bernhauer and Wagner, 1963; Smith *et al.*, 1964). The Co—S bond may then undergo reactions such as the following:

1. *Substitution of X_s by another ligand* without any change in the valency of the Co(III) ion. The possibility and position of equilibrium of these ligand substitution reactions is governed by the relevant equilibrium constants (see Table 8.7). They all appear to occur very rapidly (see Chapter 12, Section II). The sulphoxylate ion SO_2^{2-}, however, does not appear to exist free in solution, and no dissociation of sulphoxylato-cobalamin or cobinamide has been observed, nor are they attacked by cyanide in the absence of oxygen (Pratt, unpublished work). Sulphitocobalamin and cobinamide both have very high formation constants; the equilibrium constants for the substitution of H_2O by SO_3^{2-} are about 10^7 and 10^{11} respectively (see Table 8.7). These compounds can, therefore, be prepared and handled almost as easily as the analogous cyanide complexes (see, for example, Bernhauer and Wagner (1963)). It also means that they are readily formed from SO_2 in the atmosphere (Bernhauer and Wagner, 1963; Hayward *et al.*, 1965). Sulphitocobalamin, but not sulphitocobinamide, is decomposed by 1 N HCl to the aquo-complex (Bernhauer and Wagner, 1963; Dolphin and Johnson, 1965b); this presumably occurs through the intermediate formation of the cobalamin with co-ordinated SO_3H^-, since the complexes $[Co^{III}(CN)_5X]$ where $X = SO_3^{2-}$ and SO_3H^- are both known (Chen *et al.*, 1966). Isomerization of S- and N-bonded thiocyanatocobalamin occurs very rapidly (Thusius, 1968).

2. *Reduction of the cobalt ion by X_s.* The S-anions are potentially reducing agents as well as ligands and can be classified into three groups depending on their behaviour towards the cobalt ion; they seem to behave similarly in both cobalamins and cobinamides:

(a) No reduction of the cobalt(III) ion: SO_3^{2-}, $S_2O_3^{2-}$.
(b) Reduction to Co(II): HS^-, RS^-.
(c) Reduction to Co(I): SO_2^{2-}.

In both groups (b) and (c) the rate of reduction increases with pH. It has also been shown that the reduction of aquocobalamin by the thiol cysteamine requires traces of copper ions. For full details see Chapter 11, Section IV,E.

3. *Photochemical reactions.* The photolysis of aqueous solutions of aquocobalamin in the presence of thiosulphate or thiols produces cobalamin-cobalt(II). The photolysis of sulphito-cobalamin and cobinamide is complex, but probably involves the initial (and reversible) formation of the cobalt(II) complex and a radical, i.e.

$$[Co^{III}SO_3^{2-}] \underset{}{\overset{\text{light}}{\rightleftharpoons}} [Co^{II}] + SO_3^-$$

The initial step in the photolysis of p-toluenesulphinatocobalamin may be similar. For details see Chapter 14, Section II.

4. *Reduction.* The sulphite complexes are readily reduced to cobalt(I) by zinc and ammonium chloride (Bernhauer and Wagner, 1963) or borohydride (Dolphin and Johnson, 1965b). Complexes with other X_s will doubtless be reduced more easily, as their formation constants are smaller than those for sulphite (see Table 8.7).

5. *Oxidation.* Cobalt corrinoids are good catalysts for the autoxidation of thiols (RSH) to disulphides (RSSR). In alkaline solution the reaction proceeds via the formation of the cobalt(II) complex, but in neutral solution the nature of the intermediate(s) is not clear and direct reaction of O_2 with a thiolato-cobalt(III) complex cannot be excluded (see Chapter 11, Section VI). Sulphoxylatocobalamin, formed by the reaction of dithionite with aquocobalamin, is slowly attacked by O_2 to give sulphitocobalamin, but the steps involved are not known (Pratt, unpublished work). Cobalt(III) corrinoids with other S-anions such as SO_3^{2-}, $S_2O_3^{2-}$ and NCS^-, however, appear to be stable towards O_2. It has been reported that p-toluenesulphinato-cobalamin reacts with one mole of chloramine-T (p-CH_3.C_6H_4.SO_2-NHCl) to give toluene-p-sulphonyl chloride (Dolphin and Johnson, 1965b) but in view of the ready dissociation of this complex (see Chapter 8, Section IV,G) the product is probably formed by reaction with the free ligand X_s, and not with the complex. The reaction of chloramine-T with sulphito-cobalamin, as with methylcobalamin, leads to chlorination at C_{10} in the corrin ring (see Chapter 15, Section I).

6. *Alkylating agents.* A solution of aquocobalamin in the presence of excess sulphide or various thiols will react with, for example, methyl iodide to give methylcobalamin (Bernhauer *et al.*, 1963; Dolphin and Johnson, 1963, 1965b; Wagner and Bernhauer, 1964). The mechanism is obscure. In the presence of sulphide, at least, the reactive complex appears to be a cobalt(II) complex and not the thiolo-(HS$^-$)-cobalt(III) complex. Thiols and sulphide cannot be replaced by other X_s such as NCS^-, SO_3^{2-} or p-toluenesulphinate (Dolphin and Johnson, 1965b). For further details see Section I, D.

7. *β-naphthylamine.* Wagner (1965) reported that sulphitocobalamin in which the hydrogen atom on C_{10} had been replaced by either Cl or Br would react with β-naphthylamine (written $ArNH_2$ in the scheme below) in the dark to give β-naphthylsulphamic acid ($ArNHSO_3^-$) in the presence of either

1. air, which yields aquocobalamin, or
2. methyl iodide, which yields methylcobalamin

(both products retain the halogen at C_{10}). The overall reactions can be written:

$$[Co^{III}SO_3^{2-}] + ArNH_2 + \tfrac{1}{2}O_2 \rightarrow ArNHSO_3^- + [Co^{III}OH^-]$$
$$[Co^{III}SO_3^{2-}] + ArNH_2 + CH_3I \rightarrow ArNHSO_3^- + [Co^{III}CH_3^-] + H^+ + I^-$$

No details of conditions, rates or yields were given for this interesting reaction. It is possible that β-naphthylamine reacts with the sulphite complex to form a very low concentration of β-naphthylsulphamic acid and cobalt(I) in equilibrium, and that the reaction is driven to completion by removing Co(I) by the known reactions with O_2 or CH_3I, i.e.

$$[Co^{III}SO_3^{2-}] + ArNH_2 \rightleftharpoons Co^I + ArNHSO_3^-$$
$$Co^I + O_2 \text{ or } CH_3I \rightarrow \text{products.}$$

8. *Other reactions.* Various "stable yellow corrinoids" and other products of unknown composition can be formed by reactions in the presence of thiols and sulphide, but it is not known whether the co-ordinated ligand X_s is involved or not (see Chapter 15, Section II).

The above reactions leading to the formation and cleavage of the Co—S bond show some analogies to those involving the Co—C bond. The best studied S-anion is undoubtedly SO_3^{2-} and one can draw a general scheme of the types of reactions shown by sulphitocorrinoids (analogous to that drawn for organocorrinoids in the introduction to this Chapter), the letters and numbers referring to the preceding paragraphs where the reaction types are exemplified:

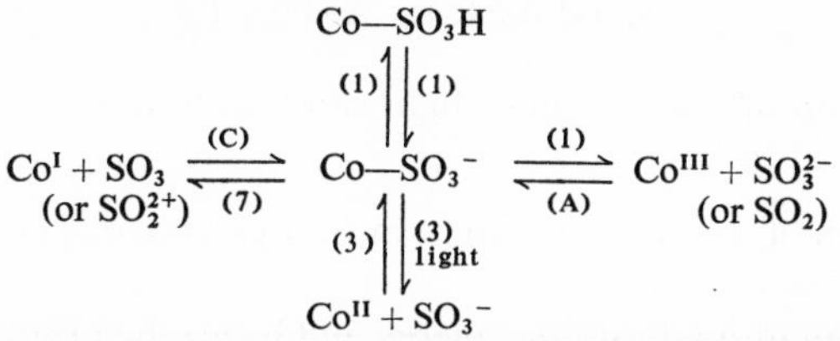

The S-anions also resemble the organo-ligands in their effect on the rest of the complex. Sulphite, the only S-anion which has been studied in any detail, usually resembles ethinyl ($HC{\equiv}C{-}$) or vinyl ($CH_2{=}CH{-}$). Compare, for example, the effect of these ligands on the u.v.-visible spectra (see Chapter 5, Section I), the equilibrium constants for ligand substitution in the *trans*-position (Chapter 8, Sections IV and V) and for the loss of co-ordinated water to give the five co-ordinate complex (Chapter 8, Section III), the polarographic half-wave potentials (Chapter 7, Section VI), the rates of ligand substitution in the *trans*-position (Chapter 12, Section II), the course of photolysis (Chapter 14, Section II) and the course of the reaction with chloramine-T (Chapter 15, Section I). The main difference between the two groups of ligands is that the Co—S bond is kinetically much more labile than the Co—C bond.

PHOTOCHEMISTRY

I. GENERAL ASPECTS

The absorption of a quantum of light can lead to one of the following net results:

1. re-emission of a quantum of light by fluorescence or phosphorescence,
2. chemical reaction or
3. degradation into vibrational energy and hence the production of heat.

No fluorescence or phosphorescence has been detected from either cyano- or dicyano-cobalamin down to 14 kK (~700 nm) (Thomson, 1969), except for an emission at 303 nm, excited at 278 nm, due to fluorescence by Bzm (Duggan *et al.*, 1957). The metal-free corrinoids, however, do fluoresce (Thomson, 1969) and also undergo photochemical reactions of an unknown character (Toohey, 1965, 1966).

A great many cobalt(III) corrinoids undergo photochemical reactions. All these reactions involve the initial breaking of a bond between the cobalt ion and an axial ligand and can be classified as either:

(A) Photoaquation, in which the ligand X (anion or base) is expelled with its full complement of electrons and replaced by H_2O without any change in the valency of the cobalt, i.e.

$$[Co^{III}X] + H_2O \xrightarrow{\text{light}} [Co^{III}OH_2] + X$$

Veer, Edelhausen, Wijmenga and Lens (1950) were the first to report that cyanocobalamin was converted into aquocobalamin by the action of light; photoaquation has subsequently been observed in other cyanocorrinoids and in ammoniacobalamin (see Section II).

(B) Photoreduction, in which homolysis occurs to give a cobalt(II) complex and a free radical, i.e.

$$[Co^{III}Y^-] \xrightarrow{\text{light}} [Co^{II}] + Y\cdot$$

Since their discovery in 1958, the coenzymes (corrinoids containing the axial ligand 5'-deoxyadenosyl) have been known to be particularly sensitive to light; but it was only three years later that Brady and Barker (1961) and Bernhauer and Müller (1961) independently discovered that the irradiation of an aqueous solution of DBC in the absence of air produced cobalamin-cobalt(II). The extreme sensitivity of the coenzymes to light was one of the reasons why they were isolated only ten years later than cyanocobalamin, even though they are by far the most abundant of the naturally occurring corrinoids. It now appears that photoreduction is the initial step in the photolysis of all organocorrinoids and has also been observed in corrinoids containing ligands such as sulphite, thiosulphate, thiols and selenocyanate (Section II).

No other types of photochemical reaction have yet been observed in cobalt corrinoids. Both aquo- and hydroxo-cobalamin and Bzm-[cobalamin]-cobalt(II) and aquo-[cobalamin(BzmH$^+$)]-cobalt(II) (i.e. $\overline{\text{B}_{12r}}$ in neutral and acid solution) are stable to light for long periods (Pratt, 1964). Cobalamin-cobalt(I) is presumably also stable to light, since it is formed to a small extent by the photolysis of certain alkylcobalamins (Yamada et al., 1966d). Reactions such as the self-reduction of hydroxocobalamin to cobalt(II) at high pH and the oxidation of cobalamin-cobalt(II) by oxygen have been shown not to be accelerated by light (Pratt, 1964).

The key questions to be answered in the photochemistry of the cobalt corrinoids are:

1. which are the photochemically active bands,
2. what are the quantum yields and what factors influence them,
3. what determines the course of the reaction (photoaquation or photoreduction).

Very little evidence relating to 1 and 2 has yet been reported, and this is considered last (Section IV). The effect of the nature of the axial ligands on the course of photolysis is discussed in Section II and the evidence for the nature of the initial and subsequent steps in the photolysis of organocorrinoids in Section III. The photochemical reactions of the cobalt corrinoids are compared with those of the iron(II) porphyrins and other organocobalt complexes in what is essentially an appendix (Section V).

To jump ahead, the main conclusions to be drawn from the experimental data presented in this chapter can be summarized as follows:

1. Photoaquation is observed when the axial ligand is CN^- or NH_3, and photoreduction when the axial ligand is any other carbanion, certain sulphur-containing anions (SO_3^{2-}, $S_2O_3^{2-}$, RS^-) and $NCSe^-$. There is a positive correlation between the effect of the ligand on the position of the γ-band in the absorption spectrum, which is in turn some measure of the amount of electron density donated to the cobalt, and the course of the photochemical reaction.

2. Both types of photolytic reaction may be reversed in the dark, at least in the case of the following two ligands:

$$[Co\text{—}CN] + H_2O \underset{dark}{\overset{light}{\rightleftharpoons}} [Co\text{—}OH_2] + CN^-$$

$$[Co\text{—}CH_3] \underset{dark}{\overset{light}{\rightleftharpoons}} [Co^{II}] + CH_3\cdot$$

3. These reactions (definitely in the case of methylcorrinoids, probably in the case of cyanocobalamin) are initiated by the absorption of a quantum of light corresponding to a π–π transition within the corrin ring.

4. The rate of photolysis of organocorrinoids (such as methylcobalamin) is accelerated by the presence of compounds (such as O_2, certain alcohols, thiols, quinones) which can rapidly react with the initially formed free radical and/or the cobalt(II) ion.

5. The photolysis of methyl-Bzm-[cobalamin] and of methyl-[cobalamin-(BzmH$^+$)] in the presence of $\overline{air}$ have quantum yields of ~0.3 and 0.3–0.5 respectively.

The main point of interest to the co-ordination chemist is probably the fact that photochemical reactions of the cobalt(III) corrinoids, like those of the iron(II) porphyrins, are initiated by the absorption of a quantum of light corresponding to an internal transition of the (equatorial) ligand, and not to d–d transitions within the metal ion or charge transfer transitions involving movement of charge between metal and ligand.

II. PHOTOAQUATION AND PHOTOREDUCTION; EFFECT OF THE LIGANDS ON THE COURSE OF THE REACTION

As already mentioned, there are two basic photochemical reactions of corrinoids, viz. photoaquation and photoreduction,

$$[Co(III)X] + H_2O \rightarrow [Co(III)H_2O] + X$$
$$[Co(III)Y^-] \rightarrow [Co(II)] + Y\cdot$$

All the experimental observations can be explained in terms of these two initial steps and the secondary reactions of the free radicals and cobalt(II) complexes.

Most of the evidence for the steps involved in photoreduction and subsequent reactions concerns methylcobalamin and 5'-deoxyadenosylcobalamin (DBC) and will be presented in Sections III,A and III,B. Here we shall survey a broader field to ascertain the effect of a wide range of ligands on the course of photolysis. Most of the experimental work has been carried out on the cobalamins. The cobinamides and other types of corrinoids will be compared at the end of the section.

There are several factors which may complicate or even prevent the observation of the initial photolytic step. Firstly, there may occur similar thermal (or dark) reactions and, unless the solutions are carefully thermostated, the observed effect of light may be due to its effect in heating the solution and accelerating a dark reaction and not to any photochemical reaction. There are, for example, dark reactions which are analogous to the photoaquation of ammoniacobalamin and the photoreduction of cysteinatocobalamin (Pratt, 1964). Secondly, substitution of the axial ligands usually occurs very rapidly and in many cases the effects of photoaquation may not be observed because equilibrium is re-established quickly; this may be the case with NCS^-. Thirdly, it appears that in photoreduction the initial homolytic step may be rapidly reversed and, unless the free radical or cobalt(II) is removed by secondary reactions or long periods of high illumination used, little or no photolysis may be observed; this appears to be the case with sulphite and methyl complexes (see below). And finally, since cobalt(II) complexes are oxidized by oxygen, photolysis in the presence of oxygen (or other reactive molecules) may prevent one from distinguishing photoreduction from photoaquation or in certain cases from observing any photochemical reaction at all.

The products of photolysis of various cobalamins in aqueous solution in the absence of oxygen are shown in Table 14.1. Additional experimental details, observations and explanatory notes are given in the notes below.

1. H_2O, HO^-. Both aquocobalamin (at pH 2) and hydroxocobalain (pH 9.3 and 14) are completely stable to light for long periods (Pratt, 1964). This clearly cannot exclude the possibility of a light-catalyzed exchange of coordinated H_2O or HO^-, which would have no effect on the spectrum. It also does not prove that photoreduction to give hydroxyl radicals does not occur, since the reverse reaction would be expected to be very fast. But, as in the case of the photolysis of the sulphite and methyl complexes (see below) or the reaction of cobalt(II) with hydrogen peroxide (see Chapter 15, Section II), one would expect some change in the spectrum, caused by the attack of hydroxyl radicals on the corrin ring, and it seems reasonable to conclude that photoreduction does not occur.

2. NH_3. The photolysis of ammoniacobalamin has been studied under nitrogen in acid solution where it is thermodynamically unstable with respect to the formation of aquocobalamin and ammonium ion (Pratt, 1964). Under

Table 14.1. *Products of the photolysis of aqueous solutions of cobalamins in the absence of oyxgen*

Ligand atom	Ligand	λ_γ (nm)	Photo-aquation	Photo-reduction	References
O	H_2O	350	−	−	c
	HO^-	357	−	−	c
N	NH_3	356	+	−	c
C	CN^-	361	>98%	0%	c, d
	$-C\equiv CH$	367	~0%	~100%	c
	$-CH=CH_2$	372	~0%	100%	c
	$-CH_3$	374	~0%	97%	c
	$-CH_2CH_3{}^b$	~375	−	+	e, f, g
	5-Deoxyadenosyl	375	~0%	101%	c
	$-COCH_3$	?	~0%	~100%	h
S	NCS^-	357	−	−	c
	SO_3^{2-}	364	?	$+^a$	c, h
	$S_2O_3^{2-}$	367	−	+	c
	RS^- (cysteinate)	370	−	+	c
	p-Toluene-sulphinate^b	?	?	$+^a$	i
Se	$NCSe^-$	371	?	+	h

λ_γ is the wavelength of the γ-band; data mainly from Table 5.1.
+ indicates reaction observed
− not observed
yields (in percent) are quoted for cobalamins with carbanions
^{a} See text.
All solutions, except those marked ^{b}, were thermostated to eliminate the effects of irradiation in raising the temperature and catalyzing any dark reaction.
Excess ligand present in all cases except cobalamins with carbanions.
References:
^{c} Pratt, 1964.
^{d} Veer *et al.*, 1950.
^{e} Dolphin *et al.*, 1964a.
^{f} Dolphin *et al.*, 1964b.
^{g} Yamada *et al.*, 1966d.
^{h} Pratt, unpublished work.
^{i} Dolphin and Johnson, 1965b.

these conditions light merely catalyses a slower, thermal reaction. No cobalt(II) was detected. It would be interesting to study the photolysis under conditions where ammoniacobalamin is stable in the dark, to see whether light can displace the dark equilibrium as it does in the case of cyanocobalamin (see below). Cooley *et al.* (1951) had previously observed that light caused the photoaquation of ammoniacobalamin, but in this case the solutions were not thermostated.

3. *Carbon-ligands.* The carbanions provide the most easily interpreted set of experimental data. They can be prepared and studied as pure compounds. The organocobalamins do not dissociate in the dark, and the formation constant of cyanocobalamin is so high that it is thermodynamically stable even at very low pH (Hayward *et al.*, 1965). One can, therefore, determine directly the relative amounts of photoaquation and photoreduction for each compound. Table 14.1 lists a range of carbanions, in which the ligand atom can have *sp*, *sp*^{2} or *sp*^{3} hybridization. The photolysis of other cobalamins with, for example, substituted methyl and ethyl ligands is mentioned in Section III,C. Corrinoids containing isocyanides (RNC) are also known (Firth *et al.*, 1969; George *et al.*, 1960), but their photolysis has not been studied. The photolysis of cyanocobalamin was first reported by Veer *et al.* (1950). They found that photolysis in air produced aquocobalamin and that the reaction was reversed on standing in the dark. The photolysis has not in fact been studied under nitrogen, but from the complete (>98%) reversibility of the reaction one can conclude that no photoreduction occurs (Pratt, 1964). Fuller details of the photolysis of the organocobalamins are given in Section III. The photolysis of methyl-, ethyl-, acetyl- and 5'-deoxyadenosyl-cobalamins in the presence of oxygen produces aquocobalamin. The rate of photolysis of 5'-deoxyadenosylcobalamin is approximately the same in the presence and absence of oxygen, while that of methyl- and ethyl-cobalamin is very markedly increased by the presence of oxygen. This can be interpreted in terms of a reversible initial photolysis to give cobalt(II) and a free radical

$$[Co(III)X^-] \underset{dark}{\overset{light}{\rightleftarrows}} [Co(II)] + X \cdot$$

The reverse reaction will occur rapidly unless the free radical and/or the cobalt(II) can react further with, for example, oxygen or, in the cases of DBC, the heterocyclic end of the ligand. The photolysis of ethinyl- and vinyl-cobalamin in the presence of air has not yet been studied.

4. *Sulphite.* The photosensitivity of sulphitocobalamin in both acid and neutral solution and of sulphitocobinamide was reported first by Bernhauer *et al.* (1962b) and Hill *et al.* (1962). Bernhauer and Wagner (1963) found that both sulphitocobalamin and cobinamide were photolyzed in the presence of air to give the corresponding aquo- or hydroxo complex. The oxygen consumption amounted to 0.35 and 0.39 mols O_2 per mol of cobalt for the cobalamin and cobinamide respectively, and in the latter case sulphate was identified as a product by infrared spectroscopy. The main reaction is clearly:

$$[Co(III)SO_3^{2-}] + H_2O + \tfrac{1}{2}O_2 \rightarrow [Co(III)OH_2] + SO_4^{2-}$$

The ease of oxidation of sulphitocobalamin to give sulphate had been reported many years previously, but no effect of light noted (Kaczka *et al.*, 1951; Smith *et al.*, 1952a). There may be a slow oxidation of sulphite to sulphate catalyzed by aquocobalamin, but it seems likely that the observed autoxidation of sulphite was in fact the photochemical reaction. It has been reported that both sulphitocobalamin (Bernhauer and Wagner, 1963; Dolphin and Johnson, 1965b; Dolphin *et al.*, 1963b) and cobinamide (Bernhauer and Wagner, 1963) are stable towards light in the absence of oxygen, but experimental details and maximum possible rates were not given. The presence of oxygen clearly has a marked accelerating effect, and in this respect the sulphite complexes are similar to the methyl complexes (see Section III,A). The reason is probably the same, namely that the initial homolysis is reversible

$$[Co(III)SO_3^{2-}] \underset{dark}{\overset{light}{\rightleftharpoons}} [Co(II)] + SO_3^- \cdot$$

and unless the $SO_3^- \cdot$ radical or the cobalt(II) complex is removed by, for example, reaction with oxygen, the sulphitocobalamin is rapidly reformed. The author reported (Pratt, 1964) that sulphitocobalamin is photolyzed in both neutral and acid solution even under nitrogen, but that the reactions were complicated and the products had not been identified. Changes in the absorption spectra were followed during the photolysis of sulphitocobalamin in the presence of a slight excess of sulphite ion in neutral de-oxygenated solution. Photolysis does occur, but the results are not readily reproducible. The spectrum shows that aquocobalamin is formed and in some, but not all, experiments bands arose at 311 and 475 nm, which disappeared on admitting air and which indicated the formation of cobalamin-cobalt(II). But the main products absorbed in the 420–470 nm region and could not be converted into dicyanocobalamin, which indicates that the corrinoid structure had been irreversibly destroyed and strongly suggests (see Chapter 15, Section II) attack by free radicals (Pratt, unpublished work). The enhancement of the rate of photolysis by the presence of oxygen, the autoxidation of sulphite to sulphate, the detection of cobalt(II) in certain cases and the destruction of the corrin ring in the absence of oxygen can all be explained on the basis of the initial reversible homolysis to give cobalt(II) and the radical anion SO_3^-. Sulphitocobalamin and cobinamide are both stable in the solid state (Bernhauer and Wagner, 1963).

5. *Thiosulphate.* This ligand provides the most clear-cut case of photoreduction among the S-anions. The photochemical reaction is accompanied by a dark reaction giving unknown products (Pratt, 1964). For the characterization of thiosulphatocobalamin see Pratt and Thorp (1966).

6. *Thiols.* The observation of any photoreduction of corrinoids in the pres-

ence of thiols is complicated by the fact that thiols reduce corrinoids to a cobalt(II) complex by a thermal (dark) reaction at a rate which increases with pH (Hill *et al.*, 1962; Peel, 1963) (see also Chapter 11, Sections IV and VI). By carefully thermostating the dark and photolyzed solutions it was possible to show that light did accelerate the reduction by cysteine when the thermal reaction was sufficiently slow, i.e. that there was a photochemical as well as a thermal reaction (Pratt, 1964). Dolphin and Johnson (1965b) observed reduction to cobalt(II) on irradiating solutions of aquocobalamin under nitrogen with the thiols glutathione, cysteine, 2-mercaptoethanol and thioglycollate. Since their solutions were not thermostated, the effect of light might have been merely to accelerate the thermal reaction by heating the solution and cannot be accepted as proof of photoreduction. It does, however, seem very likely that the photoreduction observed with cysteine would also occur with other thiols. These reductions are accompanied by other reactions leading to the destruction of the corrinoid structure (Dolphin and Johnson, 1965b). For the characterization of cysteinatocobalamin see Hill *et al.* (1970b).

7. *p-Toluenesulphinate* (p-CH_3.C_6H_4.SO_2^-). Dolphin and Johnson (1965b) reported that p-toluenesulphinatocobalamin is very similar to sulphitocobalamin in its photochemistry. It is photolyzed to give aquocobalamin in the presence of air, but is apparently stable in its absence. No test was made for the formation of products such as p-toluenesulphonic acid. As with sulphitocobalamin the initial step is probably a reversible homolysis and the reaction is listed as such in Table 14.1.

8. *Selenocyanate*. A solution of aquocobalamin in phosphate buffer pH 6 and containing M/100 KNCSe was irradiated under nitrogen at 20°. The formation of cobalt(II) was indicated by the slow rise of new absorption bands at 311 and 475 nm, which disappeared on admitting air (Pratt, unpublished work). For the characterization of selenocyanatocobalamin see Pratt and Thorp (1966).

The data on the photolysis of cobalamins with carbanions establishes the following points:

1. There are two types of photochemical reaction, viz. photoaquation and photoreduction.

2. Photoaquation can be reversible (at least in the case of the cyanide complex).

3. Photoreduction can also be reversible (at least in the case of methylcobalamin; see discussion in Section III,A).

4. Oxygen (and certain other compounds) markedly enhances the rate of photolysis of methyl- and ethyl-cobalamin (see Sections III,A and III,C).

The sulphur-anions show a parallel with the carbon-anions. Photoreduction is observed with thiosulphate and cysteine (and possibly other thiols); for reasons given above it appears that the first step in the photolysis of sulphitocobalamin is also photoreduction. The same dramatic accelerating effect of oxygen on the rate of photolysis is observed for both methyl- and sulphito-cobalamin and perhaps also for the sulphinate complex. The thiocyanate complex, on the other hand, does not undergo photoreduction at any detectable rate; photo-aquation cannot, however, be ruled out because the equilibrium would be re-established instantaneously.

It has been pointed out (Pratt, 1964) that the course of photolysis does not depend on either the nature of the ligand atom (cf. CN^- with $HC{\equiv}C^-$ and NCS^- with $S_2O_3^{2-}$) or whether the ligand is saturated or unsaturated (cf. NH_3 with CH_3^- and CN^- with $HC{\equiv}C^-$), but it does show a correlation with the position of the γ-band (see Table 14.1). Photoreduction occurs when the γ-band is situated at a wavelength longer than 361 nm (i.e. all organo-ligands, SO_3^{2-}, $S_2O_3^{2-}$, RS^-, $NCSe^-$) and photoaquation when the band occurs at shorter wavelength (NH_3, CN^-, possibly also H_2O, HO^-, NCS^-). The position of the γ-band also shows a positive correlation with the effect of the axial ligand on other properties of the complex, i.e. with their cis- and trans-effects (see summary in Chapter 18), and is some measure of the amount of charge donated by the ligand to the cobalt ion.

There is also a certain parallel between the thermal and photochemical reactions of corrinoids. For example, thermal (dark) reactions occur which are analogous to the photoaquation of ammoniacobalamin and to the photo-reduction of cysteinatocobalamin (Pratt, 1964). Some work has also been reported on the thermal decomposition of organocorrinoids and other organo-cobalt(III) complexes (for fuller details see Chapter 13, Section II,A). Pyrolysis of alkylcobalamins and other complexes in the solid state gives the same types of organic products as are obtained from the anaerobic photolysis of their solutions (Schrauzer et al., 1968b; Schrauzer and Windgassen, 1966a) and in the case of the organo-cobalt-salen complexes pyrolysis of the solid and photolysis of the solution have both been shown to give the cobalt(II) complex (Costa and Mestroni, 1967).

Very few kinetic data have been reported for these photochemical reactions. As expected, the photolysis of cyanocobalamin (in the presence of air) follows first-order kinetics, while the reverse reaction between aquocobalamin and cyanide ion in the dark follows second-order kinetics (Pratt, 1964). First-order kinetics are also observed in the photolysis of ethinyl- and vinyl-cobalamin and DBC under nitrogen but not in the case of methylcobalamin, where the rate falls as photolysis proceeds (Pratt, 1964). The anomalous kinetics of methyl-cobalamin will be discussed further in Section III,A. The photolysis of methyl-cobalamin in air, however, does show first-order kinetics when followed by the rise of the γ-band of hydroxocobalamin, even though the absence of isosbestic points shows that more than one corrinoid is involved. The half-times of these reactions, carried out under the same experimental conditions, are (from Pratt, 1964):

Ethinylcobalamin	Under nitrogen	$t_{1/2} = 25$ days
Vinylcobalamin	Under nitrogen	2.1 hours
Methylcobalamin	Under nitrogen	~20 hours
DBC	Under nitrogen	3.1 minutes
Methylcobalamin	In air	1.0 minute

These rates vary widely and show no correlation with, for example, the wavelength of the γ-band. It will be shown in Section III that the rate of photolysis is probably determined by the rate of removal of the organic radical, at least in the case of methylcobalamin and DBC and presumably also in the case of ethinyl- and vinyl-cobalamin. The photolysis in air of other cobalamins containing substituted methyl and ethyl ligands also shows first-order kinetics with relatively little variation in the rate constants (see Table 14.2).

The limited qualitative information available on the photolysis of cobinamides shows the same general pattern. Cyanoaquocobinamide undergoes photoaquation and the reaction is reversed on standing in the dark (Hayward et al., 1965). Methylcobinamide in the absence of oxygen is slowly photolyzed to give the cobalt(II) complex, but in the presence of oxygen rapidly gives the aquocobalt(III) complex (Pratt, 1964). Sulphitocobinamide, like sulphitocobalamin, is photolyzed at an appreciable rate only in the presence of oxygen (Bernhauer and Wagner, 1963). There appears to be some difference or discrepancy, however, in the case of the sulphinate complexes. Dolphin and Johnson (1965b) report that p-toluenesulphinatocobalamin is photolyzed in air to give aquocobalamin, while Bernhauer and Wagner (1963) find that both benzenesulphinato- and p-toluenesulphinatocobinamide are stable to light even in the presence of air. For examples of the photolysis of other methyl-corrinoids see Section III,A. Photochemical reactions have also been observed for cyanocobalamin in concentrated sulphuric acid (Pratt, 1964), where the corrin ring has probably been protonated (see Chapter 9, Section III), and for the sulphite complex of the chlorolactone (Dolphin et al., 1963b). It has been claimed that acetatoaquo- and chloroaquo-cobinamide are also light-sensitive (Bernhauer et al., 1962a), but the complexes concerned were not identified and in the light of our present knowledge about formation constants, rates of substitution and the effect of different ligands on the spectrum and course of photolysis, it seems unlikely that the observed reactions were due to the effect of acetate or chloride.

III. MECHANISM AND PRODUCTS OF THE PHOTOLYSIS OF ORGANOCORRINOIDS

Most work has been carried out on methylcobalamin and DBC. Methyl-cobalamin and other methylcorrinoids are treated in Section III,A, DBC and other coenzymes in Section III,B and all other organocorrinoids in Section III,C. The photolysis of these compounds when bound to protein, however, is discussed in Section III,D.

A. METHYL CORRINOIDS

Aqueous solutions of methylcobalamin are stable in the dark at room temperature in the presence or absence of oxygen, but are decomposed by light. Photolysis in the absence of oxygen is very slow and produces quantitative yields of cobalamin-cobalt(II) (Dolphin *et al.*, 1964a; Hogenkamp, 1966a; Pratt, 1964; Yamada *et al.*, 1966d). The rate of photolysis and the nature of the organic products is very dependent on the nature of other molecules in solution; the most striking, and first discovered, effect is that of oxygen.

The presence of oxygen causes a very marked increase in the rate of photolysis. Under similar conditions the half-time for photolysis of methylcobalamin decreases from about 20 hours under nitrogen to 1 minute in air, i.e. the rate increases by a factor of about 1200 (Pratt, 1964). The main corrinoid produced is aquocobalamin; but the use of methylcobalamin labelled with C^{14} in the methyl ligand provided evidence for the formation of corrinoids methylated in the organic part of the molecule (Hogenkamp, 1966a) and the spectrum of the final solution also indicated that the product was not pure aquocobalamin (Pratt, 1964). The nature of the organic products will be discussed below; they can all be explained as due to secondary reactions of an initially formed methyl radical.

The presence of cysteine(I) and homocysteine(II) during anaerobic photolysis produces S-methylcysteine(III) and methionine(IV) respectively; it is not stated whether cobalamin-cobalt(II) is formed or not (Johnson *et al.*, 1963b; Yamada *et al.*, 1966c).

$$R.S.(CH_2)_n.CHNH_2.COOH \qquad \begin{array}{ll} \text{(I) } R = H, n = 1 & \text{(III) } R = CH_3, n = 1 \\ \text{(II) } R = H, n = 2 & \text{(IV) } R = CH_3, n = 2 \end{array}$$

The addition of 1.8×10^{-3} M homocysteine approximately trebled the rate of photolysis, as judged by the amount of methylcobalamin, which remained undecomposed after a given time (Yamada *et al.*, 1966a). Photolysis in the presence of 1,4-naphthaquinone(V) produces 2-methyl-1,4-naphthaquinone-(VI), neither the conditions (O_2 or N_2) nor the corrinoid formed (cobalt(II) or (III)) are mentioned (Dolphin *et al.*, 1964a). The presence of 2.4×10^{-3} M

(V)   (VI)

p-benzoquinone approximately doubles the rate of photolysis under nitrogen; in this case the organic product was not identified (Yamada *et al.*, 1966c).

Yamada, Shimizu and Fukui (1966c) also made the interesting discovery that alcohols accelerate the photolysis of methylcobalamin to cobalamin-cobalt(II). The rate (given as the reciprocal of the half-time) was linearly dependent on the concentration of ethanol from 0 to 100% in water-ethanol mixtures. The effect of different alcohols was compared using 1 M aqueous solutions of the alcohols and the following relative rates found (reciprocal of half-times; quoted in their original paper relative to ethanol = 1): no alcohol added 1.0, methanol 16, ethanol 71, *n*-propanol 86, iso-propanol 171, tert-butanol 2.1. In addition, pinacol(VIII) was identified as a product of photolysis in the presence of isopropanol(VII), i.e.:

$$(CH_3)_2CHOH \xrightarrow{-H\cdot} (CH_3)_2\overset{\cdot}{C}OH \rightarrow H_3C-\underset{\underset{H_3C}{|}}{\overset{\overset{OH}{|}}{C}}-\underset{\underset{CH_3}{|}}{\overset{\overset{OH}{|}}{C}}-CH_3$$

(VII)   (VIII)

From the correlation between these relative rates and those for the abstraction of the α-hydrogen atom from the alcohols by known free radicals together with the observed formation of pinacol in the presence of iso-propanol they concluded that the methyl radical abstracts a hydrogen atom from the α-position of the alcohol. Methane would be expected as a major product on this scheme; no analysis was, however, made of the products derived from the methyl radical.

If the accelerating effects of the above "catalysts" are linearly related to their concentration, then comparison under the same conditions of concentration would give the following order of accelerating power:

$O_2 \gg$ homocysteine $>$ benzoquinone $\gg$ alcohols

(iso-propanol $>$ *n*-propanol, etc.) $>$ no additive.

The kinetics are interesting. Photolysis in the presence of air follows good first-order kinetics, though the absence of isosbestic points in the spectra during photolysis shows that the reaction is not simple. Under nitrogen, however, the kinetics deviate from first-order, the rate falling as photolysis proceeds (Pratt, 1964).

A considerable amount of data has been accumulated on the nature of the organic compounds produced by the photolysis of methylcobalamin in the presence and absence of oxygen. Several workers independently reported that photolysis in the presence of air yielded formaldehyde (Dolphin *et al.*, 1964a; Hogenkamp, 1964; Wagner and Bernhauer, 1964), while the much slower photolysis under about 10^{-3} mm O_2 gave a mixture of hydrocarbons (61 % ethane, 34.5% methane, 4.4% ethylene) (Dolphin *et al.*, 1964a). Subsequent work using labelled compounds by Hogenkamp ($^{13}CH_3$—Co) (1966a) and by Schrauzer, Sibert and Windgassen (CD_3—Co in H_2O, and CH_3—Co in D_2O) (1968a) revealed the formation of additional products, which could be interpreted in terms of an initial homolytic fission of the cobalt-carbon bond to give the cobalt(II) complex and a methyl radical. The radical can then react with oxygen (to give the methylperoxy radical and hence formaldehyde and formic acid), abstract hydrogen atoms from the corrin ligand or from solvent molecules ($\rightarrow$ methane), abstract methyl radicals from the corrin ligand ($\rightarrow$ ethane), dimerize ($\rightarrow$ ethane) or add to the corrin ligand ($\rightarrow$ labelled corrinoids). The ratio of methane to ethane in the anaerobic photolysis of methylcobalamin is altered by the pH, the solvent and the presence of cyanide or mercaptoethanol (Schrauzer *et al.*, 1968b).

There are two main pieces of evidence that the initial photolytic step is reversible (in the dark). Firstly, the enhancement of the rate of photolysis by compounds such as oxygen, alcohols, thiols and quinones indicates that photolysis is not the rate-determining step in their absence. Oxygen could exert its effect in more than one way, e.g. by reacting with and removing the free radical or the cobalt(II) complex, by enhancing singlet-triplet transitions etc. but the effect of alcohol can only be explained by the first mechanism and there is no reason for invoking a special mechanism for oxygen. Secondly, Schrauzer and co-workers (1968b) showed that the photolysis of methyl-bis-(dimethylglyoximato)cobalt(III) (or methylcobaloxime) in the presence of cobalamin-cobalt(II) produced some methylcobalamin, which is evidence for the reaction of cobalamin-cobalt(II) with methyl radicals. In addition, the kinetics of photolysis under nitrogen deviate from first-order and decrease as photolysis proceeds. This can be explained (Pratt and Whitear, 1971) by the increasing rate of the back reaction as the concentration of cobalamin-cobalt-(II) (and perhaps of methyl radicals) increases. We can, therefore, write:

$$\text{Co—CH}_3 \underset{\text{dark}}{\overset{\text{light}}{\rightleftharpoons}} \text{Co(II)} + \text{CH}_3\cdot$$

The quantum yield for the photolysis of aqueous solutions of methylcobalamin in the presence of air, where the photolytic step is rate-determining, by monochromatic light of wavelengths 490, 520 and 550 nm has been found to be ~0.3 (Pratt and Whitear, 1971); for further details see Section IV.

Some information is available on the photolysis of other methylcorrinoids.

Methylcobinamide and methyl-[cobalamin(BzmH$^+$)], like methylcobalamin, both undergo slow photolysis in the absence of oxygen to give the cobalt(II) complex and a much more rapid photolysis in the presence of oxygen to give the aquo-cobalt(III) complex (Pratt, 1964). Solutions of methyl-[cobalamin-(BzmH$^+$)] are photolyzed by monochromatic light with a quantum yield of 0.3–0.5 (Pratt and Whitear, 1971), which is similar to that of methylcobalamin itself; see also Section IV. Pailes and Hogenkamp (1968) have studied the effect of the nature of the second axial ligand (X) on the rate of photolysis by white light in air of methylcorrinoids and obtained the following first-order rate constants ($\times 10^4$ sec^{-1}) under their experimental conditions: X = CN$^-$, 22; pyridine, $\geqslant 16$; H$_2$O (or five-co-ordinate), ~10; imidazole, 5; NH$_3$, <4; compare also methylcobalamin at pH 8 (i.e. X = Bzm), 12.5, and at pH 1 (i.e. X = H$_2$O or five-co-ordinate), 9.5. The interesting result is that, although a change in X can radically alter the electronic state of the complex, as shown by the absorption spectrum (see Chapter 5, Section I), the rates of photolysis vary by less than an order of magnitude.

Other methylcorrinoids known to be photolabile include derivatives which differ from methylcobalamin by the substitution of the hydrogen atom on the bridge carbon atom C$_{10}$ by chlorine (Wagner and Bernhauer, 1964) and by both chlorination at C$_{10}$ and the presence of a lactone ring formed by the closing of side-chain (a) onto C$_8$ (Dolphin *et al.*, 1964a,b) and the complex formed by dissolving methylcobalamin in concentrated sulphuric acid (Pratt, 1964), where the corrin ring has probably been protonated (see Chapter 9, Section III). The methylcorrinoid in which all the side-chains terminate in tertiary alcohol groups is somewhat unusual. Photolysis in water or chloroform in the presence of air appears to give the diaquocobalt(III) complex, but in ethanol or tetrahydrofuran a stable yellow compound is produced (Wagner and Bernhauer, 1964); this yellow compound may be another example of a series of stable yellow compounds which seem to be formed as a result of attack by free radicals (see Chapter 15, Section II).

The photosensitivity of all methylcorrinoids so far studied, the enhancement of the rate of photolysis by oxygen shown for three different methylcorrinoids and the relatively small effect of any change in the axial ligand (and therefore of the electronic structure of the cobalt ion) provide strong evidence for a fundamental similarity in the photochemistry of all methylcorrinoids.

B. 5-DEOXYADENOSYLCOBALAMIN (DBC) AND OTHER COENZYMES

The photolysis of DBC is in many ways a simpler reaction than that of methylcobalamin. In the absence of oxygen photolysis gives a quantitative yield of cobalamin-cobalt(II) (Bernhauer and Müller, 1961; Brady and

Barker, 1961; Hill *et al.*, 1962; Pratt, 1964). The reaction shows good first-order kinetics and the rate is much faster than that of methylcobalamin (see Section II) (Pratt, 1964). The major organic product isolated (Hogenkamp, 1963) is 8,5′-cyclic-adenosine (I):

$$
\begin{array}{c}
\text{HO} \quad \text{OH} \\
| \qquad | \\
\text{HC}-\text{CH} \\
\text{(I)} \quad \text{HC} \quad \text{CH} \\
\text{O} \\
| \\
\text{CH}_2
\end{array}
\qquad
\begin{array}{c}
\text{N} \quad \text{N} \\
\text{N} \quad \text{N} \\
| \\
\text{NH}_2
\end{array}
$$

However, electron paramagnetic resonance spectroscopy has provided evidence for the formation of an organic free radical, so far unidentified, during the initial stages of the anaerobic photolysis of DBC both in aqueous solution and in the crystalline state (Hogenkamp *et al.*, 1963).

Photolysis in the presence of oxygen produces aquocobalamin. The rate is not significantly greater than the rate in the absence of oxygen (Brady and Barker, 1961). The organic products consist of the above cyclic nucleotide(I) and adenine-9-β-D-ribo-pento-furanosyldialdose(II), more conveniently called adenosine-5-aldehyde (Hogenkamp *et al.*, 1962):

$$
\begin{array}{c}
\text{HO} \quad \text{OH} \\
| \qquad | \\
\text{HC}-\text{CH} \\
\text{(II)} \quad \text{OHC}-\text{CH} \quad \text{CH} \\
\text{O}
\end{array}
\qquad
\begin{array}{c}
\text{N} \quad \text{N} \\
\text{N} \quad \text{N} \\
| \\
\text{NH}_2
\end{array}
$$

The formation of 8,5′-cyclic-adenosine is apparently suppressed if oxygen is bubbled through the solution during photolysis (Hogenkamp, 1964). Johnson and Shaw (1961, 1962) reported that aerobic photolysis also produced adenosine-5′-carboxylic acid, but Hogenkamp (1964) could not confirm this. Approximately 0.74 mols of oxygen, i.e. three oxidizing equivalents, are consumed per mol of DBC photolyzed (Hogenkamp, 1964); since the oxidation of cobalt(II) to cobalt(III) requires only one equivalent, two are consumed in the oxidation of the organic radicals. The experimental conditions appear to be those which would give a mixture of 8,5′-cyclic-adenosine (which would require the consumption of one equivalent) and adenosine-5′-aldehyde (three equivalents).

Anaerobic photolysis in the presence of homocysteine gave a mixture of 8,5′-cyclic-adenosine and S-adenosyl-homocysteine (Johnson *et al.*, 1963b). The effect of alcohols and other additives on the rate and nature of the products of photolysis of DBC has so far not been studied.

The most striking difference between the photolysis of DBC and of methyl-cobalamin is the absence of any significant effect of oxygen on the rate of the former. As with methylcobalamin we can postulate an initial homolysis of the cobalt-carbon bond to give cobalamin-cobalt(II) and an uncyclized free radical. The free radical end of the organic molecule can then either cyclize by attacking the heterocyclic end or react with oxygen, thiols etc. It seems that cyclization of the initially formed free radical is very rapid and that the rate-determining step is therefore the initial homolysis. This would explain why the presence or absence of oxygen does not significantly alter the rate of photolysis, though the nature of the products may be altered by competition for the free radical between the heterocycle, oxygen, thiols etc. The fate of the extra hydrogen atom in the cyclized free radical is not known. The free radical(s) detected by e.s.r. may be either or both of the initial and cyclized free radicals.

A large number of analogues of 5′-deoxyadenosylcobalamin are known which differ in the nature of the nucleoside present as the organo-ligand, the heterocyclic base of the nucleotide side-chain and the nature of the side-chains in general. All of these are photosensitive; see, for example (Hogenkamp and Oikawa, 1964; Müller and Müller 1962a; Weissbach *et al.*, 1960; Zagalak and Pawełkiewicz, 1964, 1965a,b).

Photolysis of 5-deoxyinosylcobalamin, like 5′-deoxyadenosylcobalamin, in the absence of oxygen gives cobalt(II) and a cyclic nucleoside (Johnson *et al.*, 1963a). On the other hand, photolysis of 2,3′-isopropylidene-5′-deoxy-uridinylcobalamin(III) in the absence of air gives the aquocobalt(III) complex and the cyclic product (IV). It seems reasonable that the initial step is the usual

(III)   (IV)

homolysis to give cobalt(II) and a free radical, which then cyclizes and is reduced by the cobalt(II) (Johnson *et al.*, 1964).

C. OTHER ORGANOCORRINOIDS

The photolysis of alkylcobalamins with larger alkyl groups shows features very similar to that of methylcobalamin. Photolysis in the absence of oxygen produces mainly cobalamin-cobalt(II) together with a small amount of cobalamin-cobalt(I) (see below). Qualitative information on the relative rates of photolysis under nitrogen has been obtained by Yamada, Shimizu and Fukui (1966d), who recorded the amount which remained undecomposed after a given time of irradiation. Their results, converted into percentage unphotolyzed, were as follows: methylcobalamin 10% unphotolyzed, ethyl 48, *n*-propyl 53, *n*-butyl 49, *n*-amyl 49. With the exception of methylcobalamin they are all photolyzed at rates which are the same within experimental error. Schrauzer, Sibert and Windgassen (1968a) have also reported that the anaerobic photolysis of ethylcobalamin is faster than that of methylcobalamin, in agreement with the above data.

The presence of oxygen leads to the formation of aquocobalamin and dramatically enhances the rate of photolysis in the case of ethylcobalamin and other unspecified alkylcobalamins (Dolphin *et al.*, 1964a,b, 1963a), while the presence of iso-propanol has been shown to accelerate the rate of photolysis of *n*-butyl- and *n*-amyl-cobalamin with the formation of cobalamin-cobalt(II) (Yamada *et al.*, 1966d). There is obviously a close similarity between methylcobalamin and the higher alkylcobalamins. The effects of other compounds such as thiols and quinones on the rates of photolysis have not yet been reported, though the presence of thiols alters the ratio of ethane to ethylene in the products from ethylcobalamin (see below).

There is, however, one interesting difference from methylcobalamin. Although cobalamin-cobalt(II) is the main product of photolysis in the absence of oxygen, some cobalamin-cobalt(I) is also formed in the photolysis of ethyl-, *n*-propyl-, *n*-butyl- and *n*-amyl-cobalamin (Yamada *et al.*, 1966d). Since the addition of iso-propanol increases the rate of photolysis of *n*-butylcobalamin but suppresses the formation of cobalt(I), the reaction can be interpreted in terms of an initial reversible photolysis to give cobalt(II) and a radical, which can then either lose a hydrogen atom to give an olefin by reducing the cobalt(II) to cobalt(I) or abstract a hydrogen atom from iso-propanol to give an alkane or decay by other unidentified routes (Yamada *et al.*, 1966d).

Hogenkamp and co-workers have studied the rates of photolysis in air of a range of substituted alkylcobalamins (Hogenkamp *et al.*, 1965; Hogenkamp, 1966a). The reactions produced hydroxocobalamin and followed first-order kinetics. Their rate constants are given in Table 14.2. Qualitative results on the rates of photolysis of organocobalamins and cobinamides in the presence of air have been reported by Müller and Müller (1962b) and by Zagalak (1963), who merely recorded the amount of organocorrinoid which remained undecomposed after a certain time; their results (with a few omissions) are given in Table 14.3. The most interesting conclusion which can be drawn from the data of Tables 14.2–3 is that, provided we consider only complexes in which the carbon atom has tetrahedral hybridization (and keep the other ligand constant) then there is surprisingly little variation in the rate. The small changes observed do, however, give the same order of ligands in both cobalamins and

Table 14.2. *First-order rate constants for the photolysis of alkylcobalamins in air*

Alkyl Ligand	k (sec^{-1}) $\times 10^2$
CH_3—	1.9
$CH_3.CH_2$—	3.8
$CH_3.CH_2.CH_2$—	2.7
$HOOC.CH_2$—	3.2
$CH_3OOC.CH_2$—	4.5
$HO.CH_2.CH_2$—	3.6
$CH_3O.CH_2.CH_2$—	3.5
$HOOC.CH_2.CH_2$—	2.7
$CH_3OOC.CH_2.CH_2$—	3.1
$NC.CH_2.CH_2$—	3.6
$^+H_3N.CH_2.CH_2$—	4.9
$^+(CH_3)_3N.CH_2.CH_2$—	7.0

Experimental conditions: 1.7×10^{-5} M, aqueous solutions, 25°C, 200-watt tungsten lamp at 45 cm. From Hogenkamp *et al.* 1965; Hogenkamp, 1966a.

cobinamides: ethyl > propyl, butyl > methyl > higher alkyls > 5'-deoxyadenosyl. The rate constants reported by Pailes and Hogenkamp (1968) for the photolysis in air of methylcorrinoids in which the other axial ligand was varied have already been quoted in Section III,A; for example, methylcobalamin $K = 12.5 \times 10^{-4}$ sec^{-1}, methylcobinamide 10.5×10^{-4} sec^{-1} methylcyanocobinamide 22×10^{-4} sec^{-1}. Zagalak also finds that methylcobalamin is photolyzed at a slightly faster rate than methylcobinamide (see Table 14.3B), though Müller and Müller find that methyl and deoxyadenosylcobalamin are both photolyzed about ten times faster than the cobinamides (see Table 14.3A). Qualitative observations suggest that other alkylcyanocobinamides are also much more light-sensitive than the complexes without cyanide (Firth *et al.*, 1968d; Zagalak, 1963).

Few organo-ligands have been studied, in which the co-ordinated carbon atom is not tetrahedral. Acetylcobalamin and carbethoxycobinamide (Table

14.3) provide two examples of complexes in which the carbon atom has trigonal hybridization; the former is slightly more, the latter much less, light-sensitive in air than the simple alkyl complexes. The photoreduction of ethinyl-,

Table 14.3. *Qualitative observations on the rates of photolysis of organo-corrinoids in air*

Complex	A	% Decomposed
Methylcobalamin		23
Ethylcobalamin		46
Propylcobalamin		35
Butylcobalamin		31
Amylcobalamin		28
Carboxymethylcobalamin (HOOC.CH_2—Co)		40.6
Acetylcobalamin (CH_3.CO—Co)		59
5′-Deoxyadenosylcobalamin (DBC)		15
Methylcobinamide		1.7
5′-Deoxyadenosylcobinamide		1.3
	B	
Methylcobalamin		37.7
Ethylcobalamin		63.7
n-Butylcobalamin		41.0
iso-Butylcobalamin		59.5
Methylcobinamide		30.0
Ethylcobinamide		44.9
n-Propylcobinamide		33.0
n-Butylcobinamide		34.6
iso-Butylcobinamide		37.0
n-Octylcobinamide		22.5
n-Decylcobinamide		22.0
Carbethoxycobinamide (EtO.CO—Co)		0.0[a]
5′-Deoxyadenosylcobinamide		6.6

Experimental conditions:
A: 2×10^{-5} M aqueous solutions, 22°C. 60-watt lamp at 15 cm for 115 seconds (Müller and Müller, 1962b).
B: 3.8×10^{-5} M aqueous solutions, 60-watt tungsten lamp at 25 cm. for 4 minutes (Zagalak, 1963).
[a] Photolysis observed after long exposure to sunlight.

vinyl- and acetyl-cobalamin under nitrogen has already been mentioned (Section II).

Dolphin, Johnson and Rodrigo (1964b) report that the photolysis of alkyl-cobalamins in air yields aquocobalamin and the aldehyde corresponding to oxidation of the radical, while low tensions of oxygen lead to cobalamin-cobalt(II) and a mixture of olefins and paraffins. In the case of ethylcobalamin anaerobic photolysis gave a gas which consisted of 93.5% ethylene, 3.3% ethane, 2.5% methane, together with traces of propane, propene and n-butane; no analysis was made for non-gaseous products. In the presence of air ethylcobalamin gave acetaldehyde and acetic acid, while propylcobalamin gave propionaldehyde and propionic acid (Dolphin *et al.*, 1964a). Schrauzer, Sibert and Windgassen (1968b) found that the gaseous product from the anaerobic photolysis of ethylcobalamin contained mainly ethylene (~100%); traces of ethane, butane and ethanol were also detected. The ratio of ethylene to ethane was independent of pH, but photolysis in 0.1 M KCN solutions changed the composition of the gaseous products to 75% ethylene and 25% ethane, while 1 M mercaptoethanol solutions gave 40% ethylene and 60% ethane. The anaerobic photolysis of propylcobalamin gave mainly propylene with some propane.

The organic products of photolysis have been reported for several other cobalamins. The anaerobic photolysis of carboxymethylcobalamin (Co—CH_2COOH) and 2-ethoxycarbonylethylcobalamin (Co—CH_2CH_2-COOEt) gives acetic acid (CH_3COOH) (Johnson *et al.*, 1963a) and ethyl acrylate (CH_2=CH_2COOEt) respectively (Dolphin *et al.*, 1964a). Ljungdahl and Irion (1966) carried out a more detailed investigation of the products of photolysis of carboxymethyl-cobalamin both in the presence and absence of air. A very wide range of products is formed, which can be interpreted as arising from secondary reactions of the carboxymethyl radical ($HOOC.CH_2\cdot$) such as dimerization, abstraction of a hydrogen atom, reaction with oxygen and fission of the carbon–carbon bond. The relative proportions depend on the concentration of the cobalamin as well as on the presence or absence of oxygen. The photolysis of 2,3-dihydroxypropylcobalamin (I) gave glycerol-(II) under nitrogen, a mixture of glyceraldehyde(III) and glyceric acid(IV) in the presence of oxygen, but only glyceric acid if oxygen was actually bubbled through the solution during photolysis (Yamada *et al.*, 1965).

$$
\begin{array}{cccc}
CH_2OH & CH_2OH & CH_2OH & CH_2OH \\
| & | & | & | \\
CHOH & CHOH & CHOH & CHOH \\
| & | & | & | \\
{}^{\ominus}CH_2 & \rightarrow \ CH_2OH\ + & CHO & +\ COOH \\
| & & & \\
Co^{III} & & & \\
\end{array}
$$

$$\text{(I)} \qquad \text{(II)} \qquad \text{(III)} \qquad \text{(IV)}$$

The photolysis (? in air) of acetylcobalamin (CH_3CO—Co), glycylcobalamin ($NH_2.CH_2.CO$—Co) and acetylglycylcobalamin ($CH_3CO.NH.CH_2.CO$—Co) gave acetic acid (CH_3COOH), glycine ($NH_2.CH_2COOH$) together with glycylglycine $(NH_2.CH_2.CO.NH.CH_2COOH)$ and oligopeptides, and acetylglycine $(CH_3.CO.NH.CH_2.COOH)$ respectively (Bernhauer and Irion, 1964b).

The photolysis of cobalamins with the ligands —CH$_2$Cl, —CHCl$_2$ and —CCl$_3$ has also been studied. Photolysis in an atmosphere of hydrogen yields CH$_3$Cl as a product from all three and HCl from the last two, while photolysis of Co—^{14}CHCl$_2$ under nitrogen leads to extensive incorporation of labelling into the corrinoid. It is suggested that one of the intermediates in the photolysis of Co—CHCl$_2$ may be chlorocarbene, HCCl (Kennedy et al., 1969; Wood et al., 1968a).

D. PROTEIN-BOUND ORGANOCORRINOIDS

Several workers have made the interesting observation that organo-corrinoids may be stabilized towards photolysis when bound to a protein. Taylor and Weissbach (1968) found, for example, that methylcobalamin is stable to light when bound to the enzyme N^5-methyltetrahydrofolate-homocysteine transferase (though unfortunately no minimum ratio was quoted for the rates in the presence and absence of protein) and concluded that the effect of the enzyme might be to protect the Co—C bond from O$_2$. Pailes and Hogenkamp (1968), on the other hand, concluded that the enzyme stabilized the Co—C bond by replacing Bzm by another base such as the imidazole of histidine. Babior, Kon and Lecar (1969) have studied the effect of the enzyme ethanolamine deaminase on the absorption spectra and light-sensitivity in air of several organocobalamins. Both free and bound forms of the cobalamins show the same spectra. Several cobalamins (including DBC) are readily photolyzed when bound to the enzyme to give aquocobalamin. But binding to the enzyme reduces the percent photolyzed in a given time from 97 to 93% in the case of methylcobalamin and from 98 to 65% in the case of ethyl-cobalamin (see Table II of the paper by Babior et al.) and completely stabilizes δ-(9-adenyl)-cobalamin (again no minimum ratio of rates quoted). They concluded that "the cobalt–carbon bond is actually cleaved by light but the two fragments bound tightly to the enzyme [are] constrained to remain in each other's vicinity [and] recombine immediately". The results discussed in Section III,A suggest that these conclusions are only part of the story. Photolysis will probably always be very slow (compared to the rate in aqueous solution in the presence of air) unless the initially formed free radical can undergo some further reaction very rapidly, i.e. react with some radical-acceptor in the immediate vicinity. It is not sufficient merely to prevent diffusion by tightly binding the two fragments; this may be the main factor or one of the factors in the case of δ-(9-adenyl)-cobalamin bound to the enzyme, where one can envisage the protein holding the radical by hydrogen-bonds to the adenine moiety; but it is clearly impossible in the case of methyl- and ethyl-cobalamin. Nor is it sufficient to exclude only O_2. All compounds, to which radicals can add or from which they can abstract hydrogen atoms or other radicals at a significant rate, must be excluded from the immediate vicinity of the Co—C bond; this would include amino-acids with, for example, thiol groups, aromatic and heterocyclic rings and any such groups in the organo-ligand itself.

IV. QUANTUM YIELDS AND THE NATURE OF THE ELECTRONIC TRANSITION

The absorption spectra of corrinoids have been discussed in Chapter 5. The electronic transitions which give rise to the major absorption bands from 300 nm out into the visible region correspond to four or more spin-allowed π–π transitions within the corrin ring, many of which show vibrational structure. No bands due to spin-allowed d–d transitions within the cobalt ion have yet been located, though rough estimates can be made of their probable position. Neither have any charge transfer bands been identified, except in the case of phenolatocobalamin. Spin-forbidden bands of low intensity have been observed at long wavelength in certain corrinoids, which may be spin-forbidden d–d transitions. Which of these transitions are responsible for photochemical activity in the corrinoids? And what is the quantum yield, i.e. the number of molecules photolyzed per quantum of radiation absorbed?

The following quantum yields (ϕ) have recently (Pratt and Whitear, 1971) been determined for the photolysis of methylcobalamin in water in the presence of air (to remove the cobalt(II) ions and methyl radicals) at three wavelengths spanning the $\alpha\beta$ bands ($\lambda_{max} = 520$ nm):

λ (nm)	490	520	550
ϕ	0.35 ± 0.04	0.32 ± 0.06	0.24 ± 0.05

The high and approximately constant values of ϕ show that photolysis is initiated by the absorption of a quantum of light by the intense bands due to π–π transitions within the conjugated corrin ring. Similar but less accurate values were reported (Pratt and Whitear, 1971) for the photolysis of yellow solutions of methylcobalamin in 1 N H_2SO_4, i.e. of methyl-[cobalamin-(BzmH$^+$)], by light of wavelengths spanning the first main absorption band ($\lambda_{max} = 458$ nm):

λ (nm)	436	460	500
ϕ	~0.5	~0.5	~0.3

In both cases the transfer of energy from the electronically excited corrin ring to the cobalt with consequent rupture of the cobalt–carbon bond occurs with a remarkably high efficiency. It is surprising that such a large change in the electronic structure (as evidenced by the large difference in the absorption spectra) has such a small effect on the quantum yield. It is also interesting that the rate of photolysis (by white light) in air of all organocorrinoids so far studied which contain a tetrahedral carbon atom bound to the cobalt are the same within an order of magnitude (see Table 14.2). This shows that the quantum yield is fairly high in each case and suggests that the rate-determining step in air is in fact the breaking of the cobalt–carbon bond. The slight variations in rate could be due to small differences in one or more of

1. the rate of removal of the free radical (e.g. by O$_2$) and of its reverse recombination with the cobalt(II) ion,
2. the quantum yield and
3. the absorption spectrum.

More circumstantial evidence suggests that the photoaquation of cyanocobalamin is also initiated by $\pi-\pi$ transitions within the corrin ring. Boxer and Rickards (1951) stated that monochromatic light of wavelengths 540 and 360 nm (i.e. coincident with the α and γ bands of B$_{12}$) were equally effective in causing photolysis, while Veer, Edelhausen, Wijmega and Lens (1950) provided evidence that light of wavelength in the γ-band region was effective, but did not apparently examine the region of the $\alpha\beta$ bands. No quantum yields have yet been determined for cyanocobalamin, but it can be calculated from the experimental data in Pratt (1964) (on the assumption that the rates of photolysis are temperature-independent) that cyanocobalamin is photolyzed about four times more slowly than methylcobalamin by light from a mercury lamp.

V. COMPARISON OF THE PHOTOCHEMISTRY OF COBALT CORRINOIDS AND OTHER TRANSITION METAL COMPLEXES

Almost all the work on the photochemistry of simple transition metal complexes concerns reactions in which the absorption of a quantum of light leads to a change in the electronic structure of the metal ion (d–d transition) or to a movement of charge between the metal and the ligand (charge transfer transition). Photoaquation and photoreduction are both well characterized reactions; the former tends to occur as the result of irradiating the d–d bands, the latter on irradiating the charge transfer bands. For a survey of photochemical reactions of this type see the recent reviews by Balzani et al. (1967), Wehry (1967) and Adamson (1968). With the exception of the iron porphyrin complexes, however, practically no work has been done on photochemical reactions of metal complexes due to the absorption of a quantum of light by the ligand alone.

The photochemistry of the iron porphyrin complexes began when Haldane and Smith (1896) discovered that carbon monoxide was split from carboxy-haemoglobin in daylight and that the complex was reformed in the dark. Similar reversible photolysis is shown by the CO complexes of other iron(II) porphyrins and, as in the cobalt corrinoids, the photochemically active bands are the intense absorption bands due to $\pi-\pi$ transitions within the porphyrin ligand (Appleby, 1969; Bücher and Negelein, 1941; Castor and Chance, 1959; Chance, 1953; Kubowitz and Haas, 1932; Warburg, 1949; Warburg and Negelein, 1928, 1929); the quantum yields vary between 0.25 and 1.0, depending on the complex and the solvent (Bücher and Negelein, 1941). Iron-(II) porphyrins containing cyanide (Keilin and Hartree, 1955), O_2, NO and EtNC (Gibson and Ainsworth, 1957) are also reversibly decomposed by light. No photolysis of any iron(III) porphyrin had been observed until 1968, when complexes of iron(III) aetioporphyrin I containing ethyl and p-tolyl ligands were prepared and found to be photolabile (Clarke et al., 1968).

There is obviously a close similarity in their photochemistry between the iron porphyrin and cobalt corrinoid complexes. In both groups of complexes it is the macrocyclic chromophore which absorbs the radiation and the energy can be transferred to the metal ion with consequent rupture of the bond to one of the axial ligands with a high efficiency. It would be of interest to study the photochemistry of metal complexes with other similar ligands such as the phthalocyanines.

The discovery of the organocorrinoids led to the synthesis of many other organo-cobalt(III) complexes, the majority of which have been reported as photolabile. They include complexes in which the four equatorial co-ordination positions are occupied by bidentate or tetradentate ligands such as bis-dimethylglyoxime (Schrauzer et al., 1968b; Schrauzer and Windgassen, 1966a), bis-salicylaldehyde-ethylenediamine and related Schiff bases (Costa et al., 1967; Floriani et al., 1968; Schrauzer et al., 1968b), aetioporphyrin I (Clarke et al., 1967, 1968; Dolphin and Johnson, 1965a) and phthalocyaninetetrasulphonate (Day et al., 1968). Schrauzer and co-workers have compared the gaseous products formed by the photolysis of various methyl and ethyl complexes, including the cobalamins and complexes with Schiff bases, and concluded that in all cases the initial step is the homolytic fission of the cobalt–carbon bond; similarities between these complexes were observed in the nature of the products and in the effect of added cyanide and thiols and of a change in pH (Schrauzer et al., 1968b). There is clearly also a similarity in the photo-chemical reactions of organo-corrinoids and other organo-cobalt(III) complexes.

15

REACTIONS OF THE CORRIN RING

The corrin ring can be completely destroyed by the action of strong oxidizing agents such as chlorine (Schmid *et al.*, 1953; Ellis *et al.*, 1953), permanganate, chromic acid or hydrogen peroxide (for references see Bonnett (1963)), by the prolonged action of reducing agents (Schmid *et al.*, 1953; Beaven and Johnson, 1955) and even, surprisingly enough, by ascorbic acid (Frost *et al.*, 1952). Simple cobalt(II) salts have been obtained from B_{12} by catalytic hydrogenation in boiling hydrochloric acid (Schmid *et al.*, 1953) and by degradation with ascorbic acid (Frost *et al.*, 1952). The corrin ring is, however, remarkably stable towards strongly acid and alkaline solutions. Acid catalyzes hydrogen-deuterium exchange at C_{10} (see Section I) and the corrin ring is probably protonated in liquid HF and concentrated H_2SO_4, but the ring is not irreversibly decomposed at any significant rate (see Chapter 9, Section III). Strongly alkaline conditions lead to reaction at C_8, but the conjugated system remains unaffected (see Section I and Chapter 11, Section II). Several other reactions involving attack by electrophilic and nucleophilic reagents at C_8 and C_{10} are now known; in most cases there is some evidence concerning both the reaction involved and the nature of the products formed. These reactions are discussed in Section I. Many other reactions of the corrin ring are treated together in Section II. There is no concrete evidence about the nature of the reaction or of the products in any of these cases. But there is probably some common denominator, since most of the products appear to be "stable yellow corrinoids" in which the corrin ring has been irreversibly altered in some way and many of the reactions appear to involve free radicals.

From the point of view of co-ordination chemistry the interest of these reactions lies in the evidence they provide for a kinetic *cis*-effect, whereby the nature of the axial ligand controls the position (C_8 or C_{10}) and the rate of attack on the corrin ring (e.g. in H/D exchange, attack by chloramine-T, or self-reduction followed by oxidation at C_8) and the nature of the substituent at C_{10}

influences a reaction involving the axial ligand (the reaction of co-ordinated sulphite with β-naphthylamine to give β-naphthylsulphamic acid).

These reactions are also of interest to biochemistry, both because microbial degradation of corrinoids leads to the formation of stable yellow corrinoids and because the substitution of bromine by hydrogen on C_{10} can be accomplished *in vivo*. One intriguing question is why C_{10} has not been methylated in the course of biosynthesis, when the two other bridge atoms (C_5 and C_{15}) and many of the outer carbon atoms carry methyl groups. Is this due to steric hindrance from rings B and C? Does the maintenance of an unsubstituted bridge atom have any chemical significance?

Work on the co-ordination of metal cations by metal-free corrinoids, the removal of the metal from complexes of synthetic corrinoids and attempts to remove the cobalt from naturally occurring corrinoids have all been described in Chapter 9, Section II.

I. ELECTROPHILIC AND NUCLEOPHILIC ATTACK AT C_8 AND C_{10}

The simplest reaction of the corrin ring is H/D exchange at C_{10}. This was first reported by Bonnett and Redman (1965), when studying solutions of the hexacarboxylic acid in (deutero)trifluoroacetic acid by n.m.r. spectroscopy. Further work showed that several other corrinoids underwent exchange at the C_{10} position in slightly acidified D_2O solutions (Hill *et al.*, 1968a). The following pseudo-first order rate constants were reported for exchange in aquocobalamin: 1.7×10^{-4} sec^{-1} at pD 0.95 at 23° and 2.4×10^{-4} sec^{-1} at pD 1.37 at 52°. Qualitative measurements indicated that the rate of exchange varied with the corrinoid in the order ethylcobinamide > ethylcobalamin > methylcobinamide > methylcobalamin > aquocobalamin; the half-life for exchange in ethylcobinamide at pD 5.7 was ~30 mins. It appears that exchange at C_{10} may be general for all corrinoids. The rate clearly depends on the nature of the axial ligands, but one cannot specify exactly the basis of this effect until individual rate constants have been determined for all the different species present in, for example, solutions of alkylcobalamins in acid (see Chapter 8, Section III). It should be mentioned in this connection that corrinoids dissolve in concentrated H_2SO_4 to give complexes, in which the corrin ring is probably protonated (see Chapter 9, Section III), but the site of protonation is not known.

No direct evidence has yet been obtained for H/D exchange at C_8 or any other allylic position, but reactions can occur at C_8 in alkaline solution, which may involve the loss of a proton. Todd and co-workers reported that when B_{12} is heated in alkaline solution the colour changes from red to brown (due to the formation of a cobalt(II) complex) and then on aeration back to red again (Bonnett *et al.*, 1957a). The product was shown to be the "lactam" or "dehydro-vitamin B_{12}", which differs from vitamin B_{12} only in the presence of a lactam ring fused onto ring B by the loss of the hydrogen atom at C_8 and one of the hydrogen atoms from the amide group of side-chain (c) (see Fig. 2.1). This self-reduction of the cobalt ion in B_{12} and B_{12a} is discussed in more detail in Chapter 11, Section II; it probably occurs via the initial removal of a proton from C_8 in alkaline solution to place an additional negative charge on the conjugated system, which now includes C_8, followed by reduction of the cobalt ion. It is interesting that methyl-, 5-deoxyadenosyl- and sulphito-cobalamin do not undergo this reaction under similar conditions (Wagner and Bernhauer, 1964; Wagner and Renz, 1963), while hydroxocobalamin apparently undergoes this reaction much more readily (Wagner and Bernhauer, 1964; Pratt, 1964) (see also Chapter 11, Section II). We therefore observe an interesting effect of the axial ligand on the rate of reaction at C_8, the rate decreasing in the order $X = HO^- > CN^- >$ alkyls, SO_3^{2-}. This is the order expected; as X becomes a better donor it places more negative charge on the corrin ring and thereby makes it harder to remove a proton from C_8 or conversely makes it more difficult to reduce the cobalt.

Reactions with halogenating agents were first reported in 1953. Ellis, Petrow, Beaven and Holiday (1953) studied the reaction of B_{12} with chlorine, bromine, iodine and chloramine-T (I) (see below). The action of chlorine and bromine eventually causes complete decomposition of the chromophore, but inter-mediate purple products could be obtained. Chloramine-T proved a useful reagent; it gave the same type of purple product but further reaction was much slower. No analogous reaction was observed with iodine. Schmid, Ebnöther and Karrer (1953) also reported that the action of chlorine on either B_{12} or B_{12a} produced a violet intermediate before destroying the complex; similar reactions were not observed with bromine, iodine or various acid chlorides and anhydrides. The nature of these products of halogenating reagents was clari-fied by the work of Bonnett *et al.* (1957a). The reaction of B_{12} with one mol of chloramine-T (I) at pH 4 leads to the formation of a lactone; reaction with further amounts of chloramine-T causes substitution of the hydrogen at C_{10} by chlorine. The first product was shown to be a lactone from its infrared spectrum and the effects of acid and base and it was shown by indirect means that it had a structure analogous to that of the lactam (Bonnett *et al.*, 1957a). Chloramine-T acts as a source of electrophilic chlorine (equivalent to Cl^+) and the reaction may involve the initial removal of a hydride ion from C_8 to leave a carbonium ion which then attacks the oxygen atom of the amide side-chain, followed by hydroylsis of the $C=NH_2^+$ group to $C=O$ to yield the lactone (Bonnett, 1963). The identity of the second product can be considered as estab-lished from the following results:

(1) Analysis shows the presence of one chlorine atom (Bonnett *et al.*, 1957a).
(2) The absorption spectra are similar to those of the usual cobalamins except that the bands are shifted towards longer wavelengths (see data in Table 5.5) which suggests some direct interaction between the chlorine and the conjugated ring (Bonnett *et al.*, 1957a).
(3) The proton magnetic resonance due to the hydrogen on C_{10} is missing in this derivative (Hill *et al.*, 1965b). This is the only case in which the presence of a substituent at C_{10} has been proved directly and conclusively.

$$CH_3-\langle\bigcirc\rangle-SO_2NCl^{\ominus}Na^+ \qquad \begin{array}{c} H_2C{-}CO \\ | \quad\quad NBr \\ H_2C{-}CO \end{array}$$

(I)   (II)

Reactions of this type which involve electrophilic attack at either or both of C_8 and C_{10} are listed in Table 15.1. The presence of bromine at C_{10} in some of the products can be assumed from similarities in the known reactions of N-bromosuccinimide(II) and chloramine-T (I) and in the absorption spectra of the products. The evidence for the nature and position of the substituent in the presumed cyano-[10-nitrosocobalamin] is, however, very tenuous. This compound undergoes several interesting reactions, such as reduction to a compound which may be the 10-aminocobalamin and reversible reaction with cyanide at pH 13 to give a compound with an unusual spectrum having intense bands at 442 and 358 nm (Wagner, 1965).

The following points can be made about the data in Table 15.1. The frequent occurrence of reactions at both C_8 and C_{10} means that the relative reactivity of these two positions towards a variety of reagents remains fairly constant even though the mechanisms are probably very different, e.g. elimination of hydride from the tetrahedral C_8 and addition of the electrophile to the trigonal C_{10}. But the relative rates of attack at C_8 and C_{10} are affected by the nature of the axial ligand. In all cases the presence of the better donor (CH_3^-, SO_3^{2-} etc.) as the axial ligand favours reaction at C_{10}. It would be interesting to establish this relationship quantitatively by determining the individual rate constants for reaction at C_8 and C_{10} with several different axial ligands. Hexacarboxylic acid is, unlike B_{12} and the lactam, fairly rapidly decomposed by chloramine-T (Bonnett *et al.*, 1957a); this could be due either to the effect of a change in the axial ligands (from CN^- and Bzm to CN^- and Cl^- or H_2O) or to exposing the corrin ring to further attack by removing the nucleotide side-chain. It seems at first sight that the relative rates of attack at C_8 and C_{10} by the same reagent (N-bromosuccinimide) are also affected by the nature of the solvent (see Table 15.1); this could either be a genuine direct effect or an effect on the equilibria involving potential electrophiles such as Br_2 and HOBr in addition to N-bromosuccinimide.

Table 15.1. *Some reactions of the corrin ring in cobalamins*

Reagent	Conditions[c]	Ligand X	Products[d]	Reference
Cl$_2$	B$_{12a}$ in MeOH + Cl$_2$ in CHCl$_3$	H$_2$O	Violet product (i.e. C$_{10}$—Cl)[e]	Schmid et al. (1953)
	B$_{12}$ in MeOH + Cl$_2$ in CHCl$_3$	CN$^-$	Violet product (i.e. C$_{10}$—Cl)[e]	Schmid et al. (1953)
	3 mols Cl$_2$, pH 4	CN$^-$	Purple product (i.e. C$_{10}$—Cl)[e]	Ellis et al. (1953)
Cl-T[a]	3 mols Cl-T, N/100 acetic acid	CN$^-$	Purple product (i.e. C$_{10}$—Cl)[e]	Ellis et al. (1953)
	1–3 mols Cl-T, N/250 HCl, 2 hr.	CN$^-$	(1) lactone, (2) C$_{10}$—Cl[f]	Bonnett et al. (1957a)
	1 mol Cl-T	SO$_3^{2-}$	C$_{10}$—Cl	Dolphin et al. (1963b); Wagner and Bernhauer (1964)
	1–3 mols Cl-T, N/400 HCl	CH$_3^-$	(1) C$_{10}$—Cl, (2) lactone[f]	Dolphin et al. (1964b); Wagner and Bernhauer (1964); Wagner and Renz (1963)
	1–3 mols Cl-T, N/400 HCl	5-deoxy-adenosyl	(1) C$_{10}$—Cl, (2) lactone[f]	Wagner and Bernhauer (1964); Wagner and Renz (1963)
Br$_2$	In water or glacial acetic acid	CN$^-$	Purple product (i.e. C$_{10}$—Br)[e]	Ellis et al. (1953)
	1 mol Br$_2$, acetic acid pH 4, 1 hr	CN$^-$	Lactone	Bonnett et al. (1957a)
NBS[b]	1.2 mols NBS, 0.5 N acetic acid	CN$^-$	100% lactone	Wagner (1965)
	1.2 mols NBS, 0.5 N acetic acid	CH$_3^-$	50% lactone + 50% C$_{10}$—Br	Wagner (1965)
	1.2 mols NBS, glacial acetic acid	CN$^-$	31% lactone + 48% C$_{10}$—Br	Wagner (1965)
	1.2 mols NBS, glacial acetic acid	CH$_3^-$	12% lactone + 88% C$_{10}$—Br	Wagner (1965)
I$_2$	N/20 I$_2$ (+KI), N/2 NaOH, 30 minutes	CN$^-$	Lactam	Bonnett et al. (1957a)
	N/10 I$_2$ (+KI), N/10 NaOH, 24 hours	CN$^-$	Lactone + some lactam	Bonnett et al. (1957a)
Ag$_2$O	In ethanol + pyridine, reflux	CN$^-$	Lactone and some lactam	Bonnett et al. (1957a)
NOCl	2 mols NOCl in glacial acetic acid	CN$^-$	30% lactone + 40% C$_{10}$—NO (?)	Wagner (1965)
	2 mols NOCl in glacial acetic acid	CH$_3^-$	5% lactone + 60% C$_{10}$—NO (?)	Wagner (1965)

[a] Chloramine-T, see (I).
[b] N-Bromo-succinimide, see (II).
[c] All reactions carried out at room temperature, except with Ag$_2$O.
[d] For explanation of "lactone" and "lactam" see text.
[e] The colour indicates substitution at C$_8$ but provides no evidence for or against reaction at C$_8$.
[f] Reaction first at C$_8$ (to give lactone), then at C$_{10}$ (to give the 10-chloro-lactone) or vice versa.

Wagner (1965) reports that when cyano- and methyl-[10-bromocobalamin] are treated with $NaBH_4$, Zn/CH_3COOH or H_2SO_3 the bromine atom at C_{10} is replaced by hydrogen, whereas the analogous 10-chlorocobalamins remain unchanged; growing cultures of *Propionibacterium shermanii* were also able to replace the bromine, but not the chlorine, by hydrogen. These reactions provide examples of nucleophilic attack (e.g. by H^-) on C_{10}. It would be interesting to establish whether the nature of the axial ligand affects the rate of this reaction in a sense opposite to that found for electrophilic attack at C_{10}.

Wagner (1965) has also shown that the nature of the substituent at C_{10} can affect the rate of reactions involving the cobalt ion. β-naphthylamine ($ArNH_2$) reacts with certain sulphitocorrinoids to give β-naphthylsulphamic acid according to the following scheme:

$$[Co^{III}SO_3^{2-}] + ArNH_2 \begin{cases} + O_2 \rightarrow ArNHSO_3^- + [Co^{IIII}OH^-] \\ + CH_3I \rightarrow ArNHSO_3^- + [Co^{III}CH_3^-] \end{cases}$$

The requirement for O_2 or CH_3I strongly suggests that the reaction proceeds via the reversible formation of the cobalt(I) complex, i.e.

$$[Co^{III}SO_3^{2-}] + ArNH_2 \rightleftharpoons [Co^I] + ArNHSO_3^- + H^+$$

and that the reaction is only driven to the right when the cobalt(I) complex is removed by reaction with O_2 or CH_3I. This reaction does not work with sulphitocobalamin itself, but does work with the 10-chloro- and 10-bromo-cobalamins (Wagner, 1965). It would seem that the presence of an electronegative substituent at C_{10} helps to stabilize the cobalt(I) complex.

Some interesting further insight into these reactions of the corrin ring comes from the work of Eschenmoser and his co-workers (Bormann *et al.*, 1967) on cobalt(III) and nickel(II) complexes of the totally synthetic 7,7,12,12-tetramethylcorrin ligand (the corrin ring in which the only substituents are the two pairs of methyl groups on positions 7 and 12). Dicyano-[7,7,12,12-tetramethylcorrin]-cobalt(III) will undergo acid-catalyzed H/D exchange at all three bridge carbon atoms (C_5, C_{10}, C_{15}) and there is indirect evidence that exchange occurs more rapidly at C_{15}. Base-catalyzed exchange occurs at C_8, but not at any of the other allylic positions (C_3, C_{13} or C_{17}). Base-catalyzed exchange at C_8 occurs even more rapidly in the [7,7,12,12,19-pentamethyl-corrin]-nickel(II) cation, while a proton can be removed from the C_8 position of the [7,7,12,12,19-pentamethyl, 15-cyano-corrin]-nickel(II) cation to give an uncharged complex which can be isolated in crystalline form. These results show that the methene bridge atoms C_5 and C_{15}, when they do not carry substituents as in the naturally occurring derivatives, will react similarly to C_{10} and underline the fact that C_8 is by far the most reactive of the allylic positions in the chromophore.

II. THE FORMATION OF STABLE YELLOW CORRINOIDS

A large group of reactions are known which appear to have some features in common. The products are yellow or brown and the first main band in the absorption spectrum is situated between 400 and 500 nm, i.e. at shorter wavelength than the $\alpha\beta$ bands in octahedral cobalt(III) corrinoids (see Chapter 5 Section I). But in contrast to other yellow corrinoids such as cobalamin-cobalt-(II) and the five-co-ordinate ethylcobinamide these products cannot be converted into corrinoids of the usual type (i.e. with spectra of the usual type) by the action alone or together of oxygen, hydroxide, cyanide or light. For this reason we can call them "stable yellow corrinoids". The addition of cyanide moves the first band to longer wavelength, usually ~500 nm. However, since little or no systematic study has been made of these compounds, we lack sufficient information on

(i) the nature of the reaction by which they are formed and

(ii) their absorption spectra under comparable conditions (e.g. in the presence of excess cyanide, where both axial ligands would probably be cyanide), by which to judge whether they do form a group with a common denominator or not.

Several different lines of research can be distinguished. The best characterized compounds are those produced by microbial attack on B_{12}; there is, of course, no information on the nature of the reaction involved. On the other hand, the greatest amount of information on the nature of the reaction by which some of these compounds are formed relates to the oxidation of cobalt(II) corrinoids.

The microbial degradation of B_{12} was first studied by Helgeland, Jonsen and Laland (1959, 1961) and subsequently by Pfiffner and colleagues (for references see below). Helgeland et al. found that cultures of Aerobacter aerogenes converted B_{12} into yellow or brown products, which were separated into two fractions by electrophoresis. The spectra of the two fractions showed absorption bands in water and in 0.1 N KCN as follows: Pigment I, H_2O 474 and 342 nm, KCN 500 and ~345 nm; Pigment II, H_2O 448 and ~310, KCN 482 and ~320 (see Fig. 15.1). The molar extinction coefficient of Pigment I at 474 nm was determined as 8.4×10^3 (i.e. comparable to that of the $\alpha\beta$ bands of the usual corrinoids); the ratio of intensity of the high-energy to the low-energy band was ~1 in the first pair and ~1.5 in the second pair. They suggested that their yellow compounds might have a structure analogous to that of the co-enzymes or one in which the conjugated system had been interrupted (Helgeland et al., 1961). Pfiffner et al. obtained yellow compounds from the action of cultures of several different bacteria, of which Psuedomonas rubescens attacked B_{12} the most rapidly (Scott et al., 1964). Separation of the products of the last-named reaction by electrophoresis and chromatography gave four main yellow products (which they labelled A1, A2, B1 and B2) (Burgus *et al.*, 1964). They were able to show that A1, A2 and B2 all contained cyanide as one of the ligands (infra-red; photolysis to give one mol HCN per cobalt) (Burgus *et al.*, 1965) and that the nucleotide side-chain had remained intact, but that Bzm was probably only loosely co-ordinated (Burgus *et al.*, 1964, 1965; Ing and Pfiffner, 1968). All three compounds showed very similar

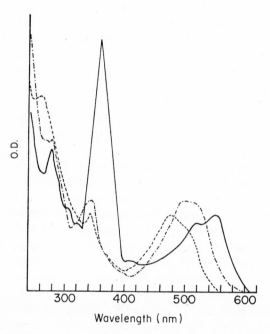

Fig. 15.1. The absorption spectrum of Helgeland, Jonsen and Laland's Pigment II in water (——) and 0.1 M KCN (·····). From Helgeland *et al.*, 1961.

absorption spectra with bands at ~490 and 325–350 of very nearly equal intensity (Burgus *et al.*, 1965). The addition of cyanide in alkaline solution moved the low-energy band to longer wavelength (wavelength not given, but see Figs 2 and 3 of Burgus *et al.* (1964). But the pigments A and B differ in their reaction with chloramine-T (Ing and Pfiffner, 1968). When the nucleotide side-chain was removed by hydrolysis the absorption spectra again showed two bands of similar intensity at 440–450 and ~310 nm (Burgus *et al.*, 1965). Pfiffner and colleages have suggested that in these yellow compounds the corrin ring has been altered in some way, e.g. by reduction, addition across one or more double bonds, introduction of a new substituent into the ring or the formation of isomers in which C_{10} carries two hydrogen atoms and C_8 (or C_{13}) has lost its hydrogen atom and is involved in the conjugated system of double bonds (Burgus et al., 1965; Ing and Pfiffner, 1968). There can be little doubt that the structure of the corrin ring in these stable yellow corrinoids differs from that in the normal corrinoids. There is no direct evidence as to the nature of this structural change, though the reaction of one of the B pigments with chloramine-T to give products whose absorption spectra showed a bathocromic shift of both bands (presumably due to chlorination at C_{10}) and whose infrared spectrum showed a band at 1780 cm^{-1} (presumably due to the formation of a lactone at C_8) (Ing and Pfiffner, 1968) suggests that neither C_8 nor C_{10} have been affected in these particular yellow corrinoids.

Some stable yellow corrinoids are formed as a by-product in the oxidation of B_{12r}. As reported in Pratt (1964), Lester Smith had isolated a yellow by-product with an absorption band at 458 nm from the aerial oxidation of B_{12r} (prepared by the catalytic reduction of B_{12}). A spectrophotometric study of the aerial oxidation of B_{12r}, prepared by the photolysis of vinylcobalamin under nitrogen, also showed the rise of a band at ~460 nm due to some product other than aquocobalamin (Pratt, 1964). Further unpublished spectrophotometric work on the oxidation of B_{12r}, prepared by controlled potential reduction in order to exclude the presence of any other potentially reactive species, showed that oxidation by 10^{-4} M H_2O_2 was much faster ($t_{1/2}$ ~5 min) than oxidation by air ($t_{1/2}$ ~30 min) and produced much more of the yellow by-product (the optical density at 460 nm was approximately equal to that of the $\alpha\beta$ bands of aquocobalamin); aquocobalamin appeared not to be attacked by H_2O_2 under the same conditions (Pratt, unpublished results). These experiments serve to narrow the range of possible reactions which have to be considered as leading to the formation of stable yellow corrinoids. The possible oxidizing agents are H_2O_2, HO_2^- and the hydroxyl radical HO. Attack may occur on the cobalt ion, the corrin ring or the side-chains; in the last case the initially formed group on the side-chain might then attack the corrin ring in a subsequent reaction. The small amount of yellow by-product formed by aerial oxidation can probably be ascribed to the subsequent reactions of H_2O_2 etc. formed in the earlier steps. One reasonable possibility is that the yellow compound is formed as a result of the attack of the hydroxyl radical on the corrin ring. This would in most cases involve an additional reaction leading to the formation of a tetrahedral carbon (or even nitrogen) atom, thereby reducing the length of the conjugated chain and causing a change in the absorption spectrum. But this suggestion has yet to be proved. Further work has also shown that the first absorption band of the yellow by-product prepared by Lester Smith may occur in the range 450–460 nm (depending on pH, etc.), but on treating with cyanide the solution becomes reddish and the absorption band moves out to 486 nm (Pratt, unpublished results).

Similar or identical compounds have been reported by several other workers when corrinoids have been reduced. Schmid, Ebnöther and Karrer (1953) were probably the first to note the formation of these yellow compounds. When solutions of B_{12} were catalytically reduced with Pt/H_2 and then reoxidized, by-products were obtained which showed an absorption band at 445–450 nm, which was shifted to 480–485 nm on being treated with cyanide. The yield of this yellow compound was increased by the presence of HCl or CO during reduction. Beaven and Johnson also obtained brown products from the aerial oxidation of the compounds formed by the reduction of B_{12} with lithium borohydride or hydrogen using a $Pd/BaSO_4$ catalyst. These brown products showed rather broad bands in the 435–450 nm region and gave reddish derivatives (spectrum not quoted) with cyanide (Beaven and Johnson, 1955). Wagner (1966) also reports the formation of yellow compounds using sodium borohydride or zinc and acetic acid as reducing agents and Friedrich and Nordmeyer (1969) isolated some stable yellow compounds from the reaction of B_{12s} with dimethyl sulphate. It is conceivable that in all these cases the stable yellow corrinoids are formed during the oxidation of the reduced corrinoids.

The formation of stable yellow corrinoids is also observed under other conditions where cobalt(II) corrinoids may occur as intermediates, e.g. in the photolysis of organocorrinoids and in the presence of bases which may promote "self-reduction". Hogenkamp reported that the photolysis of DBC in air yielded a yellow by-product which was stable to oxygen and whose absorption spectrum showed bands of approximately equal intensity at ~460 and ~330 nm. He suggested that one of the double bonds in the corrin ring had been reduced by hydrogen atoms derived from the nucleoside radical formed on photolysis (Hogenkamp, 1964); but it would now seem more likely that the yellow by-product was formed during the subsequent oxidation of the B_{12r} formed by the photolysis of DBC. Wagner and Bernhauer (1964) also found the photolysis in air of a methyl-corrinoid, in which all the side-chains are tertiary alcohols, gave a product with a spectrum resembling that of diaquo-cobinamide when carried out in water or chloroform, but a stable yellow compound with a spectrum like that of cobinamide-cobalt(II) when carried out in ethanol or tetrahydrofuran.

Yellow compounds with an absorption band at 455–463 nm, which moves to 485 nm on treating with cyanide, are also produced by the reaction of B_{12a} with γ-picoline (Pratt and Williams, 1961; Hill et al., 1962; Wagner and Bernhauer, 1964); interestingly enough, the lactam and 10-chloro-lactam analogues do not undergo this reaction. It was originally suggested that the conjugation of the corrin ring had been broken by methylation of one of the carbon atoms (Pratt and Williams, 1961; Hill et al., 1962), but recent unpublished work has shown that similar reactions may occur in the presence of other bases (HO^-, CH_3NH_2) (Pratt, unpublished work). A more likely explanation is, therefore, that the base promotes self-reduction, whereby the cobalt ion is reduced at the expense of the hydrogen atom on C_8 to give a cobalt(II) complex (see Chapter 11, Section II), which then reacts with air to give some stable yellow corrinoid. This would explain why the lactam analogues, which lack the hydrogen atom at C_8, do not undergo this reaction.

Products with increased absorption around 450 nm are also formed by the γ-radiolysis of solutions of B_{12} in phosphate buffer and in the absence of any other reagent (Sjöstedt and Ericson, 1959).

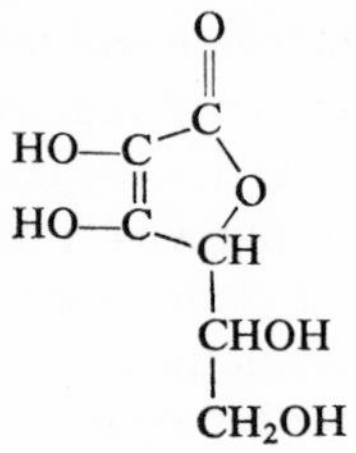

(I) 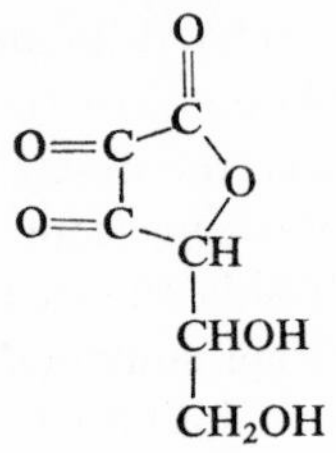   (II)

It has been known since Gakenheimer and Feller (1949) that B_{12} is destroyed by the action of ascorbic acid or vitamin C (I). This reaction has attracted considerable interest both as a simple means of analyzing for B_{12} in the presence of B_{12a} (since the latter is attacked far more rapidly) and because of the problem of the stability of corrinoids in pharmaceutical preparations, which may contain ascorbic acid. The reaction certainly involves several consecutive steps; there may even be more than one concurrent reaction. Frost et al. (1952) studied the reaction of B_{12a} with ascorbate at pH 4.5–5 in the presence of air at 65° and showed that ascorbate will completely destroy the corrinoid to release the simple aquated cobalt(II) ion. Earlier stages in the reaction show increased absorption around 480 nm (see Fig. 1 of Stapert et al. (1954)), while Rosenberg (1956) obtained a series of products from the reaction of ascorbate with B_{12} which showed greater absorption at 465 nm than B_{12}, "the most polar fraction actually (showing) greater absorption at 4650 Å than at 5300 Å". At least some of the products appear, therefore, to be fairly typical stable yellow corrinoids. B_{12a} is attacked by ascorbic acid rapidly even at room temperature and the rate increases with pH at least in the range pH 0–7 (Trenner et al., 1950). B_{12} is destroyed more slowly (Trenner et al., 1950; Frost et al., 1952; Campbell et al., 1952) and the destruction of B_{12a} is also inhibited by ligands such as CN^-, SO_3^{2-}, NO_2^-, $[Fe^{II}(CH)_6]^{4-}$ and $[Fe^{III}(CN)_6]^{3-}$, but not NCS^-, NCO^-, NH_3, histidine or various (unspecified) amino-acids, purines or pyrimidines, and is also inhibited by the presence of iron (exact form not specified) (Frost et al., 1952). Stapert et al. (1954)

found that the reaction between B_{12} and ascorbic acid required copper and was inhibited by either cyanide or diethyldithiocarbamate ion; the reaction was also catalyzed by manganese(II), molybdate and fluoride ion, but not by cobalt(II), iron(II), magnesium, zinc or iodide ions. Rosenberg (1956) studied the reaction of B_{12} with ascorbate at pH 4.7 and 76.6° and showed that the reaction was catalyzed by copper(II) ions and required either ascorbic acid (AA) or dehydroascorbic acid (DA) (II), but did not require the presence of oxygen. Approximately one mol of B_{12} was decomposed for each mol of $CuSO_4$ added; but if the copper and AA or DA were heated together for some time before the addition of B_{12}, the amount of B_{12} decomposed was decreased. It would be interesting to identify the active intermediate in this reaction. It is obviously different from the active intermediate in the reaction of B_{12r} with O_2 or H_2O_2, but the need for copper(II) ions suggests that a free radical may be involved, which could be the common denominator in the two reactions. B_{12} is also attacked by α-tocopherol, but no details of this reaction have been given (Macek and Feller, 1952).

Thiolate anions (RS^-) and HS^- can both co-ordinate to the cobalt(III) ion (see Chapter 8, Section IV) and reduce it to the cobalt(II) state (see Chapter 11, Section IV). But several other reactions have been observed, whose nature is not yet known. Kaczka et al. (1951) found that the reaction of H_2S with a solution of B_{12} in ethanol containing a drop of ammonium hydroxide gave a red, crystalline sulphur-containing product, whose spectrum was very similar to that of aquocobalamin (i.e. sulphur probably not present in the ligand) and which contained sulphur in a form which did not give a positive test for sulphide, sulphite or sulphate. Frost et al. (1952) reported that B_{12a} was destroyed by various thiols such as thioglycollic acid, cysteine, thiomalic acid and thiosorbitol as well as by ascorbic acid. Thiosorbitol approached ascorbic acid in the speed and completeness with which it attacked B_{12a}. B_{12} was destroyed much more slowly and the destruction of B_{12a} was inhibited by the addition of sulphite. No information was reported on the spectra of the products. Aronovitch and Grossowicz (1962) reported that the reaction of aquocobalamin or cyanoaquocobinamide with homocysteine or mercaptoethanol gave a yellow product with an absorption maximum at about 475 nm (see Fig. 2 of the paper by Aronovitch and Grossowicz). But, in contrast to B_{12r} which has a similar spectrum, "no reversion to the original spectrum occurred upon aeration, addition of hydrogen peroxide, or cyanide" and, in contrast to the organocobinamides, the compound was also stable to air and light. They suggested that the reaction might involve either a reduction of the cobalt together with co-ordination of the thiol or rupture of the conjugated chain. Peel (1963) made similar observations. At pH 11 thioglycollic acid reduces B_{12}, B_{12a} and cyanoaquocobinamide to the cobalt(II) complex, which can be reoxidized by air. But in neutral solution thioglycollate reacts with B_{12a} first to give a violet solution (presumably the thiolatocobalamin), which then turns yellow-brown. The yellow solution was stable to air and the first absorption maximum in the spectrum (see Fig. 6 of Peel's paper) occurred at about 490 nm. Further changes were also observed after an hour. H_2S behaves similarly to the thiols; in alkaline solution it reduces B_{12a} to B_{12r}, but in more neutral solution it reacts first to give thiolocobalamin, which then rapidly undergoes other reactions of an unknown nature (Firth *et al.*, 1969). There is also indirect evidence that H_2S will irreversibly destroy a heated solution of B_{12} (Sen, 1962). Other reactions, which do not involve simply co-ordination or reduction, have been observed between B_{12a} and thiosulphate (increased absorption around 415 nm) (Pratt, 1964) and selenourea (increased absorption around 430 nm) (Firth *et al.*, 1969). No test has been made for the possible involvement of oxygen in any of the reactions mentioned in this paragraph and there is no evidence for or against the role of free radicals. B_{12} is also destroyed by a mixture of thiamine and nicotinamide, though either alone is harmless; in this case it was shown that the reaction does not require oxygen, but no spectroscopic data were reported on the products (Blitz *et al.*, 1954).

The fact that the formation of these stable yellow corrinoids so often occurs under conditions in which free radicals are likely to be present (H_2O_2, O_2, photolysis, γ-radiolysis, thiols, copper(II) and ascorbic acid) certainly suggests attack on the corrin ring by free radicals. It would be interesting to establish this more conclusively and to elucidate the structure of one of these yellow products by X-ray analysis.

16

REACTIONS OF THE SIDE-CHAINS

Most of the simple reactions of the side-chains of corrinoids can be grouped under the headings of

(1) the conversion of the amide side-chains into carboxylic acids (i.e. hydrolysis), esters, alcohols, substituted amides etc. and
(2) the degradation of the nucleotide side-chain (i.e. hydrolysis) and the incorporation of other nucleotides.

The main aims of this synthetic and degradative organic chemistry have been

(1) to determine the structure of some of the naturally-occurring corrinoids, and
(2) to prepare derivatives in the hope (so far in vain) of finding analogues of B_{12} which are either (i) more active than B_{12} itself in the treatment of pernicious anaemia or (ii) potent antagonists which might offer the possibility of interfering with the metabolism of cancerous cells.

The relevance of this organic chemistry to the co-ordination chemistry of the corrinoids is twofold. Firstly, hydrolysis may occur as a side-reaction under the conditions where one wishes to study equilibria or reactions involving the cobalt atom or the axial ligands (for examples see below). Secondly, these reactions provide corrinoids which open up possibilities for the further study of the co-ordination chemistry, e.g. through the incorporation of various heterocyclic bases into the nucleotide side-chain (see Chapter 8, Section IV,F) or through the presence of hydrophobic side-chains which enable experiments to be carried out in aprotic solvents (for examples see below). Only the major features of the hydrolysis of the side-chains will be outlined here; for further information on the reactions of the side-chains see the reviews by Bonnett (1963), Bernhauer, Müller and Wagner (1963) and Smith (1965). Before discussing these reactions, however, it is worth emphasizing the inertness of corrinoids under certain conditions; sterile solutions of B_{12} at pH 4.5–5, for example, showed no significant change when stored at room temperature for periods of over two years (Macek and Feller, 1952).

The amide side-chains a–e and g can be hydrolyzed to carboxylic acids by the action of either acid or alkali. Under the conditions normally used the nucleotide side-chain is also hydrolyzed, but more slowly, so that corrinoids with fewer carboxylic acid groups usually retain the nucleotide side-chain. Complete hydrolysis removes the nucleotide and aminopropanol to give the heptacarboxylic acid. Mixtures of corrinoids, which differ in the number of carboxylic acid groups, are usually obtained, from which one can isolate the individual members. There are interesting differences in the rates of hydrolysis of the various amides. The same range of products is obtained from hydrolysis in mild acid or cold dilute alkali.

When B_{12} is hydrolyzed in hot concentrated alkali in the presence of air, however, the first product is the "lactam", in which a lactam ring has been fused onto ring B by the elimination of the hydrogen atom at C_8 and one of the hydrogen atoms on the amide of side-chain c (see Fig. 2.1). Further hydrolysis leads to the formation of an analogous series of carboxylic acids. The first stage in the formation of the lactam ring is a process of "self-reduction" in which the cobalt ion is reduced; this reaction is discussed in more detail in Chapter 11, Section II.

Under mildly acid conditions the aminopropanol and nucleotide side-chain is usually hydrolyzed more slowly than the amides. But under more vigorous conditions (e.g. concentrated HCl at 65° for 5 minutes) the nucleotide side-chain can be split off with little or no hydrolysis of the amides to give Factor B (or cyanoaquocobinamide). Cerium(III) hydroxide can also be used as a catalyst for the hydrolysis of both phosphate ester linkages in neutral solution. Some of the reactions of the nucleotide side-chain in acid are discussed in Chapter 13, Section II,B in connection with the rupture of the Co—C bond of the coenzymes by acid.

Certain cobalt(III) complexes are known to catalyze the hydrolysis of amides, peptides and amino-acid esters, and also the condensation of amino-acid esters to form peptide bonds (see Buckingham *et al.* (1967), Collman and Buckingham (1963), Kimura *et al.* (1970) and references therein). It would be interesting to test whether the cobalt ion in the corrinoids also catalyzes the hydrolysis of amides and peptides, in particular of the amide side-chains.

As examples of synthetic work one might mention the conversion of carboxylic acid groups of the side-chains into amides, substituted amides, esters and alcohols and the incorporation of different heterocyclic bases into the nucleotide side-chain. Some of these derivatives are of interest to coordination chemistry insofar as they allow equilibria and reactions to be observed in non-aqueous solutions. One can, for example, show that cobalt-(III) corrinoids will react with methyl magnesium iodide or lithium alkyls to give organo-cobalt(III) corrinoids by using dicyano-[cobyrinic acid heptaethyl ester] which is soluble in ether-tetrahydrofuran (Wagner and Bernhauer, 1964). And solutions of [cobyrinic acid heptamethyl ester]-cobalt(II) in benzene, but not in methanol or ethanol, will react with iodide ion to give a dimeric iodide-bridged cobalt(II) corrinoid (Werthemann, 1968) (see also Chapter 7, Section IV).

17

ENZYMATIC REACTIONS

About a dozen enzymatic reactions are now known which require corrinoids. There is every reason to suppose that others remain to be discovered. The known reactions can be classified into:

(1) reactions which involve the transfer of a methyl group and do not require 5-deoxyadenosylcorrinoids and

(2) reactions which require 5-deoxyadenosylcorrinoids and which appear to involve a hydride transfer.

None of the mechanisms of any of these reactions have yet been elucidated, though there is evidence that a $Co—CH_3$ bond is formed during the methyl transfer reactions and that the cobalt–carbon bond of the 5-deoxyadenosyl-corrinoids is broken during the reactions of the latter. These reactions will clearly become of increasing interest to organometallic chemistry as more mechanistic details are established.

In all these enzymatic reactions the corrinoids act in association with a protein. This is an example of a pattern frequently observed in enzymatic reactions. A large number of enzymes consist of a protein (called the apo-enzyme) and a smaller molecule (co-factor, coenzyme or prosthetic group), which together form the enzyme or holoenzyme. As a general rule, it is the co-factor which contains the active site(s) which determine the general types of reaction which the enzyme can catalyze, while the protein governs the specificity of the reaction and enhances the rate. All the enzymes which contain 5-deoxyadenosylcorrinoids as the co-factor, for example, appear to catalyze some type of hydride transfer reaction, but each protein confers its own specificity.

As mentioned in Chapter 2, Section III, the word "coenzyme" when used in the B_{12} field refers to 5-deoxyadenosylcorrinoids (DBC, AC, etc.). This has historical reasons but may appear somewhat confusing and illogical now, since other corrinoids may also act as coenzymes in the methyl transfer reactions; and there are, of course, many coenzymes which are not corrinoids!

Our knowledge of the enzymatic reactions is increasing rapidly, but nothing conclusive can yet be said about the co-ordination chemistry involved in the reactions. Since the situation may change rapidly and radically, it seems unnecessary to provide more than a brief summary of our present state of knowledge. Except where other references are given, all the information has been taken from the reviews by Barker (1967) and Hogenkamp (1968).

(1) Methyl transfer reactions

The known examples of these reactions are listed in Table 17.1. They do not require corrinoids in the so-called "coenzyme" form, i.e. a 5-deoxyadenosyl-

Table 17.1 *Methyl transfer reactions*

Substrates		Product
From	To	
N^5-Methyltetrahydrofolic acid (I) ⎫ Methylcobalamin^a ⎬	Homocysteine (IIa)	Methionine (IIb)
N^5-Methyltetrahydrofolic acid (I) ⎫ Various methylcorrinoids^a ⎬ CH_3OH ⎭	Various reducing agents	CH_4*
CH_3OH	$B_{12s}{}^a$	Methyl- cobalamin^{a,}*
N^5-Methyltetrahydrofolic acid (I) ⎫ Methylcobalamin^a ⎬	CO_2	CH_3COOH

^{a} Free methylcorrinoids, i.e. not bound to the apoenzyme; these are not, of course, natural substrates.
* These reactions require ATP.

(I) N^5-Methyltetrahydrofolic acid. The transferable methyl group is circled.

$$R.S.CH_2.CH_2.CHNH_2.COOH$$

(IIa) Homocysteine (R = H)
(IIb) Methionine (R = CH₃)

corrinoid. The reactions probably proceed through the intermediate formation of a methylcorrinoid. The corrinoids are all very tightly bound to the protein, which makes their study more difficult than in the case of the enzymes mentioned under (2); they probably include cobalamin, cobyric acid, 5-hydroxy- and 5-methoxybenzimidazolylcobamide derivatives. Many of the reactions listed in the Table require other co-factors (or co-catalysts). Those marked with an asterisk require adenosine triphosphate, whose function in most enzymatic reactions is to provide a source of energy to drive endothermic (or rather "endergonic") reactions. All the reactions listed in the Table were discovered in bacteria; the formation of methionine has also been shown to occur in extracts from mammalian and avian liver. Methionine and other methylthioethers ($RSCH_3$) may also be formed by non-enzymatic reactions between thiols (RSH) and methylcorrinoids (see Chapter 13, Section II,D).

(2) Reactions catalyzed by coenzymes

The so-called "isomerase" reactions are listed in Table 17.2. These reactions involve the interchange of a hydrogen atom and a larger group between two adjacent carbon atoms, as shown in the diagram attached to the Table. They require a corrinoid in the coenzyme form, i.e. a 5-deoxyadenosyl corrinoid, but in many cases different coenzymes can function with the same protein. It seems that the coenzymes are much less tightly bound to the protein in the isomerase reactions than in the methyl transfer reactions and it is consequently easier to study the mechanism of these reactions. All these reactions have been observed in bacterial extracts; methylmalonyl coenzyme A isomerase has also been observed with extracts of mammalian liver.

Tracer experiments have shown (in all reactions so far studied) that there is no incorporation of hydrogen from the solvent during the isomerase reaction, but that there is exchange of hydrogen atoms between the substrate and the C_5'-atom of the organo-ligand (i.e. the hydrogen atoms on the carbon atom which is normally co-ordinated to the cobalt) and that all the hydrogen atoms on this carbon atom become equivalent during the reaction. Other labelling experiments have demonstrated the transfer of the whole group R_2 in reactions 1, 2, 6 and 7 and have provided further information on the stereochemistry of these particular reactions.

A slightly different type of reaction involves the reduction of ribonucleoside triphosphates to 2'-deoxyribonucleoside triphosphates by various dithiols which are capable of intramolecular cyclization on oxidation (dihydrolipoate, dithioerythritol and dithiothreitol). The HO at the C_2' position of the ribose of the nucleoside is replaced by H with retention of configuration and the hydrogen atom is in this case derived from the solvent; exchange between the solvent, the hydrogen atom of the deoxyribose and the hydrogen atoms on the C_5' atom of the organo-ligand is, in fact, catalyzed by the enzyme in the presence of the dithiols obviously because the sulphur-bound hydrogen atoms exchange readily with water.

The most commonly discussed type of mechanism for these isomerase reactions involves the removal of a hydride ion from the substrate to leave a

Table 17.2. *"Isomerase" reactions requiring 5-deoxyadenosylcorrinoids*

Substrate	R_1	R_2	R_3	Product
Irreversible reactions				
Ethane-1,2-diol	H	OH	OH	Acetaldehyde
Propane-1,2-diol	CH_3	OH	OH	Propionaldehyde
Glycerol	$HOCH_2$	OH	OH	β-Hydroxypropionaldehyde
Ethanolamine	H	NH_2	OH	Acetaldehyde + NH_3
3,6-Diaminohexanoate	H	NH_2	—CH_2.$CHNH_2$.CH_2.COOH	3,5-Diaminohexanoate
Reversible reactions				
L-Glutamate	H	—$CHNH_2$.COOH	COOH	*Threo*-β-Methylaspartate
Succinyl-coenzyme A	H	—CO.SR	COOH	L-Methylmalonylcoenzyme A

$$R_1-\underset{\underset{H}{|}}{\overset{\overset{(R_2)(H)}{|}}{C}}-\underset{\underset{H}{|}}{\overset{\overset{H}{|}}{C}}-R_3 \ \rightleftharpoons \ R_1-\underset{\underset{H}{|}}{\overset{\overset{(H)(R_2)}{|}}{C}}-\underset{\underset{H}{|}}{\overset{\overset{H}{|}}{C}}-R_3$$

carbonium, oxonium or other electron-deficient ion, which undergoes re-arrangement and then picks up the hydride ion again, e.g.

$$
\begin{array}{ccccccc}
\text{OH} & & \text{OH} & & \text{OH} & & \\
| & & | & & | & & \\
\text{H--C--H} & \xrightarrow{-\text{H}^-} & \text{H--C} \overset{+}{\underset{\text{OH}}{\diagdown}} & \xrightarrow{+\text{H}^-} & \text{H--C--OH} & \xrightarrow{-\text{H}_2\text{O}} & \text{HC=O} \\
| & & | & & | & & | \\
\text{H--C--OH} & & \text{H--C} & & \text{H--C--H} & & \text{H--C--H} \\
| & & | & & | & & | \\
\text{R} & & \text{R} & & \text{R} & & \text{R}
\end{array}
$$

There is, however, evidence from u.v.-visible and e.s.r. spectroscopy that cobalt(II) corrinoids and perhaps organic radicals are formed during the steady-state of certain reactions catalyzed by DBC (Babior, 1969; Foster *et al.*, 1970; Hamilton and Blakley, 1969) and it is probably unwise to speculate too much on the mechanism as yet.

One last reaction should be mentioned—the methylation of mercury to give the very toxic dimethylmercury and methylmercury compounds. Research stimulated by incidences of poisoning by methylmercury compounds in Japan and Sweden showed that mercury was probably methylated by anaerobic bacteria and there is some suggestion that this may occur by a corrinoid-dependent methyl transfer reaction (Wood *et al.*, 1968b). Wood, Kennedy and Rosen (1968b) were able to show that methyl- and propyl-cobalamin reacted with mercury(II) ions in the presence of zinc dust to give both mono- and di-alkylated mercury; the mercury(II) ions would, however, presumably be reduced to mercury metal under these conditions, so that the reaction might in fact involve attack on the alkylcobalamin by mercury(O). It was subsequently shown at Oxford that mercury(II) ions in the absence of reducing agents will react rapidly with methylcorrinoids to give methylmercury compounds (Hill *et al.*, 1970a). More work will presumably be carried out on this rather sinister and topical reaction related to mercury pollution.

18

SUMMARY

In this final chapter we shall highlight some of the developments in the inorganic chemistry of B_{12}, which are of interest to co-ordination chemists in general.

The study of cobalt corrinoids (and of other cobalt complexes synthesized as models for the corrinoids) has, first of all, upset some of our more cherished prejudices: for example,

(1) that cobalt(III) complexes are kinetically inert (the corrinoids are not—see Chapter 12),

(2) that a compound containing a bond between a transition metal and an alkyl group is extremely unstable (the methylcorrinoids, for example, are remarkably stable towards acid, alkali and heat, though very sensitive to light; see Chapter 13, Section II and Chapter 14, Section III),

(3) that cobalt(III) complexes are six-co-ordinate (but the organo-cobalt-(III) complexes tend to be five-co-ordinate—see Chapter 8, Section III) and

(4) that the effect of changing the ligands upon the properties of the complex can be correlated with crystal field effects (if we exclude the effects of ligands upon the spectroscopic and magnetic properties of the cobalt ion, then no crystal field effects can be detected—see Chapter 6, Section III; Chapter 8, Section V; Chapter 12, Section II and below).

There are also two areas in which sufficient experimental data has been accumulated to make a more positive contribution to our knowledge and understanding of co-ordination chemistry in general:

(1) the chemistry of organo-metallic complexes containing σ-bonded organo-ligands (in contrast to the more commonly studied π-bonded ligands such as CO, olefins, cyclopentadienyl etc.) and

(2) cis- and trans-effects (the effect of changing one ligand upon the properties of the other ligands). These two areas are discussed in more detail below. One can also foresee other areas of co-ordination chemistry in which the cobalt corrinoids may make a substantial contribution, such as

(3) the photochemistry of metal complexes, initiated by internal transitions of the ligand (see Chapter 14) and

(4) the formation of metal-O_2 complexes and the mechanism of catalyzed autoxidations (see Chapter 6, Section III and Chapter 11, Sections V and VI).

The organocorrinoids are diamagnetic and can, for the sake of convenience, be considered as complexes of cobalt(III) with a co-ordinated carbanion. They almost certainly include a greater variety of σ-bonded carbanions (see, for example, Table 13.3) than any other comparable group of organometallic complexes and they include, of course, the first known naturally occurring organometallic complexes (corrinoids with the ligands 5-deoxyadenosyl, methyl and possibly carboxymethyl). They have probably also furnished the largest amount of information on the making and breaking of the metal-carbon bond and on the influence of the carbanion on the properties of the rest of the complex. This has provided a stimulus for similar work on other non-corrinoid organo-cobalt(III) complexes.

The cobalt–carbon bond in the organocorrinoids can be made and can be broken by reactions in which the transition state may correspond to

(1) Co(III) and R^- (carbanion),
(2) Co(II) and $R\cdot$ (radical) or
(3) Co(I) and R^+ (carbonium ion).

The co-ordinated organo-ligand R may also be reversibly or irreversibly modified to R'. These reaction types can be shown schematically as follows:

$$Co{-}R'$$

$$Co^I + R^+ \rightleftharpoons Co{-}R \rightleftharpoons Co^{III} + R^-$$

$$Co^{II} + R\cdot$$

Some examples of these reactions (only one axial ligand given) are:

$$Co^{III}X^- + CH_3MgBr \rightarrow Co{-}CH_3 + MgBrX$$
$$Co^I + CH_3I \rightarrow Co{-}CH_3 + I^-$$
$$Co{-}CH_3 + Hg^{2-} + H_2O \rightarrow Co^{III}OH_2 + CH_3Hg^+$$
$$Co{-}CO.CH_3 + HO^- \rightarrow Co^I + CH_3COOH$$
$$Co{-}C{\equiv}CH + H_2O \xrightarrow{H^+} Co{-}CO.CH_3$$
$$Co{-}CH_3 \underset{\longleftarrow}{\overset{\text{heat or light}}{\rightleftharpoons}} Co^{II} + CH_3.$$

It has been shown that the cobalt(I) corrinoid is one of the most powerful nucleophiles known (e.g. in reactions with alkyl halides) and that the course and rate of reaction of the Co—C bond depends on a variety of factors such as the nature of the attacking agent, the organoligand and its substituents and the ligand in the *trans*-position. These (thermal) reactions are described in Chapter 13. Most organocorrinoids are very sensitive to light and the initial step in photolysis gives the cobalt(II) ion and a radical R (see Chapter 14).

Work on the organocorrinoids has demonstrated the tremendous influence of the cobalt ion (and other ligands) on the structure and properties of the organo-ligand and vice versa. The Co—CH_2—C bond-angle in DBC, for example, is ~125°C, even though the co-ordinated carbon atom is "tetrahedral"; co-ordination to the cobalt(III) ion has caused considerable rehybridization of the usual sp^3-hybridized orbitals (see Chapter 6, Section I). And if an axial ligand such as H_2O is replaced by methyl or ethyl, this has a dramatic effect on the properties and equilibria of ligands in the other axial position; the formation constant for the substitution of H_2O by CN^-, for example, is reduced by a factor of greater than 10^{12} (see Table 8.8). This example leads us onto a fuller discussion of the interaction between ligands.

The effects of one ligand upon the properties of the other ligands in the *cis*- and *trans*-positions are termed *cis*- and *trans*-effects respectively. Experimentally one studies the effect of replacing one ligand by another on the properties of the other ligands and one can then place the ligands being changed in an order of *cis*- or *trans*-effect. One can study the effect of changing the ligand on

(1) the physical properties (bond-lengths, bond-angles, stretching force constants etc.) of the other ligands, i.e. "ground-state effects",

(2) the equilibrium constants for the addition, loss or substitution of another ligand, i.e. "thermodynamic effects" and

(3) the rates of these reactions, i.e. "kinetic effects".

For further background information see Pratt and Thorp (1969). The cobalt-(III) corrinoids have provided a fairly comprehensive and self-consistent set of data, which enables us to follow the effects of a given ligand on several different properties. The most important results can be summarized as follows. The main series of axial ligands which have been studied are H_2O, Bzm, HO^-, CN^-, $HC\equiv C^-$, $CH_2\equiv CH^-$, CH_3^- and $CH_3CH_2^-$. There is an excellent correlation between the effect of these ligands on the stretching frequency of CN^- co-ordinated in the *trans*-position (i.e. ground-state *trans*-effect), the energy of the π–π transition of the corrin ring (which can be considered as a ground-state *cis*-effect) and the equilibrium constant for the substitution of Bzm or H_2O by CN^- (thermodynamic *trans*-effect); these correlations are shown graphically in Figs 5.2 and 8.3. Other ligands can be placed in order in the series using data from the u.v.-visible spectra (see Chapter 5, Section I) and other quantitative and qualitative equilibrium constants (see Chapter 8, Sections IV and V). It is found that, in general, ligands with the more electronegative donor atoms (N, O, Cl, Br and C in CN^-) exert a "weak" cis- and trans-effect, and those with the less electronegative donor atoms (S, Se, I and C in the organo-ligands) a "strong" effect, whilst among carbanions we find the order cyanide < ethinyl < vinyl < methyl < ethyl. Replacing a "weak" ligand by a "strong" ligand means, for example, an increase in the other cobalt-ligand bond-lengths, a change in the properties of the ligands such that they approximate more to those of the free ligands, a decrease in the formation constants for the substitution of co-ordinated H_2O by more polarizable ligands and an increase in the rate of ligand substitution reactions. These orders indicate that the most important property of the ligand which determines its influence on the rest of the complex is the amount of negative charge donated to the cobalt ion via the σ-bond, i.e. its σ-donor strength. This shows a correlation with the position of the ligand in the nephelauxetic, but not the spectrochemical, series (see Chapter 5, Section I). These experimental data provide the first real test of the importance of crystal field effects in determining the chemical properties of the complex, as distinct from the physical (spectroscopic and magnetic) properties of the metal ion; the crystal field effects are not detectable.

A similar order of ligands is suggested by the more limited evidence on the effect of changing the axial ligand on the Co—N bond-lengths in the cis- and trans-positions in the cobalamins (see Chapter 6, Section III), the proton magnetic resonance of the C_{10}—H in the corrin ring (Chapter 6, Section III), the equilibrium constant for the removal of co-ordinated H_2O to give the five-co-ordinate complex (Chapter 8, Section III), the equilibrium constants for the substitution of H_2O by various other ligands (Chapter 8, Sections IV and V), the rates of ligand substitution (Chapter 12, Section II), the position of attack on the corrin ring (C_8 or C_{10}) by electrophilic reagents (Chapter 15, Section I) and even, rather surprisingly, the polarographic half-wave potentials (Chapter 7, Section VI), the course of photolysis (i.e. photoaquation or photoreduction; Chapter 14, Section II) and the cobalt coupling constant in the electron spin resonance spectra of the cobalt(II) corrinoids and their adducts with O_2 (Chapter 6, Section III). It is surprising that changes in so many different physical and chemical properties show a positive correlation.

Other cobalt(III) complexes appear to show a similar pattern of cis- and trans-effects (Pratt and Thorp, 1969), with the interesting exception that both the corrin and porphyrin ligands have a tremendous labilizing or kinetic cis-effect (Chapter 12, Section II).

As was explained in Chapter 1, Section I, the recent and rapid development in our knowledge of the co-ordination chemistry of the cobalt corrinoids, in particular of the two areas of organometallic chemistry and *cis-* and *trans*-effects, can be traced back to the work of the biochemists, X-ray crystallographers and organic chemists in isolating the B_{12} coenzyme (DBC), establishing the presence of the cobalt–carbon bond and synthesizing organo-cobalt corrinoids. It is to be hoped that work on the co-ordination chemistry may in turn help in unravelling the mechanism of the enzymatic reactions of the corrinoids and in understanding the nature of the subtle interactions between the ligands, not only in the cobalt corrinoids but in other biochemically important metal complexes such as the iron porphyrins.

APPENDIX

The main text covers the literature up to the end of 1969, together with a few more recently published papers. References are given here to several additional papers published before September 1971, which provide substantial or significant new material. The subject matter is arranged under the same section headings as in the main text.

1.I. Eschenmoser (1970) has reviewed the work of his group on the synthesis of corrinoids up to the end of 1969.

5.III. The recently determined structure of "neo-vitamin B_{12}" or "cyano-13-epicobalamin" shows that it differs from B_{12} in that epimerization has occurred at C_{13} in ring C (i.e. the propionamide side-chain now projects upwards), accompanied by a change in the direction of the slope of the $C_{12}-C_{13}$ bond relative to the plane of the corrin ring; the CD spectra of B_{12} and neo-B_{12} show considerable differences, especially below 400 nm (Bonnett *et al.*, 1971).

6.I. Complete details of the X-ray analysis of cyano-[cobalamin-5'-phosphate] or "vitamin B_{12}-5' phosphate" (Hawkinson *et al.*, 1970) and cyanoaquo-[cobyric acid] or "Factor V_{1a}" (Venkatesan *et al.*, 1971) have been given and a diagram of the structure of the metal-free 1,2,2,7,7,12,12-heptamethyl-15-cyano-corrinium bromide is given on p. 390 of Eschenmoser (1970). The structure of the so-called "iso-corrinoids" or "neo-corrinoids", which are in equilibrium with the usual form of the corrinoids in strong acid, has now been established by an X-ray analysis of "neo-vitamin B_{12}" or "cyano-13-epicobalamin", which is derived from B_{12} by epimerization at C_{13} in ring C (Bonnett *et al.*, 1971). The rapidly established equilibria ($t_{1/2} \gtrsim 20$ μsec) detected by temperature jump studies have now been observed with cobalamins containing the ligands H_2O, HO^-, N_3^-, NCS^-, SO_3^{2-} and $S_2O_3^{2-}$ (Thusius, 1971).

6.II. Thermodynamic data have been reported for the binding of B_{12} by three proteins, viz. intrinsic factor ($K = 6 \times 10^9$ M^{-1}), and transcobalamins I and II ($K \sim 3 \times 10^{11}$ M^{-1}) (Hippe and Olesen, 1971).

6.III. Brodie and Poe (1971) have studied the n.m.r. spectra of various cobalt-(III), Co(II) and Co(I) corrinoids and Bayston *et al.* (1970) have reported the e.s.r. spectra and coupling constants of additional cobalt(II) corrinoids. The n.m.r. spectrum of the coenzyme DBC has also been reported (Cockle *et al.*, 1970b).

7.III. For further e.s.r. studies of the co-ordination of axial ligands by cobalamin- and cobinamide-cobalt(II) see Bayston *et al.* (1970). The n.m.r.

spectra of certain cobalt(II) corrinoids have also been reported (Brodie and Poe, 1971).

7.V. A n.m.r. method has been used to show that B_{12s} is diamagnetic (Brodie and Poe, 1971). Schrauzer and Holland (1971) have found that the reduction of B_{12a} by zinc dust in anhydrous glacial acetic acid gives a green complex, which differs from B_{12s} in its absorption spectrum and reactions (e.g. it reacts with ethylene to form ethylcobalamin) and suggest that it may be hydridocobalamin.

7.VI. For further values of polarographic half-wave potentials see Hogenkamp and Holmes (1970).

9.I. The metal-free 1,2,2,7,7,12,12-heptamethyl-15-cyano-corrinium bromide has been studied by X-ray analysis and the structure shown in a diagram on p. 390 of Eschenmoser (1970).

11.VI. B_{12} will catalyze the reduction of the $-CCl_2-$ group by borohydride to $-CHCl-$ in compounds such as aldrin, isodrin, dieldrin and endrin (Bieniek et al., 1970). B_{12a} will catalyze the reduction of nitro-, nitroso- and azoxy-benzene by borohydride (Brearley et al., 1971).

12.II. Thusius (1971) has studied the kinetics of the forward and reverse reactions between B_{12a} and Br^-, I^-, N_3^-, NCO^-, NCS^-, SO_3^{2-} and $S_2O_3^{2-}$ and reported rate constants and activation enthalpies and entropies. He has shown that there is a linear correlation between the equilibrium constants for the substitution of co-ordinated H_2O by monobasic anions (Z) and the rate constants for the substitution of co-ordinated Z by H_2O and has concluded that ligand substitution proceeds by a limiting S_{N1} mechanism.

13.I. The Co–C bond can also be formed by the transfer of a carbanion from another organocobalt complex to the cobalt(III) corrinoid; methylcobalamin is formed in the reaction between B_{12a} and $[Me_2Co\{(DOH)(DO)pn\}]$ Costa et al., 1971).

13.II. β-Hydroxyethyl-cobalamin and cobinamide are decomposed by alkali to give acetaldehyde; 5-deoxyadenosylcobalamin (DBC) is also decomposed by strong alkali, but the product has not been identified (Schrauzer and Sibert, 1970). The methyl ligand of methylcobalamin can be removed by reaction with Tl(III), with a mixture of $PtCl_4^{2-}$ and $PtCl_6^{2-}$ or with a mixture of $AuCl_2^-$ and $AuCl_4^-$, but not with Cd(II), Pb(II) or In(III); the product is usually methyl chloride (Agnes et al., 1971a). The reaction of methylcobalamin with thioglycollic acid to give the methyl thioether has been shown to require O_2 and does not therefore proceed by the transfer of a methyl cation from the cobalt to a thiolate anion (Agnes et al., 1971b). Fukui and co-workers find that acetylcobinamide decomposes faster ($t_{1/2} = 4$ min) than acetylcobalamin ($t_{1/2} = 30$ min) in 0.05 N KOH, i.e. heterolytic fission of the Co–C bond to give the Co(I) complex is retarded by the presence of Bzm (Fukui et al., 1969).

REFERENCES

Ablov, A. V. and Palade, D. M. (1962). *Doklady Akad. Nauk. SSSR* **144**, 341.
Ablov, A. V. and Sychev, A. Y. (1959). *Russ. J. Inorg. Chem.* **4**, 1143.
Adamson, A. W. (1968). *Co-ord. Chem. Revs.* **3**, 169.
Adamson, A. W., Chiang, A. and Zinato, E. (1969). *J. Amer. Chem. Soc.* **91**, 5467.
Adler, N., Medwick, T. and Poznanski, T. J. (1966). *J. Amer. Chem. Soc.* **88**, 5018.
Agnes, G., Bendle, S., Hill, H. A. O., Williams, F. R. and Williams, R. J. P. (1971a). *Chem. Comm.* 850.
Agnes, G., Hill, H. A. O., Pratt, J. M., Ridsdale, S. C., Kennedy, F. S. and Williams, R. J. P. (1971b). *Biochim. Biophys. Acta*, **242**, 207.
Ahrland, S., Chatt, J. and Davies, N. R. (1958). *Quart Rev*, **12**, 265.
Albert, A. (1959). "Heterocyclic Chemistry", p. 143. Athlone Press, University of London.
Alicino, J. F. (1951). *J. Amer. Chem. Soc.* **73**, 4051.
Appleby, C. A. (1969). *Biochim. Biophys. Acta.* **172**, 88.
Aronovitch, J. and Grossowicz, N. (1962). *Biochem. Biophys. Res. Comm.* **8**, 416.
Ašperger, S. and Ingold, C. K. (1956). *J. Chem. Soc.* 2862.
Babior, B. M. (1969). *Biochim. Biophys. Acta* **178**, 406.
Babior, B. M. and Li, T. K. (1969). *Biochemistry* **8**, 154.
Babior, B. M., Kon, H. and Lecar, H. (1969). *Biochemistry* **8**, 2662.
Baldwin, M. E., Chan, S. C. and Tobe, M. L. (1961). *J. Chem. Soc.* 4637.
Balzani, V., Moggi, L., Scandola, F. and Carassiti, V. (1967). *Inorg. Chim. Acta Revs.* **1**, 7.
Banks, R. G. S. and Pratt, J. M. (1968). *J. Chem. Soc.* (*A*), 854.
Banks, R. G. S., Henderson, R. J. and Pratt, J. M. (1968). *J. Chem. Soc.* (*A*), 2886.
Barca, R., Ellis, J., Tsao, M. and Wilmarth, W. K. (1967). *Inorg. Chem.* **6**, 243.
Barker, H. A. (1962). *In* Proceedings of the 2nd European Symposium on Vitamin B_{12} and Intrinsic Factor, Hamburg, 1961, p. 82 (edited by H. C. Heinrich) Ferdinand Enke Verlag, Stuttgart, W. Germany.
Barker, H. A. (1967). *Biochem. J.* **105**, 1.
Barker, H. A., Weissbach, H. and Smyth, R. D. (1958). *Proc. Nat. Acad. Sci.* **44**, 1093.
Barker, H. A., Smyth, R. D., Weissbach, H., Munch-Petersen, A., Toohey, J. I., Ladd, J. N., Volcani, B. E. and Wilson, R. M. (1960a). *J. Biol. Chem.* **235**, 181.
Barker, H. A., Smyth, R. D., Weissbach, H., Toohey, J. I., Ladd, J. N. and Volcani, B. E. (1960b). *J Biol. Chem.* **235**, 480.
Barnett, R., Hogenkamp, H. P. C. and Abeles, R. H. (1966). *J. Biol. Chem.* **241**, 1483.
Basolo, F. and Pearson, R. G. (1967). "Mechanisms of Inorganic Reactions", 2nd Edn. Wiley, New York.
Bauriedel, W. R. (1956). *Iowa State Coll. J. Sci.* **30**, 321.
Bauriedel, W. R., Picken, J. C. and Underkofler, L. A. (1956). *Proc. Soc. Exptl. Biol. Med.* **91**, 377.
Bayston, J. H. and Winfield, M. E. (1967). *J. Cat.* **9**, 217.

Bayston, J. H., King, N. K., Looney, F. D. and Winfield, M. E. (1969). *J. Amer. Chem. Soc.* **91**, 2775.
Bayston, J. H., Looney, F. D., Pilbrow, J. R. and Winfield, M. E. (1970). *Biochemistry* **9**, 2164.
Beaven, G. H. and Johnson, E. A. (1955). *Nature* **176**, 1264.
Beaven, G. H., Holiday, E. R., Johnson, E. A., Ellis, B., Mamalis, P., Petrow, V. and Sturgeon, B. (1949). *J. Pharm. Pharmacol.* **1**, 957.
Beaven, G. H., Holiday, E. R., Johnson, E. A., Ellis, B. and Petrow, V. (1950). *J. Pharm. Pharmacol.* **2**, 944.
Bell, R. P. (1959). "The Proton in Chemistry", pp. 69–70. Methuen, London.
Bernhauer, K. and Irion, E. (1964a). *Biochem. Zeit.* **339**, 521.
Bernhauer, K. and Irion, E. (1964b). *Biochem. Zeit.* **339**, 530.
Bernhauer, K. and Müller, O. (1961). *Biochem. Zeit.* **334**, 199.
Bernhauer, K. and Müller, O. (1963). *Biochem. Zeit.* **337**, 366.
Bernhauer, K. and Wagner, O. (1963). *Biochem. Zeit.* **337**, 366.
Bernhauer, K., Gaiser, P., Müller, O. and Wagner, O. (1960a). *Biochem. Zeit.* **333**, 106.
Bernhauer, K., Wagner, F., Dellweg, H. and Zeller, P. (1960b). *Helv. Chim. Acta* **43**, 700.
Bernhauer, K., Wagner, F. and Zeller, P. (1960c). *Helv. Chim. Acta* **43**, 696.
Bernhauer, K., Müller, O. and Wagner, O. (1961). *In* Proceedings of the 2nd European Symposium on Vitamin B_{12} and Intrinsic Factor, Hamburg, 1961, p. 110 (edited by H. C. Heinrich). Ferdinand Enke Verlag, Stuttgart, W. Germany.
Bernhauer, K., Müller, O. and Müller, G. (1962a). *Biochem. Zeit.* **336**, 102.
Bernhauer, K., Renz, P. and Wagner, F. (1962b). *Biochem. Zeit.* **335**, 443.
Bernhauer, K., Müller, O. and Wagner, F. (1963). *Angew. Chem.* **75**, 1145.
Bernhauer, K., Müller, O. and Wagner, F. (1964). *Adv. Enzymology* **26**, 233.
Bernhauer, K., Wagner, F., Beisbarth, H., Rietz, P. and Vogelmann, H. (1966). *Biochem. Zeit.* **344**, 289.
Bernhauer, K., Vogelmann, H. and Wagner, F. (1968). *Zeit. Phys. Chem.* **349**, 1281.
Bieniek, D., Moza, P. N., Klein, W. and Korte, F. (1970). *Tetrahedron Letters* 4055.
Blitz, M., Eigen, E. and Gunsberg, E. (1954). *J. Amer. Pharm. Assoc. Sci. Ed.* **43**, 651.
Boehm, G., Faessler, A. and Rittmayer, G. (1954). *Z. Naturforschung* **9b**, 509.
Bonnett, R. (1963). *Chem. Revs.* **63**, 573.
Bonnett, R. and Redman, D. G. (1965). *Proc. Roy. Soc.* **A288**, 342.
Bonnett, R., Cannon, J. R., Clark, V. M., Johnson, A. W., Parker, L. F. J., Smith, E. L. and Todd, A. (1957a). *J. Chem. Soc.* 1158.
Bonnett, R., Cannon, J. R., Johnson, A. W. and Todd, A. (1957b). *J. Chem. Soc.* 1148.
Bonnett, R., Godfrey, J. M., Math, V. B., Edmond, E., Evans, H. and Hodder, O. J. R. (1971). *Nature* **229**, 473.
Boos, R. N., Carr, J. E. and Conn, J. B. (1953). *Science* **117**, 603.
Bormann, D., Fischli, A., Keese, R. and Eschenmoser, A. (1967). *Angew. Chem. (Internat. Ed.)* **6**, 868.
Boxer, G. E. and Rickards, J. C. (1951). *Arch. Biochem.* **30**, 382.
Brady, R. O. and Barker, H. A. (1961). *Biochem. Biophys. Res. Comm.* **4**, 373.
Brearley, A. E., Gott, H., Hill, H. A. O., O'Riordan, M., Pratt, J. M. and Williams, R. J. P. (1971), *J. Chem. Soc. (A)*, 612.
Briat, B. and Djerassi, C. (1968). *Nature* **217**, 918.
Briat, B. and Djerassi, C. (1969). *Bull. Soc. Chim. France*, p. 135.

Brierly, J. M., Ellingboe, J. L. and Diehl, H. (1953). *Iowa State Coll. J. Sci.* 27, 425.
Brierly, J. M., Ellingboe, J. L. and Diehl, H. (1955). *Iowa State Coll. J. Sci.* 30, 269.
Brink, N. G., Wolf, D. E., Kaczka, E., Rickes, E. L., Koniuszy, F. R., Wood,T. R. and Folkers, K. (1949). *J. Amer. Chem. Soc.* 71, 1854.
Brink, C., Hodgkin, D. C., Lindsey, J., Pickworth, J., Robertson, J. H. and White, J. G. (1954). *Nature* 174, 1169.
Brink-Shoemaker, C., Cruikshank, D. W. J., Hodgkin, D. C., Kamper, M. J. and Pilling, D. (1964). *Proc. Roy Soc.* A278, 1.
Brodie, J. D. (1969). *Proc. Nat. Acad. Sci.* 62, 461.
Brodie, J. D. and Poe, M. (1971). *Biochemistry* 10, 914.
Brückner, S., Calligaris, M., Nardin, G. and Randaccio, L. (1968). *Inorg. Chim. Acta* 2, 416.
Brückner, S., Calligaris, M., Nardin, G. and Randaccio, L. (1969). *Inorg. Chim. Acta* 3, 308.
Bücher, T. and Negelein, E. (1941). *Biochem. Zeit.* 311, 163.
Buckingham, D. A., Marzilli, L. G. and Sargeson, A. M. (1967). *J. Amer. Chem. Soc.* 89, 4539.
Buhs, R. P., Newstead, E. G. and Trenner, N. R. (1951). *Science* 113, 625.
Burgus, R. C., Hufham, J. B., Scott, W. M. and Pfiffner, J. J. (1964). *J. Bacteriol.* 88, 1139.
Burgus, R. C., Hufham, J. B., Scott, W. M. and Pfiffner, J. J. (1965). *Arch. Biochem. Biophys.* 110, 490.
Campbell, J. A., McLaughlan, J. M. and Chapman, D. G. (1952). *J. Amer. Pharm. Assoc. Sci. Ed.* 41, 479.
Candlin, J. P., Halpern, J. and Trimm, D. L. (1964). *J. Amer. Chem. Soc.* 86, 1019.
Castor, L. B. and Chance, B. (1959). *J. Biol. Chem.* 234, 1587.
Cavallini, D., Scandurra, R., Barboni, E. and Marcucci, M. (1968a). *F.E.B.S. Letters* 1, 272.
Cavallini, D., Scandurra, R., Barboni, E. and Marcucci, M. (1968b). *Atti Accad. Naz. Lincei, Rend. Sci. fis. mat. e nat.* 45, 390.
Chan, S. C. (1963). *J. Chem. Soc.* 5137.
Chan, S. C. and Miller, J. (1965). *Rev. Pure Appl. Chem.* 15, 11.
Chan, S. C. and Tobe, M. L. (1963a). *J. Chem. Soc.* 966.
Chan, S. C. and Tobe, M. L. (1963b). *J. Chem. Soc.* 5700.
Chance, B. (1953). *J. Biol. Chem.* 202, 397 and 407.
Chen, H. H., Tsao, M., Gaver, R. W., Tewari, P. H. and Wilmarth, W. K. (1966). *Inorg. Chem.* 5, 1913.
Clarke, D. A., Dolphin, D., Grigg, R., Johnson, A. W. and Pinnock, H. A. (1968). *J. Chem. Soc. (C)*, 881.
Clarke, D. A., Grigg, R., Johnson, A. W. and Pinnock, H. A. (1967). *Chem. Comm.* 309.
Coates, G. E. and Wade, K. (1967). "Organometallic Compounds", 3rd edn., Vol. I, p. 175. Methuen, London.
Cockle, S. A., Hill, H. A. O., Pratt, J. M. and Williams, R. J. P. (1969). *Biochem. Biophys. Acta* 177, 686.
Cockle, S. A., Hill, H. A. O. and Williams, R. J. P. (1970a). *Inorg. Nucl. Chem. Letters* 6, 131.
Cockle, S. A., Hill, H. A. O., Williams, R. J. P., Mann, B. E. and Pratt, J. M. (1970b). *Biochim. Biophys. Acta,* 215, 415.
Collat, J. W. and Abbott, J. C. (1964). *J. Amer. Chem. Soc.* 86, 2308.
Collat, J. W. and Tackett, S. L. (1962). *J. Electroanal. Chem.* 4, 59.

Collman, J. P. and Buckingham, D. A. (1963). *J. Amer. Chem. Soc.* **85**, 3039.

Conn, J. B. and Wartman, T. G. (1952). *Science* **115**, 72.

Cooley, G., Ellis, B., Petrow, V., Beaven, G. H., Holiday, E. R. and Johnson, E. A. (1951). *J. Pharm. Pharmacol.* **3**, 271.

Costa, G. and Mestroni, G. (1967). *Tetrahedron Letters* 1781.

Costa, G. and Mestroni, G. (1968). *J. Organometallic Chem.* **11**, 325.

Costa, G., Mestroni, G., Tauzher, G. and Stefani, L. (1966). *J. Organometallic Chem.* **6**, 181.

Costa, G., Mestroni, G. and Stefani, L. (1967). *J. Organometallic Chem.* **7**, 493.

Costa, G., Mestroni, G., Tauzher, G., Goodall, D. M., Green, M. and Hill, H. A. O. (1970). *Chem. Comm.* 34.

Costa, G., Mestroni, G. and Cocevar, C. (1971). *Chem. Comm.* 706.

Das, P. K., Hill, H. A. O., Pratt, J. M. and Williams, R. J. P. (1967). *Biochem. Biophys. Acta* **141**, 644.

Das, P. K., Hill, H. A. O., Pratt, J. M. and Williams, R. J. P. (1968). *J. Chem. Soc. (A)*, 1261.

Davies, M. T., Mamalis, P., Petrow, V. and Sturgeon, B. (1951). *J. Pharm. Pharmacol.* **3**, 420.

Day, P. (1967a). *Co-ord. Chem. Revs.* **2**, 109.

Day, P. (1967b). *Theor. Chim. Acta.* **7**, 328.

Day, P., Hill, H. A. O. and Price, M. G. (1968). *J. Chem. Soc. (A)*, 90.

Diehl, H. and Murie, R. (1952). *Iowa State Coll. J. Sci.* **26**, 555.

Diehl, H. and Sealock, R. R. (1952). *Record Chem. Progress Kresge-Hooker Sci. Lib.* **13**, 10.

Diehl, H., Haar, R. W. V. and Sealock, R. R. (1950a). *J. Amer. Chem. Soc.* **72**, 5312.

Diehl, H., Sealock, R. R. and Morrison, J. (1950b). *Iowa State Coll. J. Sci.* **24**, 433.

Diehl, H., Morrison, J. I. and Sealock, R. R. (1951). *Experientia* **7**, 60.

Dolbear, G. E. and Taube, H. (1967). *Inorg. Chem.* **6**, 60.

Dolphin, D. H. and Johnson, A. W. (1963). *Proc. Chem. Soc.* 311.

Dolphin, D. H. and Johnson, A. W. (1965a). *Chem. Comm.* 494.

Dolphin, D. H. and Johnson, A. W. (1965b). *J. Chem. Soc.* 2174.

Dolphin, D. H., Johnson, A. W., Rodrigo, R. and Shaw, N. (1963a). *Pure Appl. Chem.* **7**, 539.

Dolphin, D. H., Johnson, A. W. and Shaw, N. (1963b). *Nature* **199**, 170.

Dolphin, D. H., Johnson, A. W. and Rodrigo, R. (1964a). *J. Chem. Soc.* 3186.

Dolphin, D. H., Johnson, A. W. and Rodrigo, R. (1964b). *Ann. New York Acad. Sci.* **112**, 590.

Dubnoff, J. W. (1950). *Arch. Biochem.* **27**, 466.

Dubnoff, J. W. (1964). *Biochem. Biophys. Res. Comm.* **16**, 484.

Duggan, D. E., Bowman, R. L., Brodie, B. B. and Udenfriend, S. (1957). *Arch. Biochem. Biophys.* **68**, 1.

Dunitz, J. D. and Meyer, E. F. (1965). *Proc. Roy. Soc.* **A288**, 324.

Eckert, R. and Kuhn, H. (1960). *Z. Elektrochemie* **64**, 356.

Edmond, E., personal communication.

Eichhorn, G. L. (1961). *Tetrahedron* **13**, 208.

Ellenbogen, L. and Highley, D. R. (1963). *Vitamins and Horm.* **21**, 1.

Ellenbogen, L. and Highley, D. R. (1967). *J. Biol. Chem.* **242**, 1004.

Ellingboe, J. L., Morrison, J. I. and Diehl, H. (1955). *Iowa State Coll. J. Sci.* **30**, 263.

Ellis, B., Petrow, V. and Snook, G. F. (1949). *J. Pharm. Pharmacol.* **1**, 60.

Ellis, B., Petrow, V., Beaven G. H. and Holiday, E. R. (1953). *J. Pharm. Pharmacol.* **6**, 60.

Elson, E. L. and Edsall, J. T. (1962). *Biochemistry* **1**, 1.

Ericson, L. E. and Nihlén, H. (1953). *Acta Chem. Scand.* **7**, 980.

Eschenmoser, A. (1963). *Pure Appl. Chem.* **7**, 297.

Eschenmoser, A. (1970). *Quart. Rev.* **24**, 366.

Eschenmoser, A., Scheffold, R., Bertele, E., Pesaro, M. and Gschwend, H. (1965). *Proc. Roy. Soc.* **A288**, 306.

Fantes, K. H., Page, J. E., Parker, L. F. J. and Smith, E. L. (1949). *Proc. Roy. Soc.* **B136**, 592.

Felner, I., Fischli, A., Wick, A., Pesaro, M., Bormann, D., Winnacker, E. L. and Eschenmoser, A. (1967). *Angew. Chem.* (*Internat. Ed.*) **6**, 864.

Firth, R. A., Hill, H. A. O., Pratt, J. M., Williams, R. J. P. and Jackson, W. R. (1967a). *Biochemistry* **6**, 2178.

Firth, R. A., Hill, H. A. O., Mann, B. E., Pratt, J. M. and Thorp, R. G. (1967b). *Chem. Comm.* 1013.

Firth, R. A., Hill, H. A. O., Mann, B. E., Pratt, J. M., Thorp, R. G. and Williams, R. J. P. (1968a). *J. Chem. Soc.* (*A*), 2419.

Firth, R. A., Hill, H. A. O., Pratt, J. M. and Thorp, R. G. (1968b). *Anal. Biochem.* **23**, 429.

Firth, R. A., Hill, H. A. O., Pratt, J. M. and Thorp, R. G. (1968c). *J. Chem. Soc.* (*A*), 453.

Firth, R. A., Hill, H. A. O., Pratt, J. M., Thorp, R. G. and Williams, R. J. P. (1968d). ✔ *J. Chem. Soc.* (*A*), 2428.

Firth, R. A., Hill, H, A. O., Pratt, J. M., Thorp, R. G. and Williams, R. J. P. (1969). *J. Chem. Soc.* (*A*), 381.

Fischli, A. and Eschenmoser, A. (1967). *Angew. Chem.* (*Internat. Ed.*) **6**, 866.

Fleischer, E. B., Jacobs, S. and Mestichelli, L. (1968). *J. Amer. Chem. Soc.* **90**, 2527.

Floriani, C., Puppis, M. and Calderazzo, F. (1968). *J. Organometallic Chem.* **12**, 209.

Folkers, K. and Wolf, D. E. (1954). *Vitamins and Horm.* **12**, 1.

Foster, M. A., Hill, H. A. O., and Williams, R. J. P. (1970). *Biochem. Soc. Symp.* **31**, 187.

Friedrich, W. (1964). *In* "Biochemisches Taschenbuch", 2nd edn., p. 708 (edited by H. M. Rauen). Springer-Verlag, Berlin.

Friedrich, W. (1965). *Biochem. Zeit.* **342**, 143.

Friedrich, W. (1966a). *Z. Naturforsch.* **21b**, 138.

Friedrich, W. (1966b). *Z. Naturforsch.* **21b**, 595.

Friedrich, W. and Bernhauer, K. (1954). *Z. Naturforsch.* **9b**, 755.

Friedrich, W. and Bernhauer, K. (1956). *Chem. Ber.* **89**, 2507.

Friedrich, W. and Bieganowski, R. (1967). *Z. Naturforsch.* **22b**, 741.

Friedrich, W. and Königk, E. (1962). *Biochem. Zeit.* **336**, 444.

Friedrich, W. and Messerschmidt, R. (1969). *Z. Naturforsch.* **24b**, 465.

Friedrich, W. and Moskophidis, M. (1968). *Z. Naturforsch.* **23b**, 804.

Friedrich, W. and Nordmeyer, J. P. (1968). *Z. Naturforsch.* **23b**, 1119.

Friedrich, W. and Nordmeyer, J. P. (1969). *Z. Naturforsch.* **24b**, 588.

Friedrich, W., Heinrich, H. C., Königk, E. and Schulze, P. (1964). *Ann. New York. Acad. Sci.* **112**, 601.

Friedrich, W., Ohlms, H., Sandeck, W. and Bieganowski, R. (1967). *Z. Naturforsch.* **22b**, 839.

Frost, D. V., Lapidus, M., Plant, K. A., Scherfling, E. and Fricke, H. H. (1952). *Science* **116**, 119.

Fukui, S., Shimizu, S., Yamada, R. and Umetani, T. (1969). *Vitamins* **40**, 113.

Gakenheimer, W. C. and Feller, B. A. (1949). *J. Amer. Pharm. Assoc. Sci. Ed.* **38**, 660.

George, P. (1964). *In* "Oxidases and Related Redox Systems", p. 3 (edited by T. E. King, H. S. Mason and M. Morrison). Wiley, New York.

George, P., Irvine, D. H. and Glauser, S. C. (1960). *Ann. New York Acad. Sci.* **88**, 393.

Gibson, Q. H. and Ainsworth, S. (1957). *Nature* **180**, 1416.

Grassi, R., Haim, A. and Wilmarth, W. K. (1967). *Inorg. Chem.* **6**, 237.

Greenberg, S. M., Herndon, J. F., Rice, E. G., Parmelee, E. T., Gulesich, J. J. and van Loon, E. J. (1957). *Nature* **180**, 1401.

Gregory, M. E. and Holdsworth, E. S. (1955). *Biochem. J.* **59**, 335.

Grün, F. and Haas, R. (1956). *Nature* **177**, 378.

Grün, F. and Menasse, R. (1950). *Experientia* **6**, 263.

Guest, J. R., Friedman, S., Woods, D. D. and Smith, E. L. (1962). *Nature* **195**, 340.

Guest, J. R., Friedman, S., Dilworth, M. J. and Woods, D. D. (1964). *Ann. New York Acad. Sci.* **112**, 774.

Gupta, V. S. and Huennekens, F. M. (1964). *Arch. Biochem. Biophys.* **106**, 527.

Hague, D. N. and Halpern, J. (1967). *Inorg. Chem.* **6**, 2059.

Haim, A., Grassi, R. J. and Wilmarth, W. K. (1965). *In* "Mechanisms of Inorganic Reactions" (edited by R. F. Gould). Amer. Chem. Soc., Washington, U.S.A.

Haldane, J. and Smith, J. L. (1896). *J. Physiol.* **20**, 495.

Halpern, J. and Maher, J. P. (1964). *J. Amer. Chem. Soc.* **86**, 2311.

Halpern, J. and Maher, J. P. (1965). *J. Amer. Chem. Soc.* **87**, 5361.

Halpern, J.,Palmer, R. A. and Blakeley, L. M. (1966). *J. Amer. Chem. Soc.* **88**, 2877.

Hamada, S. (1961). *J. Chem. Soc. Japan* **82**, 1327.

Hambly, A. N. (1965). *Revs. Pure Appl. Chem.* **15**, 87.

Hamilton, J. A. and Blakley, R. L. (1969). *Biochim. Biophys. Acta* **184**, 224.

Hanania, G. I. H. and Irvine, D. H. (1964a). *In* Proceedings of the 8th Internat. Conf. Co-ord. Chem., Vienna, p. 418 (edited by V. Gutmann). Springer Verlag, Vienna.

Hanania, G. I. H. and Irvine, D. H. (1964b). *J. Chem. Soc.* 5694.

Hanzlík, J. and Vlček, A. A. (1969). *Chem. Comm.* 47.

Harris, R. L. N., Johnson, A. W. and Kay, I. T. (1966). *Quart. Rev.* **20**, 211.

Havemeyer, R. N. and Higuchi, T. (1960). *J. Amer. Pharm. Assoc. Sci. Ed.* **49**, 356.

Hawkinson, S. W., Coulter, C. L. and Greaves, M. L. (1970). *Proc. Roy. Soc.* **A318**, 143.

Hayward, G. C., Hill, H. A. O., Pratt, J. M., Vanston, N. J. and Williams, R. J. P. (1965). *J. Chem. Soc.* 6485.

Hayward, G. C., Hill, H. A. O., Pratt, J. M. and Williams, R. J. P. (1971). *J. Chem. Soc. (A)*, 196.

Heathcote, J. G. and Mooney, F. S. (1958). *Lancet*, p. 982.

Hedbom, A. (1960). *Biochem. J.* **74**, 307.

Hedbom, A. (1961). *Biochem. J.* **79**, 469.

Helgeland, K., Jonsen, J. and Laland, S. (1959). *Acta Chem. Scand.* **13**, 2128.

Helgeland, K., Jonsen, J. and Laland, S. (1961). *Biochem. J.* **81**, 260.

Highley, D. R., Davies, M. C. and Ellenbogen, L. (1967). *J. Biol. Chem.* **242**, 1010.

Hill, H. A. O., Pratt, J. M. and Williams, R. J. P. (1964). *Chem. Ind.* 197.

Hill, H. A. O., Pratt, J. M. and Williams, R. J. P. (1965a). *Proc. Roy. Soc.* **A288**, 352.

Hill, H. A. O., Pratt, J. M. and Williams, R. J. P. (1965b). *J Chem. Soc.* p. 2859.

Hill, H. A. O., Mann, B. E., Pratt, J. M. and Williams, R. J. P. (1968a). *J. Chem. Soc. (A)*, p. 564.

Hill, H. A. O., Morallee, K. G. Pellizer, G., Mestroni, G. and Costa, G. (1968b). *J. Organometallic Chem.* **11**, 167.

Hill, H. A. O., Pratt, J. M. and Williams, R. J. P. (1969). *Chem. in Britain*, 156.

Hill, H. A. O., Pratt, J. M., Ridsdale, S., Williams, F. R. and Williams, R. J. P. (1970a). *Chem. Comm.* 341.

Hill, H. A. O., Pratt, J. M., Thorp, R. G., Ward, B. and Williams, R. J. P. (1970b). *Biochem. J.* **120**, 263.

Hill, H. A. O., Pratt, J. M. and Williams, R. J. P., unpublished results.

Hill, J. A., Pratt, J. M. and Williams, R. J. P. (1962). *J. Theor. Biol.* **3**, 423.

Hill, J. A., Pratt, J. M. and Williams, R. J. P. (1964). *J. Chem. Soc.* 5149.

Hippe, E. and Olesen, H. (1971). *Biochim. Biophys. Acta* **243**, 83.

Hodgkin, D. C. (1958). *Fortschr. Chem. Org. Naturstoffe* **15**, 167.

Hodgkin, D. C. (1964). *In* "The Law of Mass Action; a Centenary Volume", p. 159 (edited by O. Bastiansen). Det Norske Videnskaps-Akademie, Oslo.

Hodgkin, D. C. (1965). *Proc. Roy. Soc.* **A288**, 294.

Hodgkin, D. C. (1967). *Harvey Lectures* **61**, 205.

Hodgkin, D. C., personal communication.

Hodgkin, D. C., Kamper, J., Lindsey, J., McKay, M., Pickworth, J., Robertson, J. H., Shoemaker, C. B., White, J. G., Prosen, R. J. and Trueblood, K. N. (1957). *Proc. Roy. Soc.* **A242**, 228.

Hodgkin, D. C., Pickworth, J., Robertson, J. H., Prosen, R. J., Sparks, R. A. and Trueblood, K. N. (1959). *Proc. Roy. Soc.* **A251**, 306.

Hodgkin, D. C., Lindsey, J., Sparks, R. A., Trueblood, K. N. and White, J. G. (1962). *Proc. Roy. Soc.* **A266**, 494.

Hogenkamp, H. P. C. (1963). *J. Biol. Chem.* **238**, 477.

Hogenkamp, H. P. C. (1964). *Ann. New York Acad. Sci.* **112**, 552.

Hogenkamp, H. P. C. (1966a). *Biochemistry* **5**, 417.

Hogenkamp, H. P. C. (1966b). *Fed. Proc.* **25**, 1623.

Hogenkamp, H. P. C. (1968). *Ann. Rev. Biochem.* **37**, 225.

Hogenkamp, H. P. C. and Barker, H. A. (1961). *J. Biol. Chem.* **236**, 3097.

Hogenkamp, H. P. C. and Holmes, S. (1970). *Biochemistry* **9**, 1886.

Hogenkamp, H. P. C. and Oikawa, T. G. (1964). *J. Biol. Chem.* **239**, 1911.

Hogenkamp, H. P. C., Ladd, J. N. and Barker, H. A. (1962). *J. Biol. Chem.* **237**, 1950.

Hogenkamp, H. P. C., Barker, H. A. and Mason, H. S. (1963). *Arch. Biochem. Biophys.* **100**, 353.

Hogenkamp, H. P. C., Rush, J. E. and Swenson, C. A. (1965). *J. Biol. Chem.* **240**, 3641.

Iguchi, M. (1942). *J. Chem. Soc., Japan* **63**, 634.

Ing, S. Y. S. and Pfiffner, J. J. (1968). *Arch. Biochem. Biophys.* **128**, 281.

Irion, E. and Ljungdahl, L. (1968). *Biochemistry* **7**, 2350.

I.U.P.A.C. (1958). Tentative rules for nomenclature in the vitamin B_{12} field. *In* I.U.P.A.C.'s "Nomenclature of Organic Chemistry", pp. 85–87. Butterworths, London.

I.U.P.A.C. (1960a). Definitive rules for nomenclature of inorganic chemistry, Section 7 (Co-ordination compounds), *J. Amer. Chem. Soc.* **82**, 5537.

I.U.P.A.C. (1960b). Definitive rules for the nomenclature of natural amino-acids and related substances, Section V-15, *J. Amer. Chem. Soc.* **82**, 5582.

I.U.P.A.C.–I.U.B. (1966). Commission on biochemical nomenclature. Tentative rules for the "nomenclature of corrinoids", *Biochim. Biophys. Acta* **117**, 285.

Jaselskis, B. and Diehl, H. (1954). *J. Amer. Chem. Soc.* **76**, 4345.

Jaselskis, B. and Diehl, H. (1958). *J. Amer. Chem. Soc.* **80**, 2147.

Jeffrey, G. A. and McMullan, R. K. (1967). *Progr. Inorg. Chem.* **8**, 43.
Johansen, H. and Ingraham, L. L. (1969). *J. Theor. Biol.* **23**, 191.
Johnson, A. W. (1967). *Chem. in Britain* 253.
Johnson, A. W. and Shaw, N. (1961). *Proc. Chem. Soc.* 447.
Johnson, A, W. and Shaw, N. (1962). *J. Chem. Soc.* 4608.
Johnson A. W. and Todd, A. (1957). *Vitamins and Horm.* **15**, 1.
Johnson, A. W., Mervyn, L., Shaw, N. and Smith, E. L. (1963a). *J. Chem. Soc.* 4146.
Johnson, A. W., Shaw, N. and Wagner, F. (1963b). *Biochim. Biophys. Acta* **72**, 107.
Johnson, A. W., Oldfield, D., Rodrigo, R. and Shaw, N. (1964). *J. Chem. Soc.* 4080.
Johnson, M. D., Tobe, M. L. and Wong, L. (1967). *J. Chem. Soc. (A)*, 491.
Jordan, R. B. and Sargeson, A. M. (1965). *Inorg. Chem.* **4**, 433.
Kaczka, E., Wolf, D. E. and Folkers, K. (1949). *J. Amer. Chem. Soc.* **71**, 1514.
Kaczka, E. A., Wolf, D. E., Kuehl, F. A. and Folkers, K. (1951). *J. Amer. Chem. Soc.* **73**, 3569.
Katz, J. J. (1954). *Arch. Biochem. Biophys.* **51**, 293.
Keilin, D. and Hartree, E. F. (1955). *Biochem. J.* **61**, 153.
Kennedy, F. S., Buckman, T. and Wood, J. M. (1969). *Biochim. Biophys. Acta* **177**, 661.
Kimura, E., Young, S. and Collman, J. P. (1970). *Inorg. Chem.* **9**, 1183.
Kon, S. K. and Pawełkiewicz, J. (1958). Proceedings of the 4th Internat. Congress Biochemistry, Vol. 11, p. 115.
Kratochvil, B. and Diehl, H. (1966). *Talanta* **13**, 1013.
Kubowitz, F. and Haas, E. (1932). *Biochem. Zeit.* **255**, 247.
Kuhn, H. (1959). *Fortschr. Chem. Org. Naturstoffe* **17**, 404.
Kuhn, H., Drexhage, K. H. and Martin, H. (1965). *Proc. Roy. Soc.* **A288**, 348.
Kundo, N, N, and Keyer, N. P. (1968). *Zhur. fiz. khim.* **42**, 1352.
Ladd, J. N., Hogenkamp, H. P. C. and Barker, H. A. (1960). *Biochem. Biophys. Res. Comm.* **2**, 143.
Ladd, J. N., Hogenkamp, H. P. C. and Barker, H. A. (1961). *J. Biol. Chem.* **236**, 2114.
Lalor, G. C. and Moelwyn-Hughes, E. A. (1963). *J. Chem. Soc.* 1560.
Langford, C. H. and Tobe, M. L. (1963). *J. Chem. Soc.* 506.
Latteur, J. P. (1962). "Cobalt Deficiencies and Sub-deficiencies in Ruminants". Centre d'Information du Cobalt, Brussels.
Laurence, G. S. (1956). *Trans. Faraday Soc.* **52**, 236.
Lee, L. and Schrauzer, G. N. (1968). *J. Amer. Chem. Soc.* **90**, 5274.
Legrand, M. and Viennet, R. (1962). *Bull. Soc. Chim. France*, p. 1435.
Lenhert, P. G. (1967). *Chem. Comm.* p. 980.
Lenhert, P. G. (1968). *Proc. Roy. Soc.* **A303**, 45.
Lenhert, P. G., personal communication.
Lenhert, P. G. and Hodgkin, D. C. (1961). *Nature* **192**, 937.
Lindstrand, K. (1964). *Nature* **204**, 188.
Linhard, M. and Weigl, M. (1957). *Z. Phys. Chemie, Neue Folge* **11**, 308.
Ljungdahl, L. and Irion, E. (1966). *Biochemistry* **5**, 1846.
Ljungdahl, L., Irion, E. and Wood, H. G. (1965). *Biochemistry* **4**, 2771.
Ludwick, L. M. and Brown, T. L. (1969). *J. Amer. Chem. Soc.* **91**, 5188.
Macek, T. J. and Feller, B. A. (1952). *J. Amer. Pharm. Assoc. Sci. Ed.* **41**, 285.
Mahoney, M. J. and Rosenberg, L. E. (1970). *Amer. J. Med.* **48**, 584.
March, J. (1968). "Advanced Organic Chemistry; Reactions, Mechanisms and Structure", Chapter 16. McGraw-Hill Book Co., New York.
Mason, R. and Russell, D. R. (1965). *Chem. Comm.* p. 182.

Mays, M. J. and Wilkinson, G. (1964). *Nature* **203**, 1167.

McConnel, R. J., Overell, B. G., Petrow, V. and Sturgeon, B. (1953). *J. Pharm. Pharmacol.* **5**, 179.

Melent'eva, T. A., Pekel', N. D. and Berezovskii, V. M., (1969). *Russ. Chem. Revs.* **38**, 926.

Mervyn, L. and Smith, E. L. (1964). *Progr. Ind. Microbiol.* **5**, 151.

Moore, F. M., Willis, B. T. M. and Hodgkin D. C. (1967). *Nature* **214**, 130.

Moriguchi, I. and Kaneniwa, N. (1969). *Chem. Pharm. Bull.* **17**, 394.

Morley, C. G. D., Blakley, R. L. and Hogenkamp, H. P. C. (1968). *Biochemistry* **7**, 1231.

Müller, O. and Müller, G. (1962a). *Biochem. Zeit.* **335**, 340.

Müller, O. and Müller, G. (1962b). *Biochem. Zeit.* **336**, 299.

Müller, O. and Müller, G, (1963). *Biochem. Zeit.* **337**, 179.

Nath, A., Harpold, M. and Klein, M. P. (1968). *Chem. Phys. Letters* **2**, 471.

Nihlén, H. and Ericson, L. E. (1955). *Acta Chem. Scand.* **9**, 351.

Nockolds, C. K., Ramaseshan, S., Hodgkin, D. C., Waters, T. N. M. and Waters, J. M. (1967). *Nature* **214**, 129.

Offenhartz, B. H. (1965). *Proc. Roy. Soc.* **A288**, 350.

Offenhartz, B. H. and George, P. (1963). *Biochemistry* **2**, 142.

Pailes, W. H. and Hogenkamp, H. P. C. (1968). *Biochemistry* **7**, 4160.

Pan, K. and Hsu, M. (1967). Proceedings of the 10th Internat. Conf. Co-ord. Chem. Tokyo, p. 296.

Pawełkiewicz, J., Bartosinski, B. and Walerych, W. (1960). *Bull. Acad. Pol. Sci., Class II.* **8**, 123.

Pearson, R. G., Boston, C. R. and Basolo, F. (1955). *J. Phys. Chem.* **59**, 304.

Pearson, R. G., Sobel, H. and Songstad, J. (1968). *J. Amer. Chem. Soc.* **90**, 319.

Peel, J. L. (1962a). *J. Biol. Chem.* **237**, PC263.

Peel, J. L. (1962b). *Biochem. J.* **85**, 17P.

Peel, J. L. (1963). *Biochem. J.* **88**, 296.

Perlman, D. (1959). *Adv. Appl. Microbiol.* **1**, 87.

Perlman, D. and Toohey, J. I. (1966). *Nature* **212**, 300.

Perlman, D. and Toohey, J. I. (1968). *Arch. Biochem. Biophys.* **124**, 462.

Phillips, R. (1966). *Chem. Revs.* **66**, 501.

Posey, F. A. and Taube, H. (1957). *J. Amer. Chem. Soc.* **79**, 255.

Pratt, J. M. (1964). *J. Chem. Soc.* 5154.

Pratt, J. M., unpublished work.

Pratt, J. M. and Thorp, R. G. (1966). *J. Chem. Soc.* (*A*), 187.

Pratt, J. M. and Thorp, R. G. (1969). *Adv. Inorg. Chem. Radiochem.* **12**, 375.

Pratt, J. M. and Thorp, R. G., unpublished results.

Pratt, J. M. and Williams, R. J. P. (1961). *Biochem. Biophys. Acta* **46**, 191.

Pratt, J. M. and Williams, R. J. P. (1968). *Disc. Farad. Soc.* **46**, 187.

Pratt, J. M. and Whitear, B. R. D. (1971). *J. Chem. Soc.* (*A*), 252.

Purcell, K. F. (1967). *J. Amer. Chem. Soc.* **89**, 247.

Randall, W. C. and Alberty, R. A. (1966). *Biochemistry* **5**, 3189.

Randall, W. C. and Alberty, R. A. (1967). *Biochemistry* **6**, 1520.

Rickes, E. L., Brink, N. G., Koniuszy, F. R., Wood, T. R. and Folkers, K. (1948). *Science* **107**, 396.

Rosenberg, A. J. (1956). *J. Biol. Chem.* **219**, 951.

Rossotti, F. J. C. (1960). *In* "Modern Co-ordination Chemistry", Chapter 1 (edited by J. Lewis and R. G. Wilkins). Interscience Publishers, New York, U.S.A.

Samsonov, G. V., Klikh, S. F., El'kin, G. E. and Kil'fin, G. I. (1965). *Colloid J. U.S.S.R.* **27**, 79.

Sander, E. G. and Jencks, W. P. (1968). *J. Amer. Chem. Soc.* **90**, 6154.

Schindler, O. (1951). *Helv. Chim. Acta* **34**, 1356.

Schmid, H., Ebnöther, A. and Karrer, P. (1953). *Helv. Chim. Acta* **36**, 65.

Schrauzer, G. N. (1966). *Naturwissenschaften* **53**, 459.

Schrauzer, G. N. (1968). *Acc. Chem. Res.* **1**, 97.

Schrauzer, G. N. (1969). *Ann. New York Acad. Sci.* **158**, 526.

Schrauzer, G. N. and Deutsch, E. (1969). *J. Amer. Chem. Soc.* **91**, 3341.

Schrauzer, G. N., and Holland, R. J. (1971). *J. Amer. Chem. Soc.* **93**, 4060.

Schrauzer, G. N. and Kratel, G. (1965). *Angew. Chem.* **77**, 130.

Schrauzer, G. N. and Lee, L. P. (1968). *J. Amer. Chem. Soc.* **90**, 6541.

Schrauzer, G. N. and Lee, L. P. (1970). *J. Amer. Chem. Soc.* **92**, 1551.

Schrauzer, G. N. and Sibert, J. W. (1969). *Arch. Biochem. Biophys.* **130**, 257.

Schrauzer, G. N. and Sibert, J. W. (1970). *J. Amer. Chem. Soc.* **92**, 1022.

Schrauzer, G. N. and Windgassen, R. J. (1966a). *J. Amer. Chem. Soc.* **88**, 3738.

Schrauzer, G. N. and Windgassen, R. J. (1966b). *Chem. Ber.* **99**, 602.

Schrauzer, G. N. and Windgassen, R. J. (1967a). *Nature* **214**, 492.

Schrauzer, G. N. and Windgassen, R. J. (1967b). *J. Amer. Chem. Soc.* **89**, 3607.

Schrauzer, G. N., Windgassen, R. J. and Kohnle, J. (1965). *Chem. Ber.* **98**, 3324.

Schrauzer, G. N., Deutsch, E. and Windgassen, R. J. (1968a). *J. Amer. Chem. Soc.* **90**, 2441.

Schrauzer, G. N., Sibert, J. W. and Windgassen, R. J. (1968b). *J. Amer. Chem. Soc.* **90**, 6681.

Scott, W. M., Burgus, R. C., Hufham, J. B. and Pfiffner, J. J. (1964). *J. Bacter.* **88**, 581.

Sen, S. P. (1962). *Chem. Ind.* 94.

Sidgwick, N. V. (1950). "The Chemical Elements and their Compounds", Vol. I. pp. 318–319. Clarendon Press, Oxford.

Siebert, H. (1964). *Zeit. anorg. allgem. Chemie* **327**, 63.

Silber, R. and Moldow, C. F. (1970). *Amer. J. Med.* **48**, 549.

Sillén, L. G. and Martell, A. E. (1964). "Stability Constants of Metal Ion Complexes," Chem. Soc. Special Publication No. 17.

Sjöstedt, M. and Ericson, L. E. (1959). *Acta Chem. Scand.* **13**, 1711.

Smith, E. L. (1948). *Nature* **162**, 144.

Smith, E. L. (1955). *Biochem. Soc. Symposia* **13**, 3.

Smith, E. L. (1957). Report of nomenclature commission, *in* "Vitamin B_{12} und Intrinsic Factor. 1 Europäisches Symposium, Hamburg, 1956" pp. 554–560 (edited by H. C. Heinrich). Ferdinand Enke Verlag, Stuttgart, W. Germany.

Smith, E. L. (1960). "Vitamin B_{12}", 1st edn. Methuen, London.

Smith, E. L. (1962). Report of round table discussion on nomenclature, *in* "Vitamin B_{12} und Intrinsic Factor. 2. Europäisches Symposium, Hamburg, 1961", pp. 764–768 (edited by H. C. Heinrich). Ferdinand Enke Verlag, Stuttgart, W. Germany.

Smith, E. L. (1965). "Vitamin B_{12}", 3rd edn. Methuen, London.

Smith, E. L., personal communication.

Smith, E. L. and Parker, L. F. J. (1948). *Biochem. J.* **43**, viii.

Smith, E. L., Ball, S. and Ireland, D. M. (1952a). *Biochem. J.* **52**, 395.

Smith, E. L., Fantes, K. H., Ball, S., Waller, J. G., Emery, W. B., Anslow, W. K. and Walker, A. D. (1952b). *Biochem. J.* **52**, 389.

Smith, E. L., Mervyn, L., Johnson, A. W. and Shaw, N. (1962). *Nature* **194**, 1175.

Smith, E. L., Mervyn, L., Muggleton, P. W., Johnson, A. W. and Shaw, N. (1964). *Ann. New York Acad. Sci.* **112**, 565.

Stadtman, T. C. (1967). *Ann. Rev. Microbiol.* **21**, 121.

Stapert, E. M., Ferrer, E. B. and Stubberfield, L. (1954). *J. Amer. Pharm. Assoc. Sci. Ed.* **43**, 87.

Stokstad, E. L. R. (1968). *Vit. Horm.* **26**, 443.

Tackett, S. L., Collat, J. W. and Abbott, J. C. (1963). *Biochemistry* **2**, 919.

Taylor, R. T. and Weissbach, H. (1968). *Arch. Biochem. Biophys.* **123**, 109.

Tewari, P. H., Gaver, R. W., Wilcox, H. K. and Wilmarth, W. K. (1967). *Inorg. Chem.* **6**, 611.

Thomson, A. J. (1969). *J. Amer. Chem. Soc.* **91**, 2780.

Thusius, D. (1968). *Chem. Comm.* 1183.

Thusius, D. (1971). *J. Amer. Chem. Soc.* **93**, 2629.

Tobe, M. L. (1959). *J. Chem. Soc.* 3776.

Tobe, M. L. (1966). *Record. Chem. Progress* **27**, 79.

Toohey, J. I. (1965). *Proc. Nat. Acad. Sci.* **54**, 934.

Toohey, J. I. (1966). *Fed. Proc.* **25**, 1628.

Toohey, J. I., Perlman, D. and Barker, H. A. (1961). *J. Biol. Chem.* **236**, 2119.

Trenner, N. R., Buhs, R. P., Bacher, F. A. and Gakenheimer, W. C. (1950). *J. Amer. Pharm. Assoc. Sci. Ed.* **39**, 361.

Tsiang, H. G. and Wilmarth, W. K. (1968). *Inorg. Chem.* **7**, 2535.

Veer, W. L. C., Edelhausen, J. H., Wijmenga, H. G. and Lens, J. (1950). *Biochim. Biophys. Acta* **6**, 225.

Veillard, A. and Pullman, B. (1965). *J. Theor. Biol.* **8**, 307.

Venkatesan, K., Dale, D., Hodgkin, D. C., Nockolds, C. E., Moore, F. H. and O'Connor, B. H. (1971). *Proc. Roy. Soc.* **A323**, 455.

Vitols, E., Walker, G. A. and Huennekens, F. M. (1964). *Biochem. Biophys. Res. Comm.* **15**, 372.

Wagner, F. (1965). *Proc. Roy. Soc.* **A288**, 344.

Wagner, F. (1966). *Ann. Rev. Biochem.* **35**, 405.

Wagner, F. and Bernhauer, K. (1964). *Ann. New York Acad. Sci.* **112**, 580.

Wagner, F. and Renz, P. (1963). *Tetrahedron Letters* 259.

Wallenfels, K. and Streffer, C. (1966). *Biochem. Zeit.* **346**, 119.

Wallman, J. C., Cunningham, B. B. and Calvin, M. (1951). *Science* **113**, 55.

Warburg, O. (1949). "Heavy Metal Prosthetic Groups and Enzyme Action." Oxford University Press, London.

Warburg, O. and Negelein, E. (1928). *Biochem. Zeit.* **200**, 414.

Warburg, O. and Negelein, E. (1929). *Biochem. Zeit.* **214**, 64.

Wehry, E. L. (1967). *Quart. Revs.* **21**, 213.

Weissbach, H. and Dickerman, H. (1965). *Physiol. Revs.* **45**, 80.

Weissbach, H., Toohey, J. and Barker, H. A. (1959). *Proc. Nat. Acad. Sci.* **45**, 521.

Weissbach, H., Ladd, J. N., Volcani, B. E., Smyth, R. D. and Barker, H. A. (1960). *J. Biol. Chem.* **235**, 1462.

Werthemann, L. (1968). Abhandlung, E.T.H., Zürich. Juris Druck Verlag, Zürich, Switzerland.

Wijmenga, H. G., Thompson, K. W., Stern, K. G. and O'Connell. D. J. (1954). *Biochem. Biophys. Acta* **13**, 144.

Wood, J. M., Kennedy, F. S. and Wolfe, R. S. (1968a). *Biochemistry* **7**, 1707.

Wood, J. M., Kennedy, F. S. and Rosen, C. G. (1968b). *Nature, Lond.* **220**, 173.

Woodward, R. B. (1968). *Pure Appl. Chem.* **17**, 519.

Yamada, R., Kato, T., Shimizu, S. and Fukui, S. (1964). *Biochim. Biophys. Acta* **93**, 196.

Yamada, R., Kato, T., Shimizu, S. and Fukui, S. (1965). *Biochim. Biophys. Acta* **97**, 353.

Yamada, R., Kato, T., Shimizu, S. and Fukui, S. (1966a). *Biochim. Biophys, Acta* **117**, 13.

Yamada, R., Shimizu, S. and Fukui, S. (1966b). *Arch. Biochem. Biophys.* **117**, 675.

Yamada, R., Shimizu, S. and Fukui, S. (1966c). *Biochim. Biophys. Acta* **124**, 195.

Yamada, R., Shimizu, S. and Fukui, S. (1966d). *Biochim. Biophys. Acta* **124**, 197.

Yamada, R., Shimizu, S. and Fukui, S. (1968a). *Biochemistry* **7**, 1713.

Yamada, R., Umetani, T., Shimizu, S. and Fukui, S. (1968b). *J. Vitaminology* **14**, 316.

Yamada, Y., Miljkovic, D., Wehrli, P., Golding, B., Löliger, P., Keese, R., Müller, K. and Eschenmoser, A. (1969). *Angew. Chem.* **81**, 301.

Yurkevich, A. M., Borodulina, V. I. and Preobrazhenskii, N. A. (1965). *Zhur. obshch. Khim.* **35**, 85.

Yurkevich, A. M., Rudakova, I. P. and Pospelova, T. A. (1966). *Zhur. obshch. Khim.* **36**, 850.

Yurkevich, A. M., Rudakova, I. P. and Pospelova, T. A. (1969). *Zhur. obshch. Khim.* **39**, 425.

Zagalak, B. (1963). *Acta Biochim. Pol.* **10**, 387.

Zagalak, B. and Pawełkiewicz, J. (1964). *Acta Biochim. Pol.* **11**, 49.

Zagalak, B. and Pawełkiewicz, J. (1965a). *Acta Biochim. Pol.* **12**, 103.

Zagalak, B. and Pawełkiewicz, J. (1965b). *Acta Biochim. Pol.* **12**, 219.

Author Index

Numbers in *italics* indicate the pages on which the references are listed in full

A

Abbott, J. C., 101, 104, 107, 108, 111, 195, 196, 197, *311*, *319*
Abeles, R. H., 239, 241, 245, *309*
Ablov, A. V., 216, *309*
Adamson, A. W., 63, 278, *309*
Adler, N., 145, 154, 156, 161, 199, *309*
Agnes, G., 308, *309*
Ahrland, S., 169, *309*
Ainsworth, S., 279, *314*
Albert, A., 147, 172, *309*
Alberty, R. A., 161, 215, 216, 218, *317*
Alicino, J. F., 186, 189, *309*
Anslow, W. K., 87, 98, 140, 262, *318*
Appleby, C. A., 279, *309*
Aronovitch, J., 205, 206, 208, 209, 291, *309*
Ašperger, S., 217, *309*

B

Babior, B. M. 66, 85, 177, 276, 300, *309*
Bacher, F. A., 290, *319*
Baldwin, M. E., 217, *309*
Ball, S., 87, 98, 99, 140, 176, 177, 178, 262, *318*
Balzani, V., 278, *309*
Banks, R. G. S., 109, 204, 206, *309*
Barboni, E., 154, 159, 190, 198, 199, *311*
Barca, R., 214, 216, *309*
Barker, H. A., 4, 5, 46, 98, 99, 101, 104, 135, 138, 143, 149, 161, 188, 189, 190, 236, 238, 240, 242, 243, 244, 245, 257, 270, 271, 297, *309*, *310*, *315*, *316*, *319*
Barnett, R., 239, 241, 245, *309*
Bartosinski, B., 235, *317*
Basolo, F., 211, 215, 217, *309*, *317*
Bauriedel, W. R., 141, 142, 154, 156, *309*
Bayston, J. H., 91, 92, 93, 94, 101, 103, 155, 195, 200, 202, 233, 307, *309*, *310*

Beaven, G. H., 103, 107, 109, 142, 153, 156, 186, 196, 197, 198, 199, 200, 202, 260, 280, 282, 284, 289, *310*, *312*
Beisbarth, H., 82, *310*
Bell, R. P., 150, *310*
Bendle, S., 308, *309*
Berezovskii, V. M., 6, *317*
Bernhauer, K., 4, 7, 56, 57, 74, 82, 84, 111, 117, 135, 141, 159, 161, 173, 189, 198, 200, 228, 229, 230, 231, 233, 235, 236, 239, 241, 242, 246, 247, 249, 250, 252, 253, 254, 257, 261, 262, 265, 268, 269, 276, 282, 284, 289, 293, 295, *310*, *313*, *319*
Bertele, E., 6, 183, *313*
Bieganowski, R., 53, 54, 66, 121, 122, 123, 124, 228, 229, 230, *313*
Bieniek, D., 308, *310*
Blakeley, L. M., 213, 214, *314*
Blakley, R. L., 242, 300, *314*, *317*
Blitz, M., 292, *310*
Boehm, G., 95, *310*
Bonnett, R., 5, 46, 56, 57, 66, 84, 85, 90, 193, 194, 280, 281, 282, 283, 284, 293, 307, *310*
Boos, R. N., 107, 108, 111, 112, 198, 203, 204, *310*
Bormann, D., 179, 183, 285, *310*, *313*
Borodulina, V. I., 86, 156, *320*
Boston, C. R., 217, *317*
Bowman, R. L., 67, 256, *312*
Boxer, G. E., 197, 198, 200, 278, *310*
Brady, R. O., 104, 236, 257, 270, *310*
Brearley, A. E., 308, *310*
Briat, B., 57, 61, 66, *310*
Brierly, J. M., 101, 189, 197, 204, 209, 210, 234, *311*
Brink, C., 5, 76, 77, *311*
Brink, N. G., 3, 188, 189, *311*, *317*
Brink-Shoemaker, C., 3, 71, 73, 75, 76, 81, 82, *311*

321

Subject Index

Axial ligands are tabulated separately in the Ligand Index on pp. 337–347, though selected references to a few ligands and particular corrinoids are given in the General Index.

I. GENERAL INDEX

Bold type denotes pages containing the more important tables, diagrams and structures or sections devoted mainly to the topic specified.

A

Absorption spectra (u.v.-visible), 42, 43, **44–65**, 85–9, 94–5, 98–9, **102–4**, 106–7, **108–9**, **123**, **127**, 129, **131–5**, 138, 148–9, 153–4, 156, 160–1, 165, 168, 173, **181–2**, **184–6**, 188, 192–4, 203–4, 208–9, 231, 236, 243, 246, 258, 262-5, **277–9**, 283, **286–92**, 300, 303–4, 308

bands of 5,6-dimethylbenzimidazole, 42, 59, 109, 153, 185–6

charge transfer bands, 58–9, **63–4**

d–d transitions, 58–9, 61, **64–5**, 66, 103

definition of $\alpha\beta$ bands etc., 60

extinction coefficients of B_{12} and di-cyanocorrinoids, **46**

spin-forbidden bands, **65**

theory of π–π transitions, **59–63**

typical and atypical spectra, 46–7, 53–5, 57–8, 63–4

(see also Reflection spectra)

Acid-base properties,

axial ligands, **139**, **140**, **146**, **160–2**

corrin ring 179, 181–2, **184–6**, 194–5, 281–2, 285

side-chains, 81–2, 122, 186, **187–9**

(see also 5,-6-Dimethylbenzimidazole, Equilibrium constants)

Acids,

equilibria with (see Acid-base properties)

Acids—*continued*

reactions with (see Coenzymes, Corrin ring, Hydrogen, Organo-corrinoids, Side-chains)

strong, solutions of corrinoids in, 74, 183, **184–6**, 240, 265, 269, 307

Acyl transfer, 241–2, 249–50, 275–6, 308

Alkylation,

of cobalt(I) corrinoids, 126, 193–4, **224–32**

of mercury, 39, 162, 219, **250–1**, 300

Autoxidation,

of cobalt, 101, 106, 192, 202–4, 257, 288–90

of iodide, 209–10

of thiols, 206–9

B

B_{12} (cyanocobalamin),

extinction coefficients (spectra), **46**

formula, 1

isolation, 1–3, 38–9

structure and X-ray analysis, **2–3**, **71–6**, 80–2

B_{12a} (aquo-, hydroxo-cobalamin),

pK, **139**, **140**, 142

preparation, 41

B_{12r} (see Cobalt(II) corrinoids)

B_{12s} (see Cobalt(I) corrinoids)

Biochemistry, **32–9**, **296–300**

Biosynthesis, **33–5**, 126, 158

331

II. LIGAND INDEX

The Ligand Index lists the axial ligands reported for Co(III) and Co(II) corrinoids together with a rough guide to their location in the text.

The list includes ligands known to be co-ordinated, ligands whose structure or co-ordination has not yet been fully established (e.g. SO_2^{2-}, certain nucleotide bases) and ligands postulated as reaction intermediates (e.g. CO, O-bonded SO_3^{2-}). Potential ligands which have been studied but shown not to co-ordinate (e.g. NO, ClO_4^-) are also included but enclosed in brackets. The list includes virtually all ligands named individually in the text; but there are, of course, additional ligands (e.g. certain thiols, nucleotides) which are mentioned in the literature but not referred to in the text.

The ligands are listed according to the ligand atom (H; F, Cl, Br, I; O, S, Se; N, P, As; C, Sn) and then in order of increasing negative charge (neutral bases, mono- and di-basic acids etc.). Where co-ordination may occur through more than one ligand atom (e.g. NCS^-) the ligand is listed under each ligand atom and the other possible ligand atoms given in brackets.

To avoid including an excessive number of references only the Chapter and Section, in which the particular ligand is mentioned or discussed, are given and Chapters 1–4 and 16–18 inclusive, which contain little relevant information, are omitted.

References to certain ligands (e.g. cyanide, 5,6-dimethylbenzimidazole) and corrinoids (e.g. B_{12}, cobalt(II) corrinoids, coenzymes) are also given in the General Index.

Ligand atom	Axial ligand	5	6	7
H	H⁻			V
F	F⁻			
Cl	Cl⁻	I	I	IV
Br	Br⁻	I		
I	I⁻	I, II		II, III, IV
O	O₂		III	III
	H₂O	{I, III	I, II, III	I, II, III, V, VI
	CH₃OH		III	III, IV
	Dimethylformamide		III	
	(Urea)			
	O₂⁻		III	III
	HO⁻	{I, II	I, II, III	I, III, V
	——NO₂⁻ (? N or O)——	{I, II		I
	NO₃⁻			
	(ClO₄⁻)			
	CH₃CO₂⁻	I		
	C₆H₅O⁻ (phenolate)	I, II		
S	SO₃²⁻ (O, but see also S)			
	(PO₄³⁻)			
	(Me₂S)			
	Thiourea	I		
	HS⁻			
	Thiolates (RS⁻):			
	Ethanethiol			
	2-Mercaptoethanol			
	Thioglycollic acid			
	ω-Mercaptotoluene			
	Cysteine	I		
	Cysteamine			
	Homocysteine			
	Glutathione			
	——NCS⁻ (N and S)——	{I, II	I, III	III
	HSO₃⁻			
	CH₃SO₂⁻			
	C₆H₅SO₂⁻			
	p-CH₃C₆H₄SO₂⁻			
	SO₂²⁻			
	SO₃²⁻	{I		II, VI
	S₂O₃²⁻	I, II		II

| Chapters | | | | | | | | Appendix |
8	9	10	11	12	13	14	15	dix
					I			+
IV,V								
IV,V						II	I	
IV,V								+
I,III,IV,V			VI		II			+
IV			V					
I,II,III,	I,III	I,II	I,II,III,	II	I,II,III	I,II,III	I,II	+
IV,V,VI			IV,V,VI					
I								
IV								
IV			V					
III,IV,V,		I	II,IV,VI	II	II,III	I,II,III	I,II	+
VI								
II,IV,V,							II	
VI								
IV								
IV								
IV,V	III					II		
IV,V						IV		
IV			IV	II	III			
IV								
IV								
IV,V					III			
IV,V			IV		I,III		II	
IV			IV		I			
IV			IV,VI		I	II		
IV,V			IV,VI		I	II	II	
IV					I			
IV,V			IV,V,VI		I	II		
IV			IV					
IV			IV,VI		I			
IV,V			IV,VI		I	II		
II,IV,V,				II	I,III	II		+
VI								
				II	III			
					III			
IV					III	II		
IV					I,III	II		
IV			IV		III			
I,II,III,			IV	II	I,III	I,II	I,II	+
IV,V,VI								
III,IV,V			IV		III	I,II	II	+

Ligand atom	Axial ligand	5	6	7
Se	NCSe⁻	{ I, II	I	II
	Selenourea			
N	Protonated adenine (in nucleotide side-chain)			
	NH₃	{ I		
	MeNH₂			
	EtNH₂			
	Ethanolamine			
	Piperidine			
	Amino-acids and related compounds:			
	Cysteine (S)	I		
	Glycine			
	Histidine		I	
	Lysine			
	Methionine			
	Tyrosine			
	Cysteamine (S)			
	Histamine			
	Homocysteine (S)			
	Carnosine			
	Histidylhistidine			
	Glutathione			
	Dimethylformamide (O)		III	
	(Urea)			
	Thiourea (? S)	I		
	Selenourea (Se)			
	Heterocyclic bases (underlined if part of nucleotide side-chain):			
	Adenine,		III	III
	Adenine,		III	VI
	2-methyl		III	
	5-methyl			
	2-methylthio		III	
	8-Aza-adenine			
	Benzimidazole	I	I	
	Benzimidazole,			
	5-amino			
	5-hydroxy		III	
	5-methoxy		III	
	5-methyl			

Ligand atom	Axial ligand	5	6	7
	5-nitro			
	5-trifluoromethyl			
	5,6-dimethyl		III	
	5,6-dimethyl (Bzm)	I, II, III	I, II, III	I, II, III, V, VI
	other substituents			
	Benzthiazole			
	Benztriazole			
	Guanine			
	Hypoxanthine,			
	2-methyl			
	5-methyl			
	Imidazole,	I	I	
	1-methyl			
	4,5-dimethyl			
	5,6-Imidazobenzimidazole			
	Isoquinoline		III	
	Naphthimidazole			
	Phenazine			
	Purine,			
	2,6-diamino			
	(see also Adenine)			
	Pyrazine-imidazole			
	Pyridine,	I	I, III	III
	2-methyl (α-picoline)	I	I	
	3-methyl (β-picoline)	I	I	
	4-methyl (γ-picoline)	I	I	
	Quinazoline			
	Quinoxaline			
	Uracil		III	
	(NO)			
	(CH$_3$CN)			
	HN$_3$			
	(NO$^-$)			
———	—NO$_2^-$ (? N or O)———	I, II		I
	N$_3^-$	I		
	NCO$^-$	I		
	NCS$^-$ (N and S)	I, II	I, III	III
	NCSe$^-$ (Se)	I, II	I	II
	Imidazolate (C$_3$H$_3$N$_2^-$)			
	Benzimidazolate			
	Adeninate			

| | | Chapters | | | | | | Appendix |
8	9	10	11	12	13	14	15	dix
V					II			
V					II			
I,II,III,IV,V,VI	II,III	I,II	I,II,III,IV,V,VI	II	I,II,III	I,II,III,IV	I,II	+
IV								
IV								
IV								
IV								
IV								
IV								
IV								
IV,V		I		II		III		
IV								
IV								
IV								
IV								
IV								
IV								
IV,V					II			
IV								
IV,V						III		
IV								
IV								
IV								
IV								
IV								
IV		V						
IV								
IV				II				
IV								
II,IV,V,VI							II	
IV,V				II				+
IV,V				II				+
II,IV,V,VI				II	I,III	II		+
I,II,III,IV,V						I,II		
IV,V		I						
IV								
IV								

	Chapters							Appen-dix
8	9	10	11	12	13	14	15	
IV								
IV							II	
IV							II	
IV								
			V					
IV,V			IV					
I,IV,V								
I,II,III, IV,V,VI	I,II,III	I,II	II,III,IV, V,VI	II	I,II,III	I,II,III, IV	I,II	+
I,II,III, IV,V	III	I,IV	II,III,IV, V	II	I,II,III	I,II,III, IV	I,II	+
					I	III		
			IV		I			
					I	III		
					I			
					I			
					I			
					I	III		
I,II,III,				II	I,II	II,III	I	+
IV,V								
IV,V					I,II	III		+
IV,V					II	III		
IV,V					I,II	III		
IV,V					I,II	III		
		IV			I,II			
IV,V		IV			I,II	III		
IV,V					I,II	III		
					I			
IV,V					I,II	III		
					II			
					I			
					I	III		
IV,V					I,II	III		
IV,V					I,II	III		
					II	III		
IV,V					I,II	III		
					I			
II,IV					I	III		
					I			
					I			
					I			
					I			
III,IV,V					I,II			

Ligand atom	Axial ligand	5	6	7
	—CHMeEt			
	—cyclohexyl			
	—CH=CH₂	I	II,III	II
	—CH=CHBr			
	—CH=CHCOOH			
	—CH=CHCN			
	—C≡CH	I	III	II
	—C≡CCN			
	—COCH₃	{		
	—COCH₂NH₂			
	—COCH₂NHCOCH₃			
	—COOEt			
	5-deoxyadenosyl	I,III	I,II,III	II,VI
	5-deoxyinosyl			
	5-deoxythimidyl			
	2,5-dideoxyadenosyl			
	2,3-isopropylidene-5-deoxyadenosyl			
	2,3-isopropylidene-5-deoxyuridinyl			
Sn	—SnR₃ (trialkyltin ligands)			

| | Chapters | | | | | | | Appen- |
8	9	10	11	12	13	14	15	dix
					I	III		
III,V					I,II			
I,III,IV, V			V	II	I,II,III	II	II	
					I			
					I			
					I			
I,III,IV, V			IV		I,II,III	II		
					I			
I,II,IV, V	I				I,II	II,III		+
					I,II	III		
					I,II	III		
					I,II	III		
I,II,III, IV,V,VI	I		V		I,II	I,II,III	I,II	+
						III		
IV					II			
IV					II			
IV					II			
						III		
			V					